Psychosomatic

An Introduction to Consultation–Liaison Psychiatry

Dr. James J. Amos is Associate Professor of Psychiatry in the Carver College of Medicine at The University of Iowa in Iowa City, Iowa. Dr. Amos received a B.S. degree in Distributed Studies (Zoology, Chemistry, and Microbiology) in 1985 from Iowa State University and an M.D. from The University of Iowa in Iowa City, Iowa, in 1992. He completed his psychiatry residency, including a year as Chief Resident, in 1996 at the Department of Psychiatry at The University of Iowa.

After completing residency training, Dr. Amos spent most of the time between 1996 and 2009 as a faculty clinician educator at The University of Iowa in Iowa City, Iowa. He spent a little less than a year in total in private practice, a time of enrichment that he has come to view as something of a sabbatical, where he learned a little about how the cultures of community and academic psychiatry intersect and enhance one another.

As a clinician educator, among Dr. Amos's most cherished achievements are several teaching awards and the Leonard Tow Humanism in Medicine Award. He has spent most of his career as a clinical instructor, largely in psychosomatic medicine, teaching and learning from residents in psychiatry, family medicine, internal medicine, and surgery, as well as medical students.

Dr. Robert G. Robinson is the Paul W. Penningroth Chair and Head of Psychiatry in the Carver College of Medicine at The University of Iowa in Iowa City, Iowa. Dr. Robinson received a B.S. degree in Engineering Physics in 1967 and an M.D. from Cornell University in 1971. He completed a medical internship at Montefiore Hospital and Albert Einstein Medical Center in Bronx, New York, and a year of psychiatry residency at Cornell University Medical Center, Westchester Division, in White Plains, New York. Following a two-year research associateship at the National Institute of Mental Health in the Laboratory of Neuropharmacology, he completed a residency and fellowship, including a year as Chief Resident, at the Department of Psychiatry and Behavioral Sciences, Johns Hopkins Hospital, in Baltimore, Maryland. During that time, he also was a Maudsley Exchange Resident in the Children's Department of Maudsley Hospital, Denmark Hill, London, England.

Following residency training, Dr. Robinson spent from 1977 to 1990 as a faculty member at Johns Hopkins University, School of Medicine, in the Department of Psychiatry and the Department of Neuroscience, where he rose to the rank of Professor in 1985. He was also a faculty member in the Psychiatry Department at the University of Maryland Medical School. In 1990, he moved to the University of Iowa in Iowa City, Iowa, to become Head of the Department of Psychiatry in the Carver College of Medicine, where he is also a member of the faculty of the Graduate Program in Neuroscience. In 1996, he became the Paul W. Penningroth Professor, and in 2007, the Paul W. Penningroth Chair in Psychiatry.

Dr. Robinson's research interests include a broad range of neuropsychiatric disorders associated with ischemic brain injury; animal models of mood disorders; the mechanism and emotional and behavioral manifestations of brain asymmetry; mechanism of and mood regulation in humans; mood disorders following traumatic brain injury; and the use of transcranial magnetic stimulation in the treatment of depression following stroke or vascular disease.

Throughout his career, Dr. Robinson has received 13 research grants from the National Institutes of Health (NIH), including a Research Scientist Career Award, and has received continuous funding from the NIH since 1979. He has trained 36 post-doctoral fellows in his laboratory, including seven who are now full professors.

He has published more than 390 original research articles and chapters and 5 books, including the second edition of a monograph entitled, *The Clinical Neuropsychiatry of Stroke*, which was translated into three languages. His research contributions have included pioneering work in the diagnosis, cause, and treatment of neuropsychiatric disorders following stroke; the first demonstration of treatment of depression following stroke; the identification of specific sites of brain injury associated with post-stroke depression, mania, and anxiety disorder; and identification of brain asymmetries in the physiologic and behavioral responses to brain ischemia. The work led to his receipt of the American Psychiatric Association Award for Research in 1999, as well as the Academy of Psychosomatic Medicine Research Award the same year.

Dr. Robinson is past President of the American Neuropsychiatric Association, a Fellow of the American College of Neuropsychopharmacology, and a Distinguished Fellow of the American Psychiatric Association. He is a member of the Editorial Board of eight journals. He has received the following recognitions: American Psychiatric Association Award for Research 1999; Academy of Psychosomatic Medicine Research Award 1999; American Association of Geriatric Psychiatry-Distinguished Scientist Award 2000; Raine Visiting Professor, University of Western Australia, May 2005; and the Award for Research in Geriatric Psychiatry from the American College of Psychiatrists, 2008.

Psychosomatic

A̶ ̶ ̶ ̶ ̶ ̶ ̶ ̶ ̶ ̶ ̶ ̶ n
Psy

Edited by

James J. Amos

Associate Professor of Psychiatry, Department of Psychiatry, The University of Iowa Hospitals and Clinics, Iowa City, Iowa, USA

Robert G. Robinson

Paul W. Penningroth Chair, Department of Psychiatry, University of Iowa, Iowa City, Iowa, USA

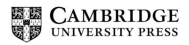

CAMBRIDGE
UNIVERSITY PRESS

CAMBRIDGE UNIVERSITY PRESS
Cambridge, New York, Melbourne, Madrid, Cape Town, Singapore,
São Paulo, Delhi, Dubai, Tokyo

Cambridge University Press
The Edinburgh Building, Cambridge CB2 8RU, UK

Published in the United States of America by
Cambridge University Press, New York

www.cambridge.org
Information on this title: www.cambridge.org/9780521106658

© Cambridge University Press 2010

First published 2010

Printed in the United Kingdom at the University Press, Cambridge

*A catalogue record for this publication is available from the
British Library*

Library of Congress Cataloguing in Publication data
Psychosomatic medicine : an introduction to consultation-liaison
psychiatry / edited by James J. Amos and Robert G. Robinson.
    p.   ;   cm.
Includes bibliographical references and index.
ISBN 978-0-521-10665-8 (pbk.)
1. Medicine, Psychosomatic.   2. Consultation-liaison psychiatry.
3. Medicine and psychology.   I. Amos, James J., 1955–
II. Robinson, Robert G. (Robert George), 1945–   III. Title.
[DNLM: 1. Psychophysiologic Disorders – diagnosis.
2. Mental Disorders – diagnosis.   3. Mental Disorders – therapy.
4. Psychophysiologic Disorders – therapy.   5. Psychosomatic
Medicine – methods.   6. Referral and Consultation.
WM 90 P9744 2010]
RC49.P787   2010
616.89 – dc22   2010004534

ISBN 978-0-521-10665-8 Paperback

We would like to dedicate this book to our families: Sena Amos and Gretchen, Jonathan, and Christopher Robinson. Without the commitment and steadfast support provided by our families, we would not have been able to carry out this endeavor. Throughout our professional careers, our families have been an abiding and sustaining source of strength, encouragement, and inspiration for which we are eternally grateful.

Contents

Preface

Since the American Board of Neurology and Psychiatry recognized psychosomatic medicine as a subspecialty, numerous important, well-written, and informative textbooks have been published. These texts have presented in-depth discussions of the broad array of disorders and issues that are confronted by the psychosomatic psychiatrist. Each year, however, more physicians who have completed their training in adult psychiatry enroll in specialty fellowship training in psychosomatic psychiatry. In addition, medical students, rotating through psychiatry, often serve on psychiatric consultation teams, or they may see inpatients or outpatients in psychiatry who have a combination of physical as well as mental disorders. This book is intended primarily for these learners, from the medical student to the resident in adult psychiatry rotating through the consultation service, to residents in combined medicine and psychiatry or family medicine and psychiatry and in geriatric psychiatry, outpatient or inpatient psychiatric residents, and to junior faculty who have just joined the psychiatry consult service. We have intentionally limited the length of each chapter in our agreement with the publisher to make this the kind of book that the clinician can carry in her pocket. And we informally gave it the name "The *Little Book of Psychosomatic Psychiatry*."

The name comes from Will Strunk's book, "*The Elements of Style*," in which he attempted to cut the vast tangle of English rhetoric down to size and write its rules and principles on the head of a pin. He hung the title "little" on his book and referred to it sardonically and with secret pride as the "the little book," always giving the word "little" a special twist, as though he were putting a spin on a ball (Essays of EB White, New York, Harper Row, 1977). Will was such a stickler for omitting unnecessary words, he was said to have made up for his own terseness by repeating himself three times, e.g., "rule 13. Omit needless words! Omit needless words! Omit needless words!" He loved the "clear, brief, bold."

This is our attempt to create the "little book of psychosomatic psychiatry." Any editor knows that something can always be said more directly using fewer words. Although we are sure that we could have been even more successful in "getting directly to the point" in this text, we have tried our best to be clear and brief. If this book is useful to those who practice the principles of psychosomatic medicine by drilling straight to the issues of patient management, and if it is right at your fingertips when you are seeing a patient, we'll count this little book a success. We'll practice what we preach, not use any more words, and hope that the consistency of chapter structure, brevity of description, and focus on patient care will make this book a useful resource in your practice of psychosomatic psychiatry.

Acknowledgements

The editors would like to thank Sherry Flanagan for her assistance in the preparation of the book and proofreading of the chapters. We would also like to thank the staff at Cambridge University Press, especially Nisha Doshi, for her assistance in helping to prepare the book for publication. Our work was supported in part by the Department of Psychiatry at The University of Iowa and grant R01-MH 065134 from the NIMH.

Contributors

Susan E. Abbey, MD
University Health Network and
Department of Psychiatry, University of
Toronto, Toronto, ON, Canada

James J. Amos, MD
Department of Psychiatry, The University
of Iowa Hospitals and Clinics, Iowa City,
IA, USA

Philip A. Bialer, MD
Psychosomatic Medicine, Beth Israel
Medical Center, New York, NY, USA

James A. Bourgeois, OD, MD
Department of Psychiatry and Behavioral
Sciences, University of California, Davis
Medical Center, Sacramento, CA, USA

Joanne A. Byars, MD
Department of Psychiatry, University of
Iowa, Iowa City, IA, USA

Jaspreet Chahal
Department of Internal Medicine,
University of Iowa, Iowa City, IA, USA

Kathy Coffman, MD
Cleveland Clinic, Cleveland, OH, USA

Mary Ann Cohen, MD
Department of Psychiatry, Mount Sinai
School of Medicine, New York, NY, USA

Catherine Crone, MD
Department of Psychiatry, Inova Fairfax
Hospital, Falls Church, VA, USA

Carlos Fernandez-Robles, MD
Psychosomatic Medicine, Massachusetts
General Hospital, Boston, MA, USA

Jess G. Fiedorowicz, MD, MS
Department of Psychiatry, University of
Iowa, Iowa City, IA, USA

Mary J. Fitz-Gerald, MD
Department of Psychiatry, Louisiana State
University Health Science Center,
Shreveport, LA, USA

Gregory Fricchione, MD
Department of Psychiatry, Harvard
Medical School, Massachusetts General
Hospital, Boston, MA, USA

Donna Greenberg, MD
Department of Psychiatry, Harvard
Medical School, Boston, MA, USA

Thomas W. Heinrich, MD
Division of Psychosomatic Medicine,
Department of Psychiatry
and Behavioral Medicine, Medical
College of Wisconsin, Milwaukee, WI,
USA

Debra R. Kahn, MD
Department of Psychiatry and Behavioral
Sciences, University of California, Davis
Medical Center, Sacramento, CA,
USA

Raheel A. Khan, DO
Department of Psychiatry, University of
California, Davis Medical Center,
Sacramento, CA, USA

Robin C. Kopelman, MD, MPH
Women's Wellness and Counseling Service,
Department of Psychiatry, University of
Iowa, Iowa City, IA, USA

Jeanne M. Lackamp, MD
Department of Psychiatry, University
Hospitals/Case Medical Center, W.O.
Walker Center, Cleveland, OH,
USA

Joseph A. Locala, MD
Division of Psychiatry and Medicine,
University Hospitals/Case Medical
Center and Department of Psychiatry,
Case Western Reserve University
School of Medicine, Cleveland, OH,
USA

Michael Marcangelo, MD
Department of Psychiatry, University of
Chicago Medical Center, Chicago, IL,
USA

Laura Marsh, MD
Departments of Psychiatry and Behavioral
Sciences and Neurology, Johns Hopkins
University School of Medicine, Baltimore,
MD, USA

Anthony C. Miller, MD
Mental Health Service Line, VA Medical
Center, Iowa City, IA, USA

Romina Mizrahi, MD, PhD
Centre for Addiction and Mental Health,
PET Centre, Toronto, ON, Canada

Megan Moore Brennan, MD
Department of Psychiatry, Psychosomatic
Medicine, Massachusetts General Hospital,
Boston, MA, USA

Maryland Pao, MD
National Institute of Mental Health,
National Institutes of Health, Bethesda,
MD, USA

John Querques, MD
Psychosomatic Medicine-Consultation
Psychiatry Fellowship Program,
Massachusetts General Hospital and
Department of Psychiatry, Harvard
Medical School, Boston, MA, USA

Davin Quinn, MD
Psychosomatic Medicine, Massachusetts
General Hospital, Boston, MA, USA

Vani Rao, MD
Department of Psychiatry and Behavioral
Sciences, Johns Hopkins University,
Baltimore, MD, USA

Robert G. Robinson, MD
Department of Psychiatry, University of
Iowa, Iowa City, IA, USA

Oludamilola Salami, MD
Department of Psychiatry and Behavioral
Sciences, Johns Hopkins University,
Baltimore, MD, USA

Sanjeev Sockalingam, MD
University Health Network and
Department of Psychiatry, University of
Toronto, Toronto, ON, Canada

Sergio E. Starkstein, MD, PhD
School of Psychiatry and Clinical
Neurosciences, University of Western
Australia, Fremantle, WA, Australia

Scott Stuart, MD
Department of Psychiatry, University of
Iowa, Iowa City, IA, USA

Adrienne Tan, MD
University Health Network and
Department of Psychiatry, University of
Toronto, Toronto, ON, Canada

Janeta Tansey, MD, PhD
Department of Psychiatry, University of
Iowa, Iowa City, IA, USA

Scott Temple, PhD
Department of Psychiatry, University of
Iowa, Iowa City, IA, USA

Alex Thompson, MD
Department of Psychiatry and Behavioral
Sciences, University of Washington
Medical Center, Seattle, WA, USA

Susan Turkel, MD
Departments of Psychiatry, Pathology and
Pediatrics, University of Southern
California Keck School of Medicine, Los
Angeles, Los Angeles, CA, USA

Michelle Weckmann, MD
Department of Psychiatry, University of
Iowa, Iowa City, IA, USA

Marcus Wellen, MD
Department of Psychiatry, Psychosomatic
Medicine, Inova Fairfax Hospital, Falls
Church, VA, USA

Thomas Wise, MD
Department of Psychiatry, Inova Fairfax
Hospital, Falls Church, VA, USA

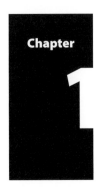

Chapter

1

The consultation process

Jeanne M. Lackamp

Introduction

Consultation psychiatrists are skilled clinicians and expert liaisons in the general hospital setting. In their roles as "med-psych detectives," consultation psychiatrists are called upon to assist in complex cases and to interact with primary teams, nursing teams, ancillary services, and patients and family members. They investigate medical/psychiatric interactions, assess psychiatric symptoms, and offer treatment recommendations. *Communication is the most crucial element of the consultation process.* Clear communication improves the process of your consultation as well as the result, by ensuring accurate, timely, and helpful interventions. This chapter strives to give residents the tools necessary to enter the world of consultation-liaison psychiatry.

First steps

Institutional and personal organization

As a member of the psychiatric consultation team, you must *know your role and maintain your identity* in your institution (1, 2). Who are the members of your team? Who carries the consult pager? What consults are appropriate for you to see (adult, pediatric, emergency room, other)? With whom do you staff new evaluations?

Being organized and having the requisite tools will prepare you to perform the duties expected of you (Table 1.1). Carry necessary items with you, and know where to access other information when needed. Finally, as noted by Wise and Rundell, "Wear a white coat – on your shoulders and in your brain" (3). Your role as a medical practitioner should be clearly and visibly evident to those who consult you, as well as to the patients you see.

Who is calling?

When a consult is called, you need to record the *name, pager number, and team affiliation of the consulting individual* (Table 1.2). This helps you in filling out your paperwork thoroughly, and ensures that you will give final recommendations to the appropriate team. If the person calling is not one of the patient's clinicians (unit clerk, nurse, social worker), ask for the appropriate contact information.

Psychosomatic Medicine: An Introduction to Consultation-Liaison Psychiatry, eds. James J. Amos and Robert G. Robinson. Published by Cambridge University Press. © Cambridge University Press 2010.

Table 1.1 Things to carry with you

Interview/assessment forms
- Departmental or personal interview guides
- MMSE, SLUMS, MoCA, etc

Psychiatric admission forms
- Voluntary
- Involuntary

Medication reference guides
Penlight
Reflex hammer
Stethoscope

Key:
MMSE = Mini-Mental State Examination (29)
SLUMS = St Louis Mental Status Examination (30)
MoCA = Montreal Cognitive Assessment (31)

Table 1.2 Important initial information

Who is calling?
- Physician name
- Physician pager number
- Physician team affiliation (e.g., internal medicine, ICU, surgery)
- Contact name/pager number for team member who should get final recommendations

What is the patient's information?
- Full name
- Age
- Gender
- Hospital number
- Specific location

What is the question?
- Formal consult question

Urgency (routine, urgent, emergent)

Who is the patient? Where is the patient?

It is important to get the *patient's full name, age, gender, hospital number,* and *hospital location* from the person who is calling the consult (Table 1.2). You want to be sure that it is appropriate for you to see the patient, and you want to find the patient quickly. It is important to note that you do not want to see the wrong patient!

Patients may change locations temporarily for testing or procedures, and at times they are transferred to other parts of the hospital for medical reasons, such as moving from the ICU to the general medical floor. When speaking to a consultee, ask how long the patient will be available in his or her current location. This will maximize your consultation time and effort.

Patients sometimes attempt to elope from hospital grounds. If you know where the patient started, you may be able to determine likely routes of egress and you can inform security personnel.

What is the consult question?

You need to know *what is prompting the consultation at this time* (Table 1.2). A statement such as, "The patient has a history of schizophrenia," is insufficient. Common consultation topics are mental health/behavioral problems and capacity evaluations; we will address these briefly. Later chapters in this handbook will address these and other frequently asked questions, elements of evaluation, and treatment recommendations (Table 1.2).

Do not limit the scope of your consultation to the initial question. Consultations for mental status changes, anxiety, depression, psychosis, and behavioral problems may evolve into consultations for delirium or other conditions. Mental flexibility is key.

Consulting teams may have identified new psychiatric symptoms or behaviors (the post-stroke patient who is voicing suicidal ideation; the post-surgical patient who is confused and pulling out intravenous lines). Consulting teams may know or suspect that the patient has a psychiatric history (the patient with schizophrenia who has been admitted for surgery and is currently NPO; the frequently admitted patient who is demanding large doses of pain medication). Consulting teams may feel that the patient would be better served on a psychiatric unit (this is particularly common in patients with suicidal ideation and mental status changes). Although consults for psychiatric transfer are common, you must *verify medical stability and appropriateness* for admission to the inpatient unit before facilitating the transfer.

Primary teams may request consultation to assess a patient's capacity – that is, to determine if the patient is able to make a particular decision (4). (Recall that "capacity" is a clinical opinion, whereas "competence" is a legal judgment.) You must know *what specific issue the patient is being asked to consider* (5). To facilitate communication, it may be helpful to ask what "ability" the team wants you to evaluate – for instance, the *ability* to understand pros/cons of treatment or treatment refusal. It is not enough to posit that patients lack capacity to make decisions simply because they disagree with their doctors (see Chapter 5).

If your role limitations preclude you from seeing a patient, or if the consult question seems better suited to another service, redirect callers appropriately. Merely refusing the consultation does not help the caller, and it can negatively impact your relationship with the consulting team. Most important, *such behavior does not help the patient.*

Although some consults may seem "inappropriate," for purposes of this chapter we will refrain from using this descriptor (6). Consult questions may be difficult to discern, or they may have "hidden agendas" (7) or "covert" motivations (8). The challenge is to *determine what you can do to help the patient and primary team.*

How acute is the consult?

Though institutional conventions vary, consults are typically described as *routine, urgent,* or *emergent. Routine* consults should be completed within 24 hours of when they are called (8). *Urgent* and *emergent* consults may require quicker action (within four hours and "as soon as possible," respectively). Asking to see a routine consult "later" is not inappropriate per se, but you must *know your department's policy* before deferring any consult. It is typically advisable to do today's work today (3).

It is considered *unprofessional* to defer consults until the next shift simply because you are tired or do not want to be bothered! This reflects poorly on you as an individual and as a team player.

Table 1.3 Information gathering

Documentation:
Notes
- Current admission
- Past admissions

Recent orders
- Activity
- Diet
- Medication (administration, discontinuation)

Vital signs and trends
Results of testing
- Laboratory results (see Table 1.4)
- Imaging results
  - Head imaging
  - Other imaging
- Electrocardiogram
- Electroencephalogram

Additional results
- Other consultations
- PT/OT evaluations
- Speech/swallowing evaluations

Patient information:
Interview and examine the patient
Obtain collateral information

Key:
OT = occupational therapy
PT = physical therapy

Next steps

You have been called to see a new patient. Your expectations are clear, and your preparation is complete. You are ready for the next steps of information gathering; these are summarized in Table 1.3.

Review documentation and results

Depending on the institution, patients may have written medical records, electronic medical records, or both. Knowing what records are available, and where different information is located, will facilitate your job as "med-psych detective."

Notes

Multidisciplinary healthcare teams include physicians, medical students, nurses, social workers, and other personnel. Review notes quickly but thoroughly to see if problems or symptoms are being documented (8). Watch for trends (confusion which worsens every evening; agitation which occurs with each dressing change). Some consultations can be averted, or significantly truncated, if you review notes carefully for details that may have been overlooked.

Records for the current admission are only part of the story – if you have access to old records, look for prior psychiatric consultations or inpatient psychiatric notes (7). Past records are especially important if the patient is unwilling or unable to participate in the interview, and/or if collateral informants are unavailable.

Table 1.4 Laboratory tests to review

Common Laboratory Tests:
- Complete blood count with differential
- Comprehensive metabolic panel including calcium, magnesium, phosphorus
- Therapeutic drug levels
- Thyroid and liver function tests
- Toxicology screens
- Urinalysis with culture/sensitivity

Additional Laboratory Tests:
- Arterial blood gas
- Blood cultures
- Cerebrospinal fluid studies
- Heavy metal screens
- Hepatitis panel
- Human immunodeficiency virus test
- Rapid plasma reagin (RPR) or Venereal Disease Research Laboratory (VDRL)
- Vitamin B12 and folate

Recent orders

Review recent orders with careful attention to *changes in activity level, diet, and medications* which correspond temporally to psychiatric symptoms. Dietary or activity restrictions can contribute to irritability; medication administration (or discontinuation) can cause behavioral and/or cognitive problems. Critically review medication lists, with awareness that non-psychiatric medications can cause psychiatric symptoms. Utilize on-line or electronic media to verify medication effects and interactions if you are unsure.

Vital signs

Vital signs out of the normal range, and vital sign trends, are important to identify because they can help you detect underlying issues. For instance, vital sign instability in a confused patient who has been hospitalized for two days might lead you to diagnose alcohol or benzodiazepine withdrawal – conditions with potentially life-threatening complications if not identified and treated promptly (9) (see Chapter 19).

Testing results (laboratory studies, imaging, electrocardiogram, electroencephalogram)

As with vital signs, abnormal laboratory studies (hyponatremia in a confused patient, hyperthyroidism in an anxious patient) may contribute to the patient's presentation. Common labs are listed in Table 1.4. If you do not see routine laboratory test results in the patient's record, or if tests have not been done in recent days, recommend them.

Imaging studies, such as head imaging revealing an acute bleed or expanding subdural hematoma, or chest imaging revealing pneumonia, may provide other medical reasons for the patient's apparent psychiatric problems. As with laboratory tests, if you feel that imaging studies may be helpful, recommend them.

Electrocardiograms (ECGs/EKGs), if available, should be reviewed and may have to be requested if not yet done during the patient's stay. Special attention should be paid to *prolongation of the corrected QT interval* (QTc), because some psychiatric medications (antipsychotics including IV haloperidol; antidepressants including citalopram) can contribute to or worsen this condition and may cause serious adverse consequences including torsades de pointes (10, 11).

Electroencephalogram (EEG) results showing seizure activity can be helpful in patients with agitation or somnolence (post-ictal phenomena), and EEG results showing diffuse slowing might be relevant in patients with ill-defined confusion (consistent with delirium). EEGs certainly are not required for every psychiatric consult, and they are not specific enough to use as a psychiatric diagnostic tool. Nonetheless, they can be helpful in certain cases, such as in helping to differentiate *general delirium* (with diffuse slowing) from *benzodiazepine/alcohol withdrawal delirium* (with faster beta wave patterns) (12). As in the above studies, recommend an EEG if the patient's case so warrants.

It is not appropriate to order every test for every patient on every occasion, in a "shotgun approach" to consulting. Use common sense! Medical acumen is a necessary part of the consultation process.

Additional results (other consultations, PT/OT evaluations, swallow studies)

Patients may see multiple consultants during their hospital stay. Review consultation notes to see if mental health issues have been noted, and/or addressed, by other teams before the time of your involvement. Neurology, palliative care, hospice, and pain management consults can be particularly illuminating.

Physical therapy (PT) and occupational therapy (OT) evaluations often comment on the patient's ability to ambulate safely and live independently. Speech and swallowing evaluations also are helpful. Inability to eat or drink properly may impact a patient's mood and cooperation with care, and may also affect what medications and routes of administration you can recommend – for example, being unable to swallow pills may necessitate liquid, intramuscular, or intravenous medications.

Interview the patient!

Psychiatric interviews in the general hospital setting are significantly different from interviews in the outpatient clinic setting. Hospitals are noisy, scary places and privacy is not easy to ensure. Roommates, visitors, nursing staff, and even maintenance personnel can infringe upon your interview! Couple the busy environment with a patient who may be struggling emotionally or cognitively, and who may not want to talk to you, and the interview becomes very challenging (13).

Basics

Before entering the room, check with the patient's nurse – is the patient going to a test? Is another consultant with the patient? Is she or he having a bedside procedure, or washing up? Is he or she finally sleeping for the first time all day? Unless you must see the patient immediately, the consult may have to be deferred temporarily. Additionally, before entering the room, make sure that you have identified any isolation or contact precautions needed (i.e., mask, gloves, or gown).

If you attempt to see a patient but are unable to do so, leave a note in the chart or page the primary team. Indicate that you attempted to do the consultation, and state when you or one of your colleagues will return. This is reassuring to the primary team, and appropriately reflects that you attempted to see the patient in a timely fashion. Notify your team that the patient wasn't seen, so another attempt can be made later.

Upon entering the patient's room, survey the scene and introduce yourself. If a 1:1 sitter is present, ask him or her to leave for the interview. If visitors are present, ask if the patient would like them to stay or leave. It is ideal to interview the patient alone, at least initially. However this is not always possible or comfortable for the patient.

Introduce yourself as a psychiatric consultant called by the primary team. Depending on the case, you may explain that it is routine for your team to be called when someone has made a suicide attempt. You may say that your team commonly visits patients who are experiencing symptoms such as low mood/confusion/insomnia. You may simply say that the team was worried and wondered if there was something you could do for the patient (14).

Ideally, the patient's team will tell him or her about the consultation before you arrive. If this doesn't happen, the patient may be surprised or upset about seeing a psychiatrist. The patient may feel ambushed (7)! Empathize with the patient, and voice a commitment to collaboration (15). Statements such as, "I wouldn't be happy about a surprise visitor either," and "Let's try to see how I can help," may set the patient at ease and facilitate the conversation.

Before launching into the formal interview, *sit down* (14). This communicates willingness to stay and listen to the patient. Offer to help the patient get comfortable for the interview (14). Raise the bed, turn down the television, and speak loudly enough for the patient to hear you. As in any psychiatric patient interview, be mindful of safety issues including the patient's proximity to the door and potentially dangerous objects in the room (e.g., metal silverware, cigarette lighters).

When starting your interview, it is both informative and polite to ask how the patient is feeling physically. Pain or fatigue may necessitate a brief initial visit, with follow-ups scheduled as the patient can tolerate. Share what you know about patients' current circumstances, so they do not have to tell their entire story, and ask how they are handling the experience of the hospitalization (14).

After establishing your identity and the reason for the interview, and after discussing the patient's medical issues, it is time to address the basic portions of the psychiatry interview (Table 1.5). Be flexible, listen closely, and follow the patient's lead (16). Adhering rigidly to a list of questions may be off-putting. Speak to patients in a manner and style to which they can relate (17). Bedside cognitive testing may be important if you suspect that the patient is having cognitive processing problems. Inform the patient that you need to ask a few standard questions, before firing away (14).

In some cases, patients are too emotionally or cognitively impaired to participate in the interview. Although sometimes described as being a "poor historian," it is less judgmental to describe the patient as "unable to contribute to the interview at this time" by virtue of emotional/cognitive impairment.

In concluding your interview, *discuss intervention options* being sure to discuss them with your attending. You may offer return visits for bedside support; you may offer medications; you may offer ancillary services such as chaplains or other therapies; you could offer the patient a list of outpatient psychiatric resources for use after discharge; you may inform patients that you will be arranging inpatient psychiatric care when they are medically stable. Tell patients that you will be calling their primary team, and tell them if and when you will return for another visit. Before exiting the room, ask if the patient needs anything (nursing assistance, refill of water pitcher), and offer to tell visitors that they can return.

Table 1.5 Elements of the mental status examination (with sample responses)

Appearance: clean, disheveled, in hospital gown, in street clothes

Psychomotor activity: retarded, agitated, restless; tremors/tics/dyskinesia/seizure activity if evident

Eye contact: poor, fair, good

Behavior: uncooperative, minimally interactive, cooperative, appropriate, pleasant

Orientation: self, location, date, circumstances

Speech: rate, tone, and amount; fluent, spontaneous; slurred or aphasic if evident; naming, repetition, comprehension

Mood: quoted in the patient's own words whenever possible

Affect: quality (appropriate/inappropriate), quantity (full-range, restricted, blunted, flat, labile), description

Thought processing: linear, future-focused, goal-directed, confused, circumstantial, tangential, loose, concrete

Thought content: psychosis (hallucinations, delusions), lethality to self/others

Bedside cognitive testing
- Memory: 3/3 registration and recall testing, remote personal history, general fund of knowledge
- Attention/concentration: serial 7's, spelling backwards
- Abstraction: idioms, similarities
- Clock-drawing test, MMSE, SLUMS, MoCA

Insight: poor, fair, good

Judgment: poor, fair, good

Key:
MMSE = Mini-Mental State Examination (29)
SLUMS = St Louis Mental Status examination (30)
MoCA = Montreal Cognitive Assessment (31)

Special cases

In some cases, communication barriers require special services. Use of professional interpretive services (via translators or phone translation systems and sign language services) is superior to using friends/family members. Friends and family may "edit" interactions between you and the patient if sensitive material is being discussed (18).

If patients are intubated, have tracheostomies, or are aphasic, creative communication may be necessary. Techniques include writing on blank paper, using word boards or computerized keyboards, and nodding/shaking head or blinking eyes for "yes" or "no."

Examine the patient

Psychiatrists typically refrain from physically examining their patients because this intimate activity can blur therapeutic lines. However, physical examinations including neurologic examinations (noting cogwheeling, rigidity, tremors, asymmetric appearance or strength, hyperreflexia, and pupil size and reactivity) can be appropriate for psychiatric consultants to perform (8). Other elements of physical examination should be done on an as-needed basis. Your exam may confirm previous physical findings, or may identify pivotal changes.

Gather collateral information

Collateral information is helpful in cases where patients are unable to communicate effectively. It is also crucial in cases where patients can communicate, but there may be concerns about truth-telling or ability to maintain safety. This includes post–suicide attempt patients now denying suicidal intention, and patients with apparent substance disorders who are minimizing their usage. Family, friends, and outpatient clinicians are common sources of collateral information. Members of the multidisciplinary team also provide key collateral information regarding the patient's status while hospitalized. Gathering data through this "expanded psychiatric interview" (19) gives a comprehensive picture of the patient.

Remember that you are allowed to obtain information from clinical care providers that the patient has seen previously, as part of care coordination. *This is allowable under HIPAA regulations* (20). Also, you can *obtain* vital information from family/friends/others, but you cannot *release* patient information unless permitted by the patient. Of course, you must not discuss any patient issues with persons to whom the information is neither relevant nor pertinent.

Interventions

Write a note

Once you have reviewed the records and interviewed the patient, you can make treatment recommendations for the patient ("consult"), and you can review basic educational concepts with the primary team ("liaison") (21). Your note is a crucial element of this process (22).

Consultation notes should be simple, devoid of "psycho-speak" terminology, modest in length, legible if handwritten, and pertinent to the consult question (7, 8). Adhere to your institution's conventions for consultation documentation. This helps primary teams identify the note visually and on the basis of location (in the "consultation" portion of the record). Document the source of your information – from the patient, from past records, from current records, or from family/others. This prevents people from assuming that your note is a record of what the patient told you himself/herself, and explains discrepancies if any.

Table 1.6 summarizes elements of your interview and consultation note. Although mental status elements of psychiatric consultation notes are much the same as other psychiatric notes, additional emphasis is placed on medical issues, medications, results of testing and other consultations, and information synthesis.

Offer treatment recommendations

It is important that recommendations are clearly detailed in the "Assessment and Recommendations" portion of your note, so primary teams understand exactly what you think needs to be done (8).

Safety first

First, you should comment upon safety issues. Primary teams may have to make adjustments in personnel or patient location if the patient needs a 1:1 sitter, so you should tell them as soon as possible about any need for sitters. If the patient is not acutely dangerous (and therefore does *not* need a 1:1 sitter), this is another helpful message for the primary team.

When patients are acutely dangerous on the open medical unit, comment on whether they might warrant an inpatient psychiatric admission. If so, this is an opportune time to comment on what issues (vital sign instability, need for intravenous medications) should be resolved before the time of psychiatry transfer. This reassures the primary team that you are

Table 1.6 Elements of the consultation interview and note

(Patient identifier: medical record sticker or electronic note tag, with name and hospital number)

Date and time of consultation

Name of consulting team attending

Names of psychiatric consultants

Patient's identifying information (first/last name, marital status, race, gender, employment status; reason for hospitalization; current hospital location)

Reason for consultation

Chief complaint (quoted in the patient's own words whenever possible)

History of present illness
- Elements of the patient's medical course (medical issues, surgical procedures, current status, progress and disposition planning)
- Symptoms that prompted the consultation

Psychiatric review of systems (including mood disorders, anxiety disorders, psychotic disorders, substance use disorders, eating disorders, somatoform disorders, cognitive disorders, lethality)

Past psychiatric history
- Age of first treatment
- Diagnosis/diagnoses
- Past medications (including efficacy, side effects, reason for discontinuation)
- Current home medications
- Current outpatient provider
- History of, and most recent, inpatient hospitalizations and suicide attempts

Past medical history, including allergies

Family medical history

Family psychiatric history

Social history
- Brief childhood/developmental information/educational level
- Employment or disability status
- Current living situation
- Marital status and social supports
- Abuse (physical, sexual, emotional), legal, and military histories

Substance use history (including caffeine, alcohol, tobacco, illicit substances, and routes of use)
- Most recent usage
- Past history of detoxification or rehabilitation
- Past history of withdrawal syndromes
- Longest sobriety
- Psychosocial problems resulting from usage

Current inpatient medications (including medications, dosages, frequency, scheduling, and any correlation between medications and psychiatric symptoms or problems)

Pertinent laboratory test results, imaging results, EKG, EEG, etc

Mental status examination (see Table 1.5)

Assessment (including brief summary/formulation of the patient's case)

Axis I-V

Recommendations
- Safety issues
- Pharmacologic and non-pharmacologic recommendations
- Laboratory studies or other studies as indicated
- Follow-up plans

Psychiatry contact information, including 24/7 pager number for emergencies

Key:
EEG = electroencephalogram
EKG = electrocardiogram

thinking ahead, and tells them what specific pieces of the medical puzzle must be addressed before the patient can be moved.

Pharmacologic interventions

Medications can be the cause and cure for myriad psychiatric issues. Identifying unnecessary and/or psychiatrically offensive medications is a significant part of consultation psychiatry. Anticholinergic medications, benzodiazepines, and narcotics are particularly "deliriogenic" in the medically ill or debilitated (23, 24). These should be minimized or avoided if possible (except for utilizing benzodiazepines in acute alcohol or benzodiazepine withdrawal syndromes) (9). See Chapters 4 and 19 for details. Commenting upon medications to be discontinued, limited, or avoided can help reduce unnecessary polypharmacy.

If you feel that psychiatric medications would benefit the patient, first check pertinent results (including pregnancy test and EKG). It is helpful to give recommendations about *specific medications, dosages, routes of administration, frequency, and indication for usage if you are recommending "PRN" dosing*. You should also alert primary teams to monitor for psychiatric medication side effects (watch for extrapyramidal symptoms or acute dystonia; monitor QTc with daily EKGs if needed; watch for anxiety or insomnia).

Non-pharmacologic interventions

Interventions other than medications can be helpful as well, including reorienting and reassuring the patient as needed, providing necessary assistive devices (including hearing aids and eyeglasses) (25), using interpretive services when needed (18), explaining procedures and communicating clearly with the patient, and having family meetings. Finally, if the primary team is going to hold an interdisciplinary team meeting, offer to attend to provide additional assistance/support.

It may be helpful to utilize psychotherapeutic interventions. Various techniques include supportive psychotherapy, interpersonal psychotherapy, and cognitive-behavioral psychotherapy. The reader is referred to several articles on brief psychotherapy at the bedside (26–28).

Ancillary resources

Some patients find it helpful, and less stigmatizing, to have *non-psychiatric services* involved in their care. These include chaplains for spiritual support, and other interventions such as relaxation, art, music, and pet therapies. Marshalling these resources shows patients that you care about their suffering, as well as about their comfort level with psychiatric interventions. Patient advocates or representatives, risk management personnel, and legal team members also may be involved if needed.

Laboratory and other studies

In this section, you can recommend laboratory, imaging, or other tests that you think might be relevant to the patient's case. Citing your rationale, and how results might direct patient care, is helpful.

Concluding remarks

At the end of your note, it is appropriate to indicate whether you will be following the patient routinely, peripherally, or not at all. In all cases, you need to include *contact information* so that the primary team can reach psychiatry personnel 24/7 if they need assistance. If you will not be seeing the patient again, or if you are signing off on a long-term case, it is both politically and medically wise to offer that the primary team can call anytime if new or acute psychiatric needs arise.

Communicate directly with the consulting team

You should find a member of the consulting team when you have completed the consult, to directly relay your recommendations. The primary team will know immediately that you have seen the patient and have made recommendations, and they can ask questions and request clarification from you personally. This is an improvement over merely seeing the patient, writing a note, and vacating the premises. Presenting yourself as willing to answer questions and discuss the case will show the primary team that you are invested in the collaborative (*liaison*) process.

Return for follow-up visits and recommendations as needed

One-time consultations may include capacity evaluations, safety assessments before the time of discharge, or assessments which lead directly to psychiatric admission. More complicated issues require frequent, even daily, follow-up. Anytime you are following a patient, the rules of medical record documentation apply. *Be sure to leave progress notes in the appropriate portion of the medical record* (7). Follow up on your previous recommendations, and make new ones when indicated. If you cannot locate a patient on a particular day, leave a note to that effect in the chart so that the primary team knows that you have attempted to see the patient (and so they do not think that you have forgotten them).

Along with the patient's medical acuity and psychiatric needs, remember that you were consulted by a primary team of clinicians who were worried about the patient. Therefore, consider the patient's mental health needs, as well as the primary team's comfort, before signing off. Always offer re-consultation if needed.

References

1. Abram HS. Interpersonal aspects of psychiatric consultations in a general hospital. Psychiatry Med. 1971;2:321–6.

2. Abramson R. Liaison psychiatrist as priest or bartender. J Am Soc Psychosom Dent Med. 1978;25(1):20–7.

3. Wise MG, Rundell JR. Effective psychiatric consultation in a changing health care environment. In: Wise MG, Rundell JR, editors. Clinical manual of psychosomatic medicine: a guide to consultation-liaison psychiatry. Washington (DC): American Psychiatric Publishing, Inc; 2005. p. 1–10.

4. Ganzini L, Volicer L, Nelson W, Derse A. Pitfalls in assessment of decision-making capacity. Psychosomatics. 2003;44(3): 237–43.

5. Elliott RL. Psychiatric consultations in medical settings. Part II: clinical strategies. Dir Psychiatry. 2003;23(3): 31–41.

6. Kucharski A, Groves JE. The so-called "inappropriate" psychiatric consultation request on a medical or surgical ward. Int J Psychiatry Med. 1976–77;7(3): 209–20.

7. Rowe CJ, Billings RF, Pohlman ER, Silver IL. Pitfalls and pratfalls in consultation-liaison psychiatry in a general hospital. Can J Psychiatry. 1988;33(4):294–8.

8. Elliott RL. Psychiatric consultations in medical settings. Part I: an introduction. Dir Psychiatry. 2003;23(2):17–28.

9. Myrick H, Anton RF. Clinical management of alcohol withdrawal. CNS Spectr. 2000; 5(2):22–32.

10. Zemrak WR, Kenna GA. Association of antipsychotic and antidepressant drugs with Q-T interval prolongation. Am J Health Syst Pharm. 2008;65(11):1029–38.

11. Kanjananthai S, Kanluen T, Chareonthaitawee P. Citalopram induced torsade de pointes, a rare life threatening side effect. Int J Cardiol. 2008;131(1): e33–4.

12. Trzepacz PT, Meagher DJ. Delirium. In: Wise MG, Rundell JR, editors. Clinical manual of psychosomatic medicine: a guide to consultation-liaison psychiatry. Washington (DC): American Psychiatric Publishing, Inc; 2005. p. 91–130.

13. Wise MG, Rundell JR. Mental status examination and other tests of brain function. In: Wise MG, Rundell JR, editors. Clinical manual of psychosomatic medicine: a guide to consultation-liaison psychiatry. Washington (DC): American Psychiatric Publishing, Inc; 2005. p. 11–27.

14. Yager J. Specific components of bedside manner in the general hospital psychiatric consultation: 12 concrete suggestions. Psychosomatics. 1989;30(2):209–12.

15. Knesper DJ. My favorite tips for engaging the difficult patient on consultation-liaison psychiatry services. Psychiatr Clin North Am. 2007;30(2):245–52.

16. Henry GW. Some modern aspects of psychiatry in general hospital practice. Am J Psychiatry. 1929;9(3):481–99.

17. Viederman M. The therapeutic consultation: finding the patient. Am J Psychother. 2006;60(2):153–9.

18. Phelan M, Parkman S. How to work with an interpreter. Br Med J. 1995; 311(7004):555–7.

19. Meyer E, Mendelson M. Psychiatric consultations with patients on medical and surgical wards: patterns and processes. Psychiatry. 1961;24(3): 197–220.

20. Simon RI, Schindler BA, Levenson JL. Legal issues. In: Levenson JL, editor. Textbook of psychosomatic medicine. Washington (DC): American Psychiatric Publishing, Inc; 2005. p. 37–53.

21. Oken D. Liaison psychiatry (liaison medicine). Adv Psychosom Med. 1983; 11:23–51.

22. Alexander T, Bloch S. The written report in consultation-liaison psychiatry: a proposed schema. Aust N Z J Psychiatry. 2002;36: 251–8.

23. Pisani MA, Murphy TE, Araujo KL, Slatum P, Van Ness PH, Inouye SK. Benzodiazepine and opioid use and the duration of intensive care unit delirium in an older population. Crit Care Med. 2009; 37(1):177–83.

24. Agostini JV, Leo-Summers LS, Inouye SK. Cognitive and other adverse effects of diphenhydramine use in hospitalized older patients. Arch Intern Med. 2001; 161(17):2091–7.

25. Inouye SK, Bogardus ST Jr, Williams CS, Leo-Summers L, Agostini JV. The role of adherence on the effectiveness of nonpharmacologic interventions: evidence from the delirium prevention trial. Arch Intern Med. 2003;163(8):958–64.

26. Griffith JL, Gaby L. Brief psychotherapy at the bedside: countering demoralization from medical illness. Psychosomatics. 2005;46(2):109–16.

27. Muskin PR. The combined use of psychotherapy and pharmacotherapy in the medical setting. Psychiatr Clin North Am. 1990;13(2):3 41–53.

28. Viederman M. Active engagement in the consultation process. Gen Hosp Psychiatry. 2002;24(2):93–100.

29. Folstein MF, Folstein SE, McHugh PR. "Mini-mental state." A practical method for grading the cognitive state of patients for the clinician. J Psychiatr Res. 1975; 12(3):189–98.

30. Tariq SH, Tumosa N, Chibnall JT, Perry MH 3rd, Morley JE. Comparisons of the Saint Louis University mental status examination and the mini-mental state examination for detecting dementia and mild neurocognitive disorder – a pilot study. Am J Geriatr Psychiatry. 2006; 14(11):900–10.

31. Nasreddine ZS, Phillips NA, Bedirian V, Charbonneau S, Whitehead V, Collin I, et al. The Montreal Cognitive Assessment, MoCA: a brief screening tool for mild cognitive impairment. J Am Geriatr Soc. 2005;53(4): 695–9.

Chapter 2

Assessing capacity in the medically ill: I don't want to!

Mary J. Fitz-Gerald

Typical consult question

Please assess competency in this patient

The patient, Ms. A., a thirty-four year old female with end-stage renal disease, was admitted several days before the consult with multiple electrolyte abnormalities due to non-compliance with dialysis and medications. During her hospital stay, she refused dialysis or left before treatment was completed. Though hyperkalemic, she refused to follow the renal diet. She spoke rationally on the phone, but would ignore her physicians' questions. When the team attempted to discharge her against medical advice, Ms. A. refused to leave the hospital. The nephrology team requested the psychiatry consult for competency evaluation.

During the psychiatric interview, Ms. A. was sullen and uncooperative. She responded to only some of the questions and repeated, "I'm not crazy!" Ms. A. did tell the consult team that she was the mother of five school-aged children, but she didn't know who was watching the children while she was in the hospital, or even if they were currently in school. Ms. A. traveled and lived between two cities approximately two hundred miles apart. When asked why she was refusing dialysis, Ms. A. didn't answer. She told us to contact her physician in the other city. According to the paperwork faxed from this physician, he'd discharged her from his care because of non-compliance. She'd been discharged from dialysis centers around the city for the same reason. Ms. A. announced she'd talk to us if the hospital attorney (not her attorney) was present. When the attorney arrived, she refused to speak.

Background

Patient autonomy and physician beneficence are two aspects of twenty-first century medical ethics. In some countries and in years past, beneficence was the primary aspect of medical ethics. Today, patient autonomy has assumed greater importance. Informed consent allows for patient autonomy. Assessment of capacity to make medical decisions correlates the concepts of patient autonomy and physician beneficence, and is an important factor in current medical practice (1).

Physicians make at least an informal decision on a continual basis regarding the patient's ability to give informed consent. Prescribing medicines or recommending follow-up to a patient assumes that he has the ability to understand the instructions. Physicians assess capacity any time consent is signed for a medical procedure, treatment, or advance directives. Any physician may be asked about a patient's ability to drive or handle finances. Patients who

Psychosomatic Medicine: An Introduction to Consultation-Liaison Psychiatry, eds. James J. Amos and Robert G. Robinson. Published by Cambridge University Press. © Cambridge University Press 2010.

are confused, refuse treatment, or suffer from mental illness may raise red flags for the attending physician. At these times, a consultant psychiatrist may be contacted to formally evaluate the patient for capacity to make medical decisions. In spite of the frequency of formal and informal capacity assessment, numerous fallacies exist about capacity determination (2).

Misconceptions

The difference between *competency* and *capacity* is a common misconception, and the terms, *competency* and *capacity*, are often used interchangeably in consult requests. *Competency,* a legal decision, refers to the ability to handle personal affairs and make decisions. Only a judge may declare a person incompetent for either specific functions or global incompetence. Individuals are presumed competent; the burden of proof lies with the individual alleging incompetence of the patient. A determination of *capacity,* ability to make an informed decision, may be made by any licensed physician. The terms *competency* and *capacity* are used interchangeably if all parties acknowledge that the decision is not a legal one, but is specific to the procedure or activity specified (3).

Capacity is often considered an "all-or-none" phenomenon, and this may be the most common fallacy (2). In addition to the ability to give consent, other aspects of capacity include the ability to care for self independently at home or to make financial decisions. Issues may arise regarding ability to leave against medical advice or refuse treatment.

All of these decisions require an assessment and an evaluation of risks and benefits to the patient. A patient may have the ability to make some decisions and not others. One tool physicians utilize to assess capacity is a risk versus benefit analysis. Procedures involving minimal risk with high potential gain require a lower standard of understanding and capacity than procedures with higher risk require. For example, an individual may have the capacity to agree to a lumbar puncture in a case of suspected meningitis, but may lack the capacity to refuse the lumbar puncture or to leave against medical advice if meningitis is suspected. In this instance, the benefits of the lumbar puncture far outweigh any risks. Conversely, the risks of leaving against medical advice in a patient with an unstable medical condition may outweigh the benefits the patient specifies for his professed decision to leave against medical advice. This sliding scale approach has drawbacks, but presents a practical manner by which to allow the patient autonomy when possible (4, 5).

Another fallacy is that many believe that any decision made regarding capacity is permanent (2). Clinicians should realize that the capacity to make decisions fluctuates with the patient's condition. A delirious individual may initially lack the capacity to agree to a procedure, but may regain the ability as his orientation and mental status improve. Also, the reverse is true. An individual may initially have the capacity to agree to procedures, but may lose the capacity if his condition deteriorates (6). The physician should analyze the patient's ability to make decisions with every procedure; failure to do so increases liability and can decrease patient trust in the relationship. Furthermore, the clinician's responsibility is to help the patient regain capacity if at all possible, and the psychiatric consultant may be invaluable in this regard.

Studies show that physicians are more apt to question a patient's ability to refuse recommended treatment than to question if the patient has the ability to consent to the recommendations (7). Part of the evaluation of capacity analyzes the *process* that the patient utilizes to reach a decision. Many clinicians assess the final decision only, and not the patient's rationale for the decision (2). A patient may agree with the physician's recommendations and may even voice risks, benefits, and alternatives to the proposed treatment. Yet, the patient may still lack capacity if conditions exist which impair capacity. For example, studies show that up to 52% of patients with schizophrenia have faulty capacity to make medical decisions (8). Suicidal ideation and depression may cause a patient to refuse life-saving treatment (9).

Reasons for evaluation

Studies show that requests for capacity evaluations fall into several categories. Farnsworth (6) examined 90 requests for competency between 1983 and 1986. The largest percentage (approximately half) consisted of a request to evaluate the patient's ability to function independently on discharge. The next most common reason for evaluation was competency to refuse medical treatment. Seventeen percent of evaluations were requested to determine if the patient was able to give informed consent. Requests to leave against medical advice prompted 5% of the consults (6).

The most common diagnoses which prompt request for capacity evaluation include dementia and delirium. Other diagnoses include substance abuse, affective disorders, personality factors, and psychotic disorders. It is interesting to note that the diagnosis also affected the reason for consult. Of the consults evaluating ability to give informed consent, one-fourth had a diagnosis of schizophrenia. The most frequent reason for the consult in patients with organic mental disorder was ability to return home (6).

Myers and Barrett (10) examined 100 retrospective and 100 prospective requests for capacity evaluation. They identified three major categories. The first group was hospitalized because of self-injury and then either refused treatment, or desired discharge. The second group was composed of the elderly or others with cognitive deficits. The third group consisted of individuals with personality characteristics and difficult management issues. Similar concerns were found by Mebane and Rauch (11).

Legal issues

Ms. B., an eighteen year old G_1P_0, was admitted to a Louisiana hospital at twenty-four weeks gestation in diabetic ketoacidosis and acutely psychotic. She had a history of insulin-dependent diabetes mellitus and schizoaffective disorder and was non-compliant for both illnesses. The obstetric and psychiatric consult teams felt that involuntary hospitalization was necessary for the protection of mother and baby. The judge agreed with the petition. At thirty-four weeks gestation the obstetric team petitioned the court to allow for any necessary surgical obstetric intervention.

Because informed consent is one of the major issues in competency evaluation, we must note that there are exceptions to the need for informed consent. Some states have laws which limit the ability to give consent to medical treatment for certain groups of patients. For instance, patients who are involuntarily committed for mental illness in Louisiana may not give consent for major surgery without a court order. Even if the patient does have the capacity to make a decision and agrees with the procedure, a judicial ruling is necessary. In the case above, Ms. B. was aware of the possibility of a cesarean delivery, knew the risks and benefits, and was agreeable should the occasion arise. Because of her involuntary commitment status, however, the court hearing was necessary to provide consent (12). An informal study conducted by the author among house staff and faculty in her institution revealed that many non-psychiatrists were not aware of this requirement.

Other exceptions exist. For individuals who lack capacity to give informed consent or who have previously been found legally incompetent, consent is obtained from a legally acceptable substitute decision-maker. Another exception can be seen in the case where immediate emergency treatment is necessary to save life or limb, or to prevent serious harm. The risk must be imminent and due to the patient's condition, and the physician must document the emergent need and the inability to obtain consent from the individual or an alternate consenter (13).

Two other rationales for lack of informed consent are commonly accepted. With therapeutic privilege, the psychiatrist determines that complete disclosure to meet the requirements of informed consent would be harmful to the patient. The last is when a patient has waived his right to obtain full information (13). Studies conflict on how much information patients actually want about treatments (14–16).

Maladaptive denial

Mr. C., a sixty-two year old male, was admitted to the hospital with a gangrenous great toe. A chart review showed that his psychiatric history was negative, but he'd had a diagnosis of diabetes mellitus for several years and had been non-compliant with treatment and follow-up. Though a former nursing assistant, he denied that he had diabetes. He refused amputation because "I don't need it." The surgery was done with surrogate decision-maker consent on an emergent basis. Mr. C. then refused treatment for his diabetes saying, "There are plenty of people out there walking around with sugars higher than mine and they're not on medicines!"

As stated above, the process the patient utilizes to make a decision is more important than the actual decision. Denial, a defense mechanism utilized to avoid unpleasant effects by denying aspects of reality (17), can be helpful for patients in some cases. For instance, a person with cancer may minimize the seriousness of his condition and believe that all will be well if he exercises, follows the doctor's recommendations, meditates, etc. In this case, denial doesn't interfere with treatment and provides a psychological benefit to the patient.

A condition known as *maladaptive denial* is sometimes seen in patients referred for capacity evaluation. Because of denial of illness and consequences, the patient lacks the insight to make treatment decisions (18). Denial of illness may occur even if the patient declares that he knows that he has the disease and knows the consequences. Anyone who has treated substance abusers realizes that some may voice the words, but their actions don't correlate with the words. The legal system has recognized that *maladaptive denial* of illness may impair the capacity of an individual to make medical decisions (18).

Work-up

The consult for competency is often requested on an emergent basis (11). The initial assessment, as with any request for psychiatric consultation, involves discussion with the requesting physician. What is the physical condition of the patient? Why does the physician question the patient's ability to make a decision about his/her care? Has the physician discussed with the patient and family recommended treatment options, alternatives, risks, and benefits? What does the physician expect the consultant psychiatrist to address? To question the patient, the psychiatrist must have a firm grasp of the nature of the physical condition and available treatments; the other questions help the consultant understand the relationship between the physician and the patient.

An interview for competency/capacity includes a chart review, history, and mental status exam, as well as questioning of the patient related to the ability to give consent for the procedure. The psychiatrist develops rapport with the patient by introducing himself and discussing his role. Open-ended questions provide valuable information about the patient's perception of his illness and his perception of his treatment. Often, miscommunication between parties prompts the consult request, and the consultant psychiatrist utilizes his liaison role to facilitate agreement (19).

Capacity to make medical decisions includes the ability to communicate a choice, understand relevant information, appreciate the situation and its consequences, and compare choices (20). Additional aspects include voluntariness and consistency of the decision. An interview with the patient will reveal his ability to understand his physical condition and the proposed treatments. Questions should also address the patient's stated desires. Family sometimes consciously or unconsciously influences the patient's decision. If the treating physician isn't coercing the patient, influence by the family is likely unavoidable and doesn't negate the validity of the consent (20).

Mr. D. is a nineteen year old male, status post motor vehicle collision. As a result of the accident, he sustained a traumatic brain injury and fracture of his ankle. Infection from the fracture led to osteomyelitis. The patient agreed to an amputation of his foot; he knew the risks and benefits of the procedure and alternatives to treatment. On the surface the patient appeared to have the capacity to give informed consent to the procedure. Yet, during the routine mental status exam questioning, Mr. D. reported that he was hearing voices from the television and the voices were telling him to have an amputation.

Mr. E. is a sixty year old male with a history of cardiovascular disease and recent onset of confusion and fatigue. He was admitted for work-up and was found to have hemoglobin of 5.9 grams per deciliter. Mr. E.'s Mini-Mental State Examination score was 15. He refused a blood transfusion, stating that he was a Jehovah's Witness and he didn't believe transfusions were God's will. He maintained his beliefs during multiple interviews and despite family opposition.

Low Mini-Mental State Examination (MMSE) scores do not automatically signify that the patient lacks the capacity to make a decision regarding treatment (1). The MMSE measures cognitive ability. Cognitive ability and capacity are not identical. In the case of Mr. D., he had an acceptable MMSE score of 28, but delusions interfered with the ability to give consent. In spite of his low MMSE score, Mr. E. gave a valid rationale on repeat questioning and appeared to have the competency to refuse the blood transfusion.

Additional assessments facilitate competency evaluations (6). A physical therapist can give an objective view of physical abilities. An individual who is unable to ambulate in any fashion based on physical therapy evaluation is usually unable to live alone and unassisted. Nursing notes identify problematic behavior or confusion. Occupational therapists evaluate the patient's ability to care for basic needs independently. Neuropsychological testing pinpoints and assesses cognitive deficits. These ancillary support personnel are especially helpful in performing capacity evaluations for financial management, driving, and ability to live independently.

Clinical decision-making and treatment

Analyzing information obtained from the interview, patient collateral, and ancillary services help the psychiatrist or treating physician make a decision regarding competency and possible treatments. A variety of other factors impinge upon an individual's medical decision-making capacity. Fear and uncertainty after an unexpected diagnosis of a life-threatening illness may cause a knee-jerk negative reaction to treatment recommendations. Power struggles between the patient and the physician may prompt treatment refusal or a request to leave against medical advice. Conflicting advice from different medical specialists may cause confusion. These events may occur in addition to the all too common cultural or language barriers. Female physicians sometimes hear, "I don't listen to no woman!" Studies show that common reasons for treatment refusal are denial of seriousness of illness, mistrust of team, fear of pain, and a belief that treatment was futile (19).

The danger is that initial refusal by the patient will lead to anger and rejection by the treatment team. Psychiatric consultation facilitates discussion between the patient and the treatment team. The psychiatrist functions as a sounding board for the patient and the team to individually air their frustrations. Allowing the patient time to react to the change in physical status helps to improve cooperation. Katz et al. showed that up to 50% of patients who initially refused treatment later accepted it (19).

What about patients who can speak but refuse to participate fully in the interview, as in the case of Ms. A.? Psychiatrists have little difficulty assessing catatonic or psychotic patients who refuse to speak. If the patient is not obviously psychotic and apparently is only oppositional, a decision about capacity is problematic. Sometimes the patient will agree to speak with others. If the patient still refuses to talk, the consultant and the treating physician should assess the risk to the patient caused by treatment refusal. In cases of high risk where the patient continues to refuse to answer questions or to receive appropriate treatment in spite of numerous attempts, requests, and explanations, one should proceed as though the patient lacks capacity and obtain substitute decision-making (21).

We were unable to locate Ms. A.'s relatives to discuss treatment options until the time of the initial court hearing. After the first hearing, the patient cooperated with psychological testing, which showed paranoid schizophrenia and a cognitive disorder, not otherwise specified, moderate. During a repeat court hearing, the judge committed Ms. A. to outpatient dialysis treatment and to the community health center. She was started on a low dose of an antipsychotic. Ms. A. continued to miss an occasional outpatient dialysis treatment, but the treatment team decided to not pursue additional court intervention unless she became gravely ill as the result of failure to cooperate with treatment.

Mentally ill patients are not incompetent to make medical decisions solely on the basis of that illness. Because psychosis may affect the ability to make medical decisions (see earlier), appropriate medication will improve the patient's disposition. Recognition and treatment of delirium, which is a frequent cause of incapacity (6) and is often misdiagnosed (22), may affect the patient's ability to cooperate with treatment. Studies show, however, that treatment for depression may not affect an individual's desire for treatment (23).

Some individuals are deemed competent, refuse treatment, and suffer deleterious effects. Some individuals are deemed incompetent, receive treatment, and suffer deleterious effects. Both novice and experienced clinicians can suffer doubts about their role in the capacity decision. Autonomy is a legal and moral imperative, and none of us has the ability to predict the future.

In summary, guidelines exist to help the consultant psychiatrist make a decision about the capacity of individuals. Furthermore, the psychiatrist has an important role in improving communication, handling difficult relationships, and improving capacity for patients with psychiatric impairments. Yet, capacity examination is an inexact science, and is a prime example of the art of psychiatry.

References

1. Etchells E, Katz MR, Shuchman M, Wong G, Workman S, Choudhry NK, et al. Accuracy of clinical impressions and Mini-Mental State Exam scores for assessing capacity to consent to major medical treatment: comparison with criterion-standard psychiatric assessments. Psychosomatics. 1997;38(3):239–45.

2. Ganzini L, Volicer L, Nelson W, Derse A. Pitfalls in assessment of decision-making capacity. Psychosomatics. 2003;44(3): 237–43.

3. Resnick PJ, Sorrentino RN. Forensic considerations. In: Blumenfield M, Strain JJ, editors. Psychosomatic medicine. Philadelphia (PA): Lippincott Williams & Wilkins; 2006. p. 91–106.

4. Gutheil TG, Appelbaum PS. Clinical handbook of psychiatry and the law. 2nd ed. Philadelphia (PA): Lippincott Williams & Wilkins; 2000.

5. Drane JF. Competency to give an informed consent, a model for making clinical assessments. JAMA. 1984;252(7):925–7.

6. Farnsworth MG. Competency evaluations in a general hospital. Psychosomatics. 1990;31(1):60–6.

7. Weinstock R, Copelan R, Bagheri A. Competence to give informed consent for medical procedures. Bull Am Acad Psychiatry Law. 1984;12(2):117–25.

8. Grisso T, Appelbaum PS. The MacArthur Treatment Competence Study, III: abilities of patients to consent to psychiatric and medical treatments. Law Hum Behav. 1995;19(2):149–74.

9. Wear AN, Brahams D. To treat or not to treat: the legal, ethical and therapeutic implications of treatment refusal. J Med Ethics. 1991;17(3):131–5.

10. Myers B, Barrett CL. Competency issues in referrals to a consultation-liaison service. Psychosomatics. 1986;27(11): 782–8.

11. Mebane AH, Rauch HB. When do physicians request competency evaluations? Psychosomatics. 1990; 31(1):40–6.

12. Louisiana. R.S. 2002;28:2.

13. Simon RJ. Legal and ethical issues. In: Wise MG, Rundell JR, editors. The American Psychiatric Publishing textbook of consultation-liaison psychiatry: psychiatry in the medically ill. 2nd ed. Washington (DC): American Psychiatric Publishing; 2002. p. 167–86.

14. Strull WB, Lo B, Charles G. Do patients want to participate in medical decision-making? JAMA. 1984;252:2990–4.

15. Cassileth BR, Zupkis RV, Sutton-Smith K, March V. Information and participation preferences among cancer patients. Ann Intern Med 1980;92(6):832–6.

16. Ende J, Lewis K, Ash A, Moskowitz MA. Measuring patients' desire for autonomy: decision making and information-seeking preferences among medical patients. J Gen Intern Med. 1989;4(1):23–30.

17. Freud A. The ego and the mechanisms of defense. In: Writings of Anna Freud. Vol 2 (rev ed). New York: International Universities Press; 1967.

18. Simon RI, Schindler BA, Levenson JL. Legal issues. In: Levenson JL, editor. Textbook of psychosomatic medicine. Arlington (VA): American Psychiatric Publishing Co; 2005. p. 37–53.

19. Katz M, Abbey S, Rydall A, Lowy F. Psychiatric consultation for competency to refuse medical treatment: a retrospective study of patient characteristics and outcome. Psychosomatics. 1995;36(1): 33–41.

20. Group for the Advancement of Psychiatry Committee on Medical Education. A casebook in psychiatric ethics. New York: Brunner/Mazel; 1990. p. 15–7.

21. Hurst SA. When patients refuse assessment of decision-making capacity: how should clinicians respond? Arch Intern Med. 2004; 164(16):1757–60.

22. Cole MG. Delirium in elderly patients. Am J Geriatr Psychiatry. 2004;12(1):7–21.

23. Lee M, Ganzini L. The effect of recovery from depression on preferences for life-sustaining therapy in older patients. J Gerontol. 1994;49(1):M15–21.

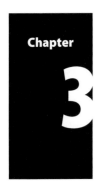
The difficult patient encounter: understanding what just happened

Raheel A. Khan and Mary J. Fitz-Gerald

Typical consult question

"We need help with a sixty-four year old professional male with end-stage renal disease on hemodialysis. He has been kicked out of all other dialysis centers due to his obnoxious behavior. He hollers and berates the staff and may be banned from our state operated unit. Is there anything that can be done to manage his behavior?"

Often, a consult, as above, is called in by members of a frustrated and perplexed team who are desperately seeking a solution for their "difficult" patient. The psychiatric consultant is asked to swoop in and "deal" with this patient because the primary team can no longer do so. It is important for the consultant to understand not only the underlying causes of the patient's behavior, but also the emotions generated in the treating staff, if a successful resolution is to be achieved.

Background

When students are asked why they enter into medicine, a common theme involves helping others and contributing to the welfare of humanity. However, after even a few years of clinical practice, many physicians will readily admit to experiences of anger, frustration, inadequacy, and, occasionally, strong negative reactions towards patients (1). Indeed, studies have demonstrated that up to 15% of patients are labeled as difficult by their physicians (2).

Difficult patients are those who present with the following (1, 2):

- Vague and generalized somatic symptoms
- Depression
- Anxiety
- Medication non-compliance
- A personality disorder
- Excessive demands and repeat visits

It is important to remember that medical illness and hospitalization can be very stressful, even for the most well adjusted individuals. First, experiencing a medical illness severe enough to require admission is universally considered a narcissistic injury. Patients must re-examine their own self-views and address any feelings of invulnerability to illness that they may have had, while also confronting the impermanence of life. This may lead the patient to feel "defective, weak, and less desirable" (3). Second, being in a hospital is very uncomfortable, forcing a patient to endure both body exposure, in thin flimsy gowns, and constant

Psychosomatic Medicine: An Introduction to Consultation-Liaison Psychiatry, eds. James J. Amos and Robert G. Robinson. Published by Cambridge University Press. © Cambridge University Press 2010.

personal and bodily intrusions. Finally, patients are separated from their normal comfortable environments and social supports yet are expected to accept a certain degree of dependency on their caregivers (3).

However, despite these factors, not all patients are difficult patients, and not all difficult patients require a psychiatric consultant. Patients who evoke strong emotional reactions such as "aversion, fear, despair, or malice" in their caregivers are the ones who require the urgent frustrated consults described previously (4). Often, but not always, these patients have personality disorders which explain the strong emotions they engender. To help patients and teams manage these complicated situations, it is vital that the consultant understand what constitutes a personality structure (e.g., coping styles, defense mechanisms), as well as the emotions experienced by the primary team (countertransference) (3, 5). Through an understanding of these psychodynamic factors, the well-informed consultant can manage even the most demanding "hateful" patients (4).

Work-up

Often, the work-up in these situations involves pattern recognition and a keen sense of one's own reaction to the patient, which can provide valuable clues to the diagnosis.

Personality types

All humans have a personality, that is, a combination of characteristics that predisposes them to think, feel, and behave in certain ways, in varied situations. Both inborn, *temperament*, and environmentally influenced, *character*, traits sculpt each individual's personality (6). A disorder of personality occurs when an individual uses a personality style that is "rigid, extreme, maladaptive, or damaging to self or others" and results in impairment in interpersonal, social, or occupational domains (5).

However, as stated previously, not all difficult patients have personality disorders (PD) or vice versa. Thus, it is useful to examine the concept of personality types, which exist on a continuum with personality disorders (Table 3.1). Under stressful situations, individuals may regress and display personality styles inconsistent with their typical behavior, or may display extremes of typical behavior. It is important to note that many patients will not fit neatly into a distinct personality style, but will display features from multiple categories. However, a basic understanding of each of these styles will help the consultant understand how a patient might be experiencing his illness and will help the consultant to recognize any countertransference feelings that may arise (3, 5, 6).

Coping styles

Another important aspect of personality is how one copes. Classically, coping has been defined as how an individual manages and attempts to alter a stressful situation. This can be problem-focused or emotion-focused. Examples of problem-focused coping are seeking information, planning, and taking action; emotion-focused coping can involve focusing on positive aspects of the situation, mental or behavioral disengagement, and seeking emotional support from others (7). Healthy copers generally use a combination of problem- and emotion-focused coping to deal with a specific stressor and use different strategies for varied situations. They are optimistic, practical, flexible, and composed; they consider possible

Table 3.1 Personality types/disorders and countertransference reactions

Personality Type	Associated Personality D/O	Countertransference Reaction
Needy-clingy	Dependent PD Histrionic PD	Initially – powerful and needed Later – depleted, irritated, angry Avoid/withdraw
Orderly-controlled	Obsessive-compulsive PD	Initially – admire diligence Later – frustrated, battle to control, "battle of wills"
Timid-apprehensive	Avoidant PD	Annoyed and frustrated by patient's weakness
Dramatizing-emotional	Histrionic PD	Initially – flattered, seduced, aroused, wish to rescue Later – depleted, angry, attempt to avoid
Masochistic	Borderline PD Antisocial PD (certain types)	Overwhelmed, helpless, filled with self-doubt
Cold-deceitful	Antisocial PD	Feel used, uncover lies, punish
Superior-critical	Narcissistic PD	Enjoy working with important person (if famous) Desire to "put in place," devalue. Or may feel inferior
Guarded-suspicious	Paranoid PD	Defensive, feeling accused
Distant-aloof	Schizoid PD	Desire to break through No connection to patient Detached, removed
The odd patient	Schizotypal PD	Break through the oddness Detached, removed

Table 3.2 Coping styles

Coping Style	Description
Confrontative	Hostile or aggressive efforts to alter a situation
Distancing	Efforts to mentally detach self from a situation
Self-controlling	Attempting to regulate one's feelings or actions
Seeking social support	Attempting to seek emotional support or information from others
Accepting responsibility	Accepting a personal role in the problem
Escape-avoidance	Efforts to escape/avoid a problem or situation, both cognitively and behaviorally
Planful problem solving	Attempting to come up with solutions to alter a situation
Positive re-appraisal	Re-framing a situation in a more positive light

outcomes and emphasize immediate problems. Poor copers are passive, deny excessively, and hold rigid and narrow views. They often are unable to make decisions, but paradoxically they have moments of impulsivity and unexpected compliance (8).

Although hundreds of coping styles are described, a well-studied categorization of coping utilizes the Ways of Coping Questionnaire–Revised, which defines eight distinct subsets (3, 7, 8) (Table 3.2). Closely related to how one copes with medical illness, is how the individual views his illness, also known as illness behavior. Adaptive coping occurs when patients view illness as a challenge, strategy, or value. Conversely, poor coping is associated with the view of illness as an enemy, punishment, weakness, relief, or irreparable loss (3).

Table 3.3 Commonly used defense mechanisms

Defense Mechanism	Description
Mature	
Humor	Emphasizing the amusing or ironic aspects of the conflict or stressors
Sublimation	Channeling unacceptable impulses into more constructive activities
Suppression	Intentional exclusion of material from consciousness
Neurotic	
Displacement	Transfer of unacceptable thoughts, feelings, or desires from one object to a less threatening substitute
Isolation of affect	Separation of painful idea/event from feelings associated with it
Rationalization	Inventing a socially acceptable and logical reason why one is not bothered
Reaction formation	Going to the opposite extreme to overcompensate for unacceptable impulses
Repression	Involuntary forgetting of a painful event
Immature	
Acting out	Performing an action to express unconscious emotional conflicts; usually antisocial in nature
Devaluation	Exaggerated negative qualities of others
Idealization	Overestimating the desirable qualities of self or others
Passive aggression	Indirect and passive expression of anger towards others
Projection	Attribution of own unacceptable desires/impulses to another person
Regression	Reversion of personality to a lower level of expression
Splitting	Separating people and actions into categories of all good and all bad
Psychotic	
Projective identification	Projecting a negative aspect of the self onto another and then coercing the other into identifying with the projected emotion
Psychotic denial	Failing to recognize obvious implications or consequences of a thought, act, or situation

Defense mechanisms

Whereas coping styles are primarily consciously applied behavioral actions, defense mechanisms are largely unconscious, psychological processes used by patients to deal with reality and to maintain self-image. Defenses are used by all individuals to protect the self from anxiety and to provide refuge from a situation with which one cannot currently cope. Healthy individuals usually use different defenses throughout their lives, whereas pathological use occurs when persistent use of certain defenses leads to maladaptive behavior that affects one's physical and/or mental health (3, 5). Additionally, there appears to be a strong relationship between coping styles and defense mechanisms, both healthy and unhealthy (9).

Typically, defenses are ranked within an adaptive hierarchy: psychotic, immature, neurotic, and mature (3, 5) (Table 3.3). Defenses most often used by "difficult patients" fall under the immature category; these are characteristic of the cluster B personality disorders (antisocial, borderline, histrionic, and narcissistic). Often, these defenses are irritating to others as this defense style transmits patients' "shame, impulses, and anxiety to those around them" (3). Neurotic defenses, which can also be maladaptive, are experienced more privately and usually do not annoy others because they do not distort reality as much. Simply stated, immature defenses make others suffer, while neurotic defenses cause the self to suffer (3).

This is an important concept for the consultant to learn as it will allow for anticipation of and methods to deal with the resultant behavior, and will prevent personal insult from these actions (5, 10). For example, awareness of splitting will allow the consultant to be astute for signs of division in the medical staff as "all good" or "all bad" caregivers, or potential conflicts between the consultant and staff. Awareness of the potential for idealizing/devaluing will allow for an understanding of the glowing praises, followed soon by harsh criticizing that is likely to occur (10). Although interpretations of these defenses may be helpful for the consultant and the primary team, direct confrontation of the patient in the acute setting may be dangerous. As mentioned previously, these defenses are generally unconscious, and improper interpretation and confrontation will not lead to an epiphany of understanding in these patients. Conversely, further escalation of angry, oppositional behavior is likely to occur (10, 11).

Countertransference

As crucial as it is to understand the patient-driven components of a "difficult encounter," physician factors also contribute. For example, does the physician adhere to a doctor- versus patient-centered approach, meaning how closely does he follow a strict medical model versus a more psychosocial approach? Additionally, a physician's ability to tolerate uncertainty and his willingness to take risks play a role in determining which patients he will find difficult to treat (2, 11).

However, perhaps the most important physician factor in these encounters is the countertransference that occurs in the care of difficult patients. Classically, countertransference was explained as reactions to a patient that represent the past life experiences of the clinician. For example, a frail elderly woman is given extra attention by a physician because she reminds him of his mother, or a young diabetic patient is scolded for non-compliance because the nurse's own child is diabetic and non-compliant (5). Recently, countertransference has come to encompass all feelings and attitudes of clinicians towards the patient, both physician- and patient-originated (5, 12).

These patient-originated physician reactions are the types of reactions that Groves classically described as "aversion, fear, despair, or even…malice" (4). However, these negative reactions are not the only types of countertransference, nor are they the only types of feelings that should be a matter of concern. Patients who generate strong positive emotions must be watched closely as this may predict later devaluation, or may potentially lead to significant boundary violations on the part of the clinician, in an effort "to do everything possible" for the patient (4, 5, 13). Each personality type and disorder engenders its own set of countertransference feelings in clinicians. Being aware of these emotions allows the clinician to attain better understanding to and provide better care for the patient (5, 6) (Table 3.1).

The "Hateful" Patient

As previously mentioned, patients can be difficult patients for various reasons (e.g., agitated delirium). However, few patients are as mystifying to primary teams as the "hateful patient," the quintessential difficult patient. In his seminal article "Taking Care of the Hateful Patient" (4), Groves introduced four distinct interpersonal styles that evoked "helplessness in the helper": Dependent Clingers, Entitled Demanders, Manipulative Help-Rejecters, and

Table 3.4 The hateful patient

The Hateful Patient	Associated Personality	Defense Mechanisms	Coping Styles	Countertransference
Dependent Clingers	Dependent Histrionic	Regression Passive aggression Idealization	Excessively seeking social support	Power and special Depleted, exhausted Wish to escape
Entitled Demanders	Narcissistic	Self-idealization Devaluing Projection Splitting	Confrontational	Fearful of reputation Enraged about demands Ashamed, inferior
Manipulative Help-Rejecters	Borderline	Splitting Projective identifying Idealizing/devaluing	Escape-avoidance Seek social supports	Anxiety overlooking illness Irritation/frustration Depression/self-doubt
Self-Destructive Deniers	Antisocial (or any cluster B)	Primitive denial Acting out Devaluing	Distancing Escape-avoidance	Enraged/malice Wish the patient were dead

Self-Destructive Deniers (4). Each of these can be linked to a classic personality style or disorder, with unique coping styles, defense mechanisms, and countertransference reactions (Table 3.4).

Dependent Clingers

As described by Groves, Dependent Clingers are "overt in their neediness" and have "repeated cries...for all forms of attention imaginable" (4). They appear completely unable to solve problems on their own or to self-soothe, continually seeking assistance from others (3). Classically, these patients resemble those with a dependent personality disorder, although histrionic patients, who can demonstrate a "pervasive childlike dependence" and regress in the context of medical illness, may also present in this manner (3, 5).

A forty-five year old male with a history of peripheral vascular disease who recently underwent a below the knee amputation is now crying and sobbing on the unit. He becomes highly anxious and despondent when there is not somebody in the room with him, calling for the nurses incessantly. When family is present, he requires their constant attention, requesting they feed him, help him drink liquids, and even blow his nose, despite full upper extremity mobility.

This patient has regressed in the context of his acute stress, acting in a very childlike manner. Although it is not obvious here, passive aggression and idealization are very common in Dependent Clingers. They are using maladaptive coping styles such as excessive use of seeking social support, while not accepting any responsibility and not using positive reappraisal (3, 5). It is not surprising that such patients engender a "sense of weary aversion" in their caregivers (4). Initially, however, physicians may feel flattered, and even a sense of specialness and power, with a strong desire to care for or rescue the patient. This is short-lived, however, and soon the depletion and bottomless need for attention begin (4, 5).

Entitled Demanders

If there is one word to describe these patients, it is "narcissistic." They present as arrogant, vain, critical, devaluing, and demanding and are easily recognized. Yet, despite this superior attitude, their goal is the same as that of the Clinger, to receive the "inexhaustible attention" of the treating team and to avoid the "terror of abandonment" (3–5).

"A fifty-six year old male is admitted to the hospital secondary to AIDS complications. Throughout the hospitalization, he is belligerent and belittling to the staff and physicians, including the junior members of the psychosomatic service. He is pleased to hear that his case is 'unique,' requiring the director of the psychosomatic service to meet him personally. Upon arrival of the director, the patient immediately comments, 'you have a lot of guts wearing that outfit. How much is it worth? $100? $1000? You could feed a hundred starving children in Africa for your one outfit. I hope you can live with yourself.'"

It is difficult not to be repulsed by the innate sense of deservedness and superiority these patients exude. Often there is a strong desire to confront such patients, to "put them in their place" and prove that they are no more special than the next patient. However, this attitude of grandiosity, self-idealization, and devaluing is defensive, protecting against the core of low self-esteem and preserving the patient's own sense of self (4, 5). The medical illness, which is a narcissistic injury for anyone, is a death blow for the narcissistic patient, leaving him dejected, deflated, and demeaned. To cope with this, he will be overtly confrontational while exhibiting little self-control or problem solving (3, 5).

Manipulative Help-Rejecters

These patients are truly paradoxical. On one hand, they appear to seek treatment by constantly coming to care providers, but on the other, they will sabotage or reject treatment solutions that are offered to them. As described by Groves, they appear "almost smugly satisfied, they return again and again…to report that, once again, the regimen did not work" (4). Having a masochistic personality style, they attempt to maintain a relationship with their physicians through the constant reappearance or worsening of their illness (3).

A sixty-eight year old female who recently left AMA from another hospital presents to the emergency department for worsening edema of her lower extremities. Upon further evaluation, she is found to have significant congestive heart failure and is admitted. During her admission, she is initially cooperative with the primary team, but as her condition improves, she becomes belligerent and hostile with the staff, complaining that her water has too much ice in it, the coffee is not served on time, and the nurses are not looking at her properly. Indignant, she demands to leave the hospital AMA, stating that she will get better care elsewhere. When records are obtained from the other hospital, it is discovered that a similar scenario occurred there.

Why would a person return again and again to a hospital only to leave before his illness is treated? As stated previously, it is the illness, not the treatment, that is important. Often, such patients have learned that only when they are suffering will others pay attention, and their illness becomes a manifestation of that desire (3). Although somatoform and factitious disorder patients can easily fall under this category, the most classic illness using this style is borderline personality disorder. Described as "hostile dependents," these patients can be demanding and clinging at the same time (5). Using such defenses as splitting, projectively identifying, and idealizing/devaluing, these patients generate in the primary team anger, exhaustion, and feelings of being manipulated (5, 10). Using excessive escape-avoidance and immature efforts to seek social supports, these individuals have limited ability to accept responsibility, problem-solve, or conduct positive re-appraisal (3).

Self-Destructive Deniers

Although denial is typically considered an immature defense, its use is not always self-destructive. Some patients use denial to cope with a new medical illness, to protect them from the enormity of a situation. This type of denial will help individuals come to terms with their new condition in a way that is not overwhelming or detrimental (3, 4). The Self-Destructive Denier is not such a person. Much like the Manipulative Help-Rejecter, the illness is sacrosanct for these patients. As described by Groves, they "seem to glory in their own destruction…appear to find their main pleasure in furiously defeating the physician's attempts to preserve their lives" (4).

A thirty-six year old male with end-stage liver disease has frequent re-admissions to the hospital for altered mental status. Despite his worsening status, he continues to drink heavily and uses other illicit substances. With each admission, he requests a liver transplant but then angrily reacts when he is advised that abstinence is a requirement for transplant consideration. He is hostile and belligerent with the staff, threatening them on multiple occasions.

Gaining an understanding of these patients can be very difficult. Often, physicians may wonder, "Why does this patient keep returning?" or "Why won't he just die?" This may in turn evoke shame or guilt in the caregivers, which can lead to worsening despair and hatred (1, 4). Although, such patients can have any personality disorder, cluster B, a specific subset of the antisocial personality disorder, fits this style well. Antisocial individuals are typically characterized as lying, deceitful, lacking empathy, and exploitive of others (5, 13). However, it should be noted that such patients can also have a complete disregard for the self, may have very low self-esteem, and are prone to substance abuse (5, 13). Their acting out, devaluing, and substance use serve as ways to distance and escape-avoid from a world that they feel holds nothing for them (1, 4, 5).

Clinical decision-making and treatment

Behavioral management

As has been mentioned previously, successfully working with such patients requires gaining a better understanding of them. Recognizing the defense mechanisms and coping styles that an individual patient is using will allow the consultant and the primary team to approach these difficult situations in a different and more constructive manner. Appreciating that often a patient's hostility, belligerence, or manipulation is a maladaptive manifestation of the need for the physician to be the "inexhaustible mother" will allow greater empathy to develop (4).

Keys to management of the difficult patient include the following (5, 13, 14):

- Ensure that the basic needs of the patient (privacy, food, etc.) are being met. Included in this is an attempt to maintain consistent staff.
- Attempt to understand and empathize with the patient and acknowledge the real stresses in the current situation.
- Accept the patient's limitations by not directly confronting immature defenses or poor coping styles.
- Set firm limits on unreasonable expectations by consistently declaring that "in order to provide the best medical care possible…" However, reasonable requests, or approximations thereof, should not be refused.

Table 3.5 Common symptoms to treat in hateful patients

	1st line	2nd line	Avoid

Depression/anxiety	SSRIs
	SNRIs
	Mirtazapine
	Bupropion
	Hydroxyzine
		Lithium
		Aripiprazole
		Bipolar depression:
		    Quetiapine
		    Lamotrigine
			Stimulants
			TCAs and MAOIs
			    (lethal in OD)
			Benzodiazepines

Insomnia	Mirtazapine Trazodone Melatonin/ramelteon Hydroxyzine	Zolpidem Eszopiclone Quetiapine	Benzodiazepines Opiates
Irritability/impulsivity	Divalproex Quetiapine Olanzapine Risperidone	Lamotrigine Aripiprazole Ziprasidone First-generation antipsychotics Oxcarbazepine Carbamazepine Lithium	Benzodiazepines Opiates

Key:
MAOIs = monoamine oxidase inhibitors
OD = overdose
SNRIs = serotonin-norepinephrine reuptake inhibitors
SSRIs = selective serotonin reuptake inhibitors
TCAs = tricyclic antidepressants

- Do not directly confront the patient's entitlement or rage.
- Gently discuss any irrational fears about the illness or treatment that the patient may have, and assess his ability for reality testing (i.e., ensure that a transient psychosis is not occurring).
- Acknowledge and empathize with the primary team's countertransference. Discuss with team members the universality of these emotions.
- Use psychopharmacology when appropriate.

Psychopharmacology

Despite limited evidence for the use of psychotropic medications in personality disorders, they still can have some benefit. First, it should be remembered that despite having a primarily Axis II condition, difficult patients are likely to have Axis I conditions as well. Mood and anxiety disorders are common for such individuals, as are periods of transient psychosis. Additionally, impulsivity and anger are often cited problems, and mood stabilizers and antipsychotics provide some reported benefit for these symptoms. Because of the propensity of these patients for substance abuse and suicide attempts, use of medications with high addictive potential and those that are lethal in overdoses should be minimized (Table 3.5) (5, 13).

The difficult patient can present in many ways, but perhaps the most frustrating and hard to understand are the type that Groves described as the "hateful patient" (4). Such patients are a conundrum to their primary treatment providers, leading to significant chaos, confusion, and outright hostility among care providers. The psychiatric consultant is called in to make these patients "go away," or at the very least to make them "compliant and easy to deal with." However, even for the specialist, this is no easy task; only by having a deeper understanding of these patients' personality structures (defense mechanisms and coping styles) and an appreciation of clinician countertransference will the consultant begin to make some headway into these very difficult situations.

References

1. Strous RD, Ulman AM, Kotler M. The hateful patient revisited: relevance for 21st century medicine. Eur J Intern Med. 2006;17(6):387–93.

2. Jackson JL, Kroenke K. Difficult patient encounters in the ambulatory clinic. Arch Intern Med. 1999;159(10):1069–74.

3. Groves MS, Muskin P. Psychological responses to illness. In: Levenson J, editor. Textbook of psychosomatic medicine. Washington (DC): American Psychiatric Publishing, Inc; 2005. p. 67–88.

4. Groves JE. Taking care of the hateful patient. N Engl J Med. 1978;298(16):883–7.

5. Feinstein RE. Personality traits and disorders. In: Blumenfield M, Strain JJ, editors. Psychosomatic medicine. Philadelphia: Lippincott Williams & Wilkins; 2006. p. 843–65.

6. Miller MC. Personality disorders. Med Clin North Am. 2001;85(3):819–37.

7. Penley JA, Tomaka J, Wiebe JS. The association of coping to physical and psychological health outcomes: a meta-analytic review. J Behav Med. 2002;25(6):551–603.

8. Sclozman SC, Groves JE, Weisman AD. Coping with illness and psychotherapy of the medically ill. In: Stern TA, Fricchione GL, Cassem NH, et al., editors. Handbook of general hospital psychiatry. Philadelphia: Mosby; 2004. p. 61–8.

9. Bouchard G, Theriault VJ. Defense mechanisms and coping strategies in conjugal relationships: an integration. Int J Psychol. 2003;38:79–90.

10. Stoudemire A, Thompson TL. The borderline personality in the medical setting. Ann Intern Med. 1982;96(1):76–9.

11. Smith S. Dealing with the difficult patient. Postgrad Med J. 1995;71(841):653–7.

12. Ozmen M. Transference and countertransference in medically ill patients. Turk Psikiyatri Derg. 2007;18(1):1–7.

13. Groves JE. Difficult patients. In: Stern TA, Fricchione GL, Cassem NH, et al, editors. Handbook of general hospital psychiatry. Philadelphia: Mosby; 2004. p. 293–312.

14. Groves JE. Management of the borderline patient on a medical or surgical ward: the psychiatric consultant's role. Int J Psychiatry Med. 1975;6(3):337–48.

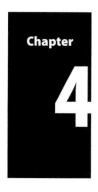

Psychopharmacology in the medically ill

Sanjeev Sockalingam, Adrienne Tan, and Susan E. Abbey

Typical consult questions

(1) *"Is it okay for Mr. Jones with schizophrenia to be treated with an atypical antipsychotic, now that he's been newly diagnosed with decompensated liver cirrhosis?"* (2) *"Mrs. Smith has always relapsed when her SSRI was stopped, but we need to use linezolid – does it preclude the use of all SSRIs?"* (3) *"Mr. Wilson has not been participating in physiotherapy after his cardiac surgery – do you think he would benefit from an antidepressant?"*

Developing an approach to psychopharmacology in psychosomatic medicine patients

Polypharmacy in the medically ill is often the rule rather than the exception.

Relevant psychopharmacologic principles

1. Diagnostic clarity is paramount. The PM fellow must understand both the underlying psychiatric disorder and co-morbid medical conditions. Clinicians should consider whether optimization of medical management or removal of potentially complicating medications is possible before initiating psychopharmacologic treatment.
2. Target symptoms for proposed pharmacologic treatments should be identified.
3. Clinicians should consider possible drug interactions in vulnerable patient populations (e.g., anticholinergic effects of tricyclic antidepressants may exacerbate pre-existing cognitive impairment in the elderly). Careful consideration of the cytochrome P450 (CYP450) system is paramount to minimizing drug-drug interactions (Table 4.1).
4. Pharmacologic parsimony is the ideal. Medications with favorable actions or side effects may be selected in specific scenarios (e.g., the oncology patient suffering from depression, nausea, weight loss, and sleep disturbance may benefit from pharmacodynamic properties of mirtazapine that address these symptoms).
5. Psychopharmacology with the medically ill is shared with geriatric psychiatry – start low, go slow – but remember don't stop until you have given an agent a full trial, unless side effects are limiting.
6. Drug information pharmacists at your institution and medical liaison officers from pharmaceutical companies may be very helpful in challenging cases.

Psychosomatic Medicine: An Introduction to Consultation-Liaison Psychiatry, eds. James J. Amos and Robert G. Robinson. Published by Cambridge University Press. © Cambridge University Press 2010.

Table 4.1 Psychotropic drug pharmacokinetics (2, 41–43)

Medication	Major CYP450 Inhibition or Induction	Dose Adjustment in Hepatic Disease	Dose Adjustment in Renal Disease
Anticonvulsants			
Gabapentin (Neurontin) / Pregabalin (Lyrica)	–	–	+++
Valproic acid (Depakote, Depakote ER, Depakene, Depacon, Divalproex, Epival)	Mild-moderate inhibitor 2C9, 2C19, and UGT	+++ (in children)	–
Carbamazepine (Tegretol, Carbatrol)	3A4 inhibition within first 1–2 weeks Potent 3A4 induction	+	+/–
Oxcarbazepine (Trileptal)	Mild 3A4 induction	–	–
Lamotrigine (Lamictal, Labileno, Lamictin)	–	+	+
Topiramate (Topimax, Epitomax, Topamac, Topamax)	–	–	++
Lithium	–	–	+++
Antipsychotics			
Haloperidol (Haldol)	Moderate inhibition of 3A4 and 2D6	–	–
Risperidone (Risperdal, Consta)	Mild inhibition of 2D6 and 3A4	+	++ (active metabolite)
Paliperidone (Invega)	–	–	++
Olanzapine (Zyprexa, Olasek, Ziprexa)	–	+	–
Quetiapine (Seroquel, Seroquel XR)	–	+	–
Ziprasidone (Geodon, Zeldox)	–	–/+	–/+
Aripiprazole (Abilify)	–	–	+
Clozapine (Clozaril, Leponex)	–	+	–
Antidepressants			
SSRIs			
Fluoxetine (Prozac, Prozac Weekly, Sarafem)	Potent inhibitor of 2D6 Mild to moderate inhibition of 1A2, 2B6, 2C9, 2C19, and 3A4 *Can be considered "pan-inhibitor" of P450	+++	–

(cont.)

Table 4.1 (*cont.*)

Medication	Major CYP450 Inhibition or Induction	Dose Adjustment in Hepatic Disease	Dose Adjustment in Renal Disease
Paroxetine (Paxil, Paxil CR, Pexeva)	Potent inhibitor of 2B6 and 2D6 Mild inhibitor of other P450 enzymes	++	++
Sertraline (Zoloft)	Dose-dependent inhibition of 2D6 Moderate inhibitor of 2B6 and 2C19 Mild inhibitor of 1A2 and 3A4	++	–
Fluvoxamine (Luvox)	"Pan-inhibitor" of P450 enzymes, like fluoxetine Potent inhibitor of 1A2, 2C19 Mild to moderate inhibitor of 2B6, 2C9, 2D6, 3A4	++	–
Citalopram (Celexa)	Mild inhibition of 2D6	+	++
Escitalopram (Lexapro, Cipralex)	Pharmacokinetic features essentially the same as citalopram	+	++
SNRIs			
Venlafaxine (Effexor, Effexor XR)	Mild inhibition of 2D6	++	+
Desvenlafaxine (Pristiq)	Mild inhibition of 2D6	+	+
Duloxetine (Cymbalta)	Moderate to potent inhibitor of 2D6	Not recommended for use in patients with substantial alcohol abuse, chronic liver disease, or hepatic insufficiency	++ Avoid in severe renal insufficiency, CrCl <30 ml/min
Atypical Antidepressants			
Bupropion (Wellbutrin, Wellbutrin SR, Wellbutrin XL, Zyban, Buproban)	Moderate to potent inhibitor of 2D6	++	++
Mirtazapine (Remeron, Remeron SolTab)	–	++	++
Trazodone	–	++	+/–
Nefazodone (Serzone)	Potent inhibitor of 3A4	*Drug withdrawn because of reported cases of hepatotoxicity, some generic forms still available in United States	

Table 4.1 *(cont.)*

Medication	Major CYP450 Inhibition or Induction	Dose Adjustment in Hepatic Disease	Dose Adjustment in Renal Disease
"Classic" Antidepressants (TCAs and MAOIs)			
TCAs	*In general TCAs are considered P450 inhibitors		
Tertiary Amines			
Amitriptyline (Elavil) *Demethylated to nortriptyline	1A2, 2C19, 2D6	++	–
Clomipramine (Enafranil) *Demethylated to desmethyl-clomipramine	2D6, 1A2, 2C19	++	+/–
Imipramine (Tofranil, Tofranil PM) *Demethylated to desipramine	2C19, 2D6, 1A2, 3A4	++	–
Doxepin (Sinequan) *Demethylated to desmethyldoxepin	1A2, 2C19	++	–
Trimipramine (Surmontil) *Demethylated to desmethyltrim-ipramine	–	++	
Secondary Amines			
Desipramine (Norpramin)	2D6, 2C19	++	+
Nortriptyline (Aventyul, Pamelor)	2D6, 2C19	++	–
Protriptyline (Vivactil)	–	++	+/–
MAOIs	*Possible inhibition of P450 enzymes, data lacking		
Irreversible			
Isocarboxazid (Marplan)	2D6, 2C19	++	–
Phenelzine (Nardil)	2D6, 2C19	++	–
Tranylcypromine (Parnate)	2C19, 2D6, 2A6, 2C9	++	–
Reversible Inhibitor of MAO-A (RIMA)			
Moclobemide (Manerix, available in Canada)	2C19, 2D6, 1A2		–

(cont.)

Table 4.1 (cont.)

Medication	Major CYP450 Inhibition or Induction	Dose Adjustment in Hepatic Disease	Dose Adjustment in Renal Disease
Anxiolytics/Hypnotics			
Benzodiazepines	*No known inhibition or induction		
Alprazolam (Xanax, Xanax XR, Niravam)		++	–
Chlordiazepoxide (Librium)		+++	++
Clonazepam (Klonopin, Klonopin wafer, Rivotril, Clonapam)		++	–
Diazepam (Valium, Diastat, Diastat AcuDial, Vivol, E Pam, Diazemuls)		+++ Avoid in acute or severe liver disease	–
Lorazepam (Ativan)		+	++
Midazolam (Versed)		+++	–
Oxazepam (Serax)		–	–
Temazepam (Restoril)		–	–
Triazolam (Halcion)		++	–
Other/Non-benzodiazepine Anxiolytics/ Hypnotics	*In general, none are P450 inhibitors, all are partially or completely dependent on 3A4 for metabolism.		
Zaleplon (Ambien, Ambien CR)		?	+
Zolpidem (Sonata, Starnoc)		++	++
Zopiclone (Imovane, available in Canada)		++	?
Eszopiclone (Lunesta)		++	?
Chloral hydrate (Aquachloral Supprettes, Somnote)	Inducer of CYP450 enzymes	++	?
Ramelteon (Rozerem)		++	–
Buspirone (BuSpar, Vanspar)		+ Not recommended for use with severe hepatic impairment	+ Not recommended for use with severe renal impairment

Table 4.1 *(cont.)*

Key:
− No known induction/inhibition or no dose adjustment required
+ Mild dose adjustment
++ Moderate dose adjustment
+++ Significant dose adjustment
+/− Inconclusive
CrCl = creatinine clearance
CYP450 = cytochrome P450
SNRIs = serotonin-norepinephrine reuptake inhibitors
SSRIs = selective serotonin reuptake inhibitors
TCAs = tricyclic antidepressants
UGT = uridine-5′-diphosphate glucuronosyltransferase

Pharmacodynamics and pharmacokinetics

Pharmacodynamics refers to "the effect of the drug on the body" and the activity of the drug at receptor sites. Pharmacokinetics refers to "the body's effect on the drug," which includes absorption, metabolism, distribution, elimination, and protein binding. Sequelae of medical disease may result in end-organ damage and disrupt pharmacokinetic processes.

Drug absorption is influenced by disruptions in the absorption site, such as reduced blood flow, loss of surface area, changes in pH, and destruction of gastric mucosal integrity. Increased gastric absorption occurs with an empty stomach, and the rate of absorption is increased with parenteral versus oral drug administration. Furthermore, orally administered drugs are susceptible to the effects of first-pass metabolism; sublingual, topical, and rectal drug administrations have reduced first-pass effects.

Metabolism or **biotransformation** occurs in the liver and the gut wall. Nearly all psychotropics, with the exception of lithium, topiramate, and gabapentin, are dependent primarily on hepatic metabolism. Biotransformation occurs in two phases: Phase I involves oxidation, hydrolysis, or reduction; phase II involves conjugation (glucuronidation, acetylation, and sulfation). In patients with severe liver impairment, glucuronidation is preserved and drugs that rely solely on phase II biotransformation, such as lorazepam, are preferred. Phase I oxidation uses the CYP450 monooxygenase system, and nearly 90% of human drug oxidation occurs in the enzymes 1A2, 3A4, 2C9, 2C19, 2D6, and 2E1 (1). Potent inhibitors of CYP450 isoenzymes can elevate active drug metabolites and cause significant adverse effects (Table 4.2). Moreover, impairment in hepatic function can decrease drug metabolism, and standardized measures of liver disease, such as the Child-Pugh score, can inform the need for dose reduction.

Volume of distribution is the total amount of drug in the body in proportion to the plasma concentration of the drug. Drug distribution is increased by several factors, including reduced hepatic blood flow, fluid retention, reduced protein binding, serum pH, lipid solubility, and drug ionization. Psychotropic drugs, with the exception of lithium, are lipophilic and have a large volume of distribution caused by absorption into fatty tissue.

Most psychotropics are highly protein bound and are influenced by fluctuations in protein levels. Specific drug-binding proteins include albumin and globulin, which generally bind to acidic (e.g., valproic acid) and basic (e.g., tricyclic antidepressant [TCA]) psychotropic drugs, respectively. Several medical illnesses, such as pneumonia, liver cirrhosis, and renal failure, are associated with low albumin levels and require drug dose reductions to account for higher

Table 4.2 Examples of drug-drug interactions in medically ill

Non-Psychotropic Drug Classes	Interaction	Examples of Psychotropic Drug Interaction
Antimicrobial/ Antiviral		
Protease inhibitors (e.g., ritonavir)	Metabolized by CYP3A4 Inhibit CYP3A4	Can increase levels of CYP3A4 metabolized psychotropics (e.g., alprazolam, quetiapine, trazodone) Reduce protease inhibitor drug levels with carbamazepine
Antifungals (e.g., itraconazole, ketoconazole)	Inhibit CYP3A4	Can increase levels of CYP3A4 metabolized psychotropics (e.g., alprazolam, quetiapine, trazodone)
Ciprofloxacin	Inhibits CYP1A2	Increases levels of clozapine and olanzapine
Linezolid	Nonselective reversible MAOI	Serotonin syndrome when co-administered with SSRI
Erythromycin (Clarithromycin)	Inhibits CYP3A4	Can increase levels of CYP3A4 metabolized psychotropics (e.g., alprazolam, quetiapine, trazodone)
Rifampin	Induces CYP3A4 & 2B6	Can reduce levels of psychotropics metabolized by CYP3A4 (e.g., alprazolam, quetiapine, trazodone) and CYP2B6 (e.g., bupropion)
Cardiac		
Warfarin	Highly protein bound	Displaced by highly bound psychotropics (e.g., valproic acid)
Diltiazem	Inhibits CYP3A4 (mild-moderate)	Can increase levels of CYP3A4 metabolized psychotropics (e.g., alprazolam, quetiapine, trazodone)
Amiodarone	Inhibits 2C19, 2D6, and 3A4	Can increase TCA (tertiary amines) and paroxetine/ fluoxetine drug levels
Immunosuppressants		
Cyclosporine	Inhibitor of CYP3A4 (mild-moderate)	Can increase levels of CYP3A4 metabolized psychotropics (e.g., alprazolam, quetiapine, trazodone)
Tacrolimus	Inhibitor of CYP3A4 (mild-moderate)	Can increase levels of CYP3A4 metabolized psychotropics (e.g., alprazolam, quetiapine, trazodone)
Analgesics		
Tramadol	Metabolized by CYP2D6	Paroxetine and fluoxetine can increase drug levels due to CYP2D6 inhibition
Meperidine	Inhibits serotonin transporter	Co-administration with MAOI can lead to serotonin syndrome
Anticonvulsants		
Phenytoin	Inducer of CYP3A4	Can reduce levels of psychotropics metabolized by CYP3A4 (e.g., alprazolam, quetiapine, trazodone)
Gastrointestinal		
Omeprazole, Lansoprazole	Weak inhibitor of CYP1A2	Can lower clozapine levels

Table 4.2 (*cont.*)

Non-Psychotropic Drug Classes	Interaction	Examples of Psychotropic Drug Interaction
Substances		
Caffeine	Predominantly metabolized by CYP1A2	Can increase clozapine through competitive inhibition, decreases lithium levels
Nicotine	Potent induced CYP1A2	Can lower clozapine and olanzapine levels

* Excludes lorazepam, oxazepam, temazepam

free drug levels. Routine laboratory drug levels do not differentiate between free and bound drug levels. In this case, drug dosing should be based on response and tolerability as per clinical assessment.

Elimination is determined primarily by renal function, which is estimated by calculating creatinine clearance. Few psychotropic drugs require significant dose adjustments in patients with dialysis.

Classes of medications

Anticonvulsants

Although anticonvulsants are used in psychiatry for stabilization of bipolar disorder, alcohol withdrawal, and aggression, medically ill patients may also receive these drugs during treatment for epilepsy, neuropathic pain, and migraines (Table 4.1).

Gabapentin and pregabalin

Gabapentin and pregabalin are often used for treating neuropathic pain and symptoms of anxiety symptoms, specifically, generalized anxiety disorder. However, they have limited efficacy as mood stabilizers. Gabapentin and pregabalin act on the alpha-2-delta component of voltage-gated calcium channels. Common side effects include sedation, dizziness, and edema. See Table 4.1 for dosage adjustments.

Valproic acid

Valproic acid is commonly used in psychiatric settings as a mood stabilizer in bipolar disorder and has demonstrated benefit in managing alcohol withdrawal and refractory agitation (2, 3). Valproic acid is theorized to inhibit voltage-gated sodium channels and possibly calcium channels, resulting in reduction of glutamate activity and enhancement of gamma-aminobutyric (GABA) effects. It is metabolized primarily through glucuronidation and mitochondrial-β-oxidation. Adverse effects of valproic acid include hair loss, weight gain, sedation, and transient increases in liver enzymes. Divalproex sodium is associated with fewer gastrointestinal side effects as compared with sodium valproate and valproic acid. Rare reports of hepatotoxicity, pancreatitis, thrombocytopenia, and other coagulopathies have been associated with valproic acid. With regard to valproic acid–induced hepatotoxicity, cases are limited to young children and patients on multiple anticonvulsants. Pediatric patients and patients with mental retardation appear to be at greatest risk of valproic acid–induced hyperammonemia (4). Moreover, valproic acid can cause polycystic ovarian syndrome in approximately 10% of bipolar patients receiving valproic acid for mood stabilization (5).

Carbamazepine and oxcarbazepine

Carbamazepine is orally administered and acts through voltage-gated sodium channels in a similar manner to valproic acid. Oxcarbazepine is not the metabolite of carbamazepine but an inactive prodrug that is converted into eslicarbazepine, the active form. Carbamazepine and oxcarbazepine can cause central nervous system side effects, specifically, sedation, muscle weakness, ataxia, and visual disturbances. In addition, carbamazepine is associated with bone marrow suppression and may result in transient leukopenia and, rarely, aplastic anemia. Oxcarbazepine and, to a lesser extent, carbamazepine can cause the syndrome of inappropriate antidiuretic hormone secretion (6). Although benign skin rashes occur in approximately 10% to 15% of patients treated with carbamazepine, Stevens-Johnson syndrome (SJS) occurs in rare instances.

Lamotrigine

Lamotrigine has utility in bipolar disorder, specifically, in the acute depressive and maintenance phases. It acts on voltage-gated sodium channels and reduces the release of glutamate. Most anticonvulsants can cause benign rashes in up to 20% of cases; however, lamotrigine can cause potentially life-threatening rashes, specifically, SJS and toxic epidermal necrolysis, which occur in 0.1% of adults and in 1% to 2% of children. In comparison with carbamazepine, lamotrigine has a lower risk of blood dyscrasias (7). Last, lamotrigine is metabolized primarily by UDP-glucuronosyltransferase (UGT) 1A4, which is inhibited by valproic acid. Therefore, concurrent valproic acid use requires lower dosing and slower titration of lamotrigine.

Topiramate

Although results with topiramate as a mood stabilizer in bipolar disorder have been inconclusive, it is approved for treating migraines and is an anticonvulsant. It causes weight loss in 6% to 16% of treated patients and may be beneficial in managing weight gain related to medical illness or medications (8). Approximately 70% of topiramate is excreted unchanged in the urine. Rapid dose titration and higher doses of topiramate have been associated with greater cognitive deficits predominantly in verbal processing, which may limit its tolerability and may reduce compliance (9) (Box 4.1).

> **Box 4.1 Clinical Pearls – Mood Stabilizers**
>
> - Gabapentin, pregabalin, and topiramate are renally excreted and require significant dose modification in renal disease.
> - Be cognizant of the effect of hypoalbuminemia on highly protein-bound drugs (e.g., valproic acid), specifically, the increase in free drug levels. Standard serum drug levels do not differentiate the amount of free versus bound drug.

Lithium

Lithium has multiple systemic effects and can precipitate or exacerbate underlying medical illness. Lithium is commonly associated with gastrointestinal distress, tremor, headache, weight gain, and dermatologic side effects, such as acne or exacerbation of psoriasis. Cardiac changes secondary to lithium are often benign. An ECG is recommended before lithium is started, and patients with pre-existing sinus node dysfunction should be screened before starting lithium therapy. Hypothyroidism occurs in approximately 30% of patients on long-term lithium therapy, with female and elderly patients at highest risk (10, 11).

Defects in urine concentration due to decreased sensitivity of the collecting tubule to antidiuretic hormone occur with lithium treatment. Symptoms of polyuria and polydipsia can progress to nephrogenic diabetes insipidus in up to 55% of patients on long-term lithium treatment, and approximately 5% to 10% of these patients will develop persistent symptoms (12).

Recent literature from 14 separate studies reported a prevalence of 15% for reduced glomerular filtration rate (GFR) associated with long-term lithium therapy (13). Therefore, it has been recommended that increasing creatinine levels (1.6 mg/dl or >140 mmol/L) or reduced GFR warrants the use of expert consultation to reassess the risk of continued lithium treatment (14).

Because of lithium's reliance on renal excretion, several medications that alter renal function can impact lithium levels. Angiotensin-converting enzyme inhibitors, non-steroidal anti-inflammatory drugs, and thiazide diuretics can increase lithium levels, resulting in lithium toxicity. In contrast, medications that decrease lithium levels, including carbonic anhydrase inhibitors, xanthenes, and osmotic diuretics (e.g., mannitol), may precipitate a relapse in mood symptoms in patients previously stabilized on lithium (Box 4.2).

Box 4.2 Clinical Pearls – Lithium

- Lithium levels should be measured 4 to 5 days after a dose change to assess steady state.
- Lithium toxicity can range from mild toxicity (ataxia, coarse tremor, mild confusion, nausea, diarrhea) to severe toxicity (hyperreflexia, epileptic seizures, cardiovascular collapse, coma).
- If required, lithium can be given in a single dose post dialysis to patients with end-stage renal disease, as it will be removed with each dialysis treatment.

Antidepressants

Antidepressant use within the psychiatric setting has greatly expanded to include treatment of eating disorders, premenstrual dysphoric disorder, chronic aggression and impulsivity, and impulse control disorders, just to name a few of the growing uses of antidepressants. As in the psychiatric setting, medically ill patients are most often prescribed antidepressant medications for the management of depression and anxiety disorders. However, they are also used "off label" in the medical setting to treat some somatoform disorders (e.g., hypochondriasis), chronic fatigue syndrome, and chronic pain syndromes such as diabetic neuropathy or fibromyalgia, or for less common indications such as neurocardiogenic syncope, when other standard treatments prove ineffective.

MAOIs and TCAs

Monoamine oxidase inhibitors (MAOIs) and TCAs, although shown to be effective for anxiety and depressive disorders, are limited in their use in the medically ill because of tolerability and the potential for serious adverse effects. Although MAOIs are not known to have any effects on cardiac conduction, they do have high potential for causing orthostatic hypotension. In addition, dose-related activation (restlessness, anxiety, agitation, and aggressivity) can occur, especially with tranylcypromine. Restriction of tyramine-rich foods and avoidance of concomitant use of sympathomimetic agents (e.g., ephedrine, salbutamol) are also required because of the risk of hypertensive crisis. Finally, there is also a risk of precipitating a serotonin syndrome when MAOIs are used with other psychotropic and non-psychotropic medications with serotonergic properties. In general, a two-week washout period is recommended when the switch is made from an MAOI to another antidepressant medication, to allow the MAO to regenerate.

With regard to TCAs, they are commonly used "off label" in the medical setting to treat chronic pain (especially amitriptyline and nortriptyline) and insomnia (in low doses), and as migraine headache prophylaxis. Because of antagonism at cholinergic muscarinic receptors, TCAs can have both central and peripheral effects. Central effects include confusion, delirium, and hallucinations; peripheral effects consist of dry eyes and mouth, constipation, urinary hesitancy or retention, and blurred vision. Moreover, as a result of antagonism at a variety of receptors, TCAs are known to have significant cardiovascular effects (15). Anticholinergic activity of TCAs can lead to tachycardia. TCAs are class I antiarrhythmics and are known to prolong QRS and PR intervals. In general, TCAs are contraindicated in patients with ischemic heart disease, in cases of heart block, and post myocardial infarction (MI).

SSRIs and SNRIs

Selective serotonin receptor inhibitors (SSRIs) and serotonin-norepinephrine receptor inhibitors (SNRIs) are two of the most commonly prescribed antidepressant medications because of their tolerability and effectiveness. Although all six of the currently available SSRIs work through serotonin reuptake inhibition, each has unique pharmacologic properties (e.g., presence of active metabolites, differing elimination half-lives). Commonly reported adverse effects include gastrointestinal symptoms, activation/nervousness or sedation, and sexual dysfunction. From a medical perspective, SSRIs have been shown to have a relatively benign cardiac profile – they do not slow cardiac conduction or cause orthostatic hypotension, and they are rarely lethal in overdose (unlike the TCAs); however, they have been reported to cause bradycardia. SSRIs may reduce platelet aggregation, which may have salubrious effects in cardiac disease, but they may also increase the risk of gastrointestinal bleeding, a risk that has also been demonstrated with the SNRI, venlafaxine (16). SSRIs are known to lead to hyponatremia, presumably caused by stimulation of inappropriate antidiuretic hormone secretion (i.e., SIADH). SSRIs and SNRIs both have the potential on their own or in conjunction with other serotonergic medications to produce serotonin syndrome (Box 4.3).

SNRIs include venlafaxine, desvenlafaxine, and duloxetine. Venlfaxine, the first SNRI marketed in the United States, produces more potent inhibition of serotonin (5-HT) at lower doses, with moderate norepinephrine (NE) reuptake inhibition at higher (>150 mg) dosages. A dose-related increase in blood pressure has also been reported. The immediate-release formulation of venlafaxine has been eclipsed by the extended-release (XR) formulation because of greater tolerability, predominantly, decreased nausea. Especially with sudden discontinuation from high dosages, venlafaxine is associated with potentially severe withdrawal reactions. Desvenlafaxine is the active metabolite of venlafaxine. Both venlafaxine and desvenlafaxine have been shown to be efficacious in reducing vasomotor symptoms in menopause and have been associated with hormonal manipulations secondary to chemotherapy. Duloxetine is a potent inhibitor of serotonin and norepinephrine throughout the dose range and may have a lower incidence of hypertension and less severe withdrawal reactions than

---

Box 4.3 Serotonergic Syndrome (17, 30)

- Rare but potentially fatal complication of therapy with serotonergic agents – most commonly, serotonergic psychotropic medications (SSRIs, SNRIs, mirtazapine, trazodone, TCAs, MAOIs, bupropion) – but the roles of "medical" medications (e.g., meperidine, dextromethorphan, sibutramine, tramadol) and "recreational" drugs (e.g., cocaine, NMDA, Ecstasy, amphetamines) also must be considered
- Typically occurs soon after another serotonergic medication is started, increased, or added to another serotonergic medication
- Diagnostic symptoms – fever, autonomic dysregulation, neurologic symptoms, and mental status changes

Recent diagnostic criteria – four major or three major + two minor symptoms (30)

Mental (cognitive and behavioral) Symptoms

Major – confusion, coma, semi-coma, elevated mood
Minor – agitation, nervousness, insomnia

Autonomic Symptoms

Major – fever, hyperhidrosis
Minor – tachycardia, tachypnea, dyspnea, diarrhea, low or high blood pressure, or labile blood pressure

Neurologic Symptoms

Major – myoclonus, rigidity, hyperreflexia, tremors, chills
Minor – impaired coordination, akathisia, mydriasis

- Autonomic instability and hyperthermia are the major causes of morbidity and mortality.
- Ensure that infectious and other medical causes of symptoms are excluded.
- No characteristic laboratory abnormalities
- Management includes discontinuing all serotonergic medications and supportive care, at times requiring ICU care. In refractory cases, consider use of serotonin antagonist, cyproheptadine.

Key:
MAOIs = monoamine oxidase inhibitors
NMDA = N-methyl-D-aspartic acid
SNRIs = serotonin-norepinephrine reuptake inhibitors
SSRIs = selective serotonin reuptake inhibitors
TCAs = tricyclic antidepressants

---

venlafaxine. It has been shown to be efficacious in painful syndromes such as diabetic neuropathy and possibly fibromyalgia.

Other/atypical antidepressants

The serotonin antagonist reuptake inhibitor (SARI) trazodone is commonly used for sleep because of sedating properties. It has minimal anticholinergic effects and is known to increase slow-wave (stage 3 and 4) sleep. With higher doses (>200 mg), arrhythmias have been reported. In addition, priapism is an uncommon but potentially serious side effect associated with the use of trazodone in men. Bradycardia has been reported with nefazodone, although use of this medication has generally fallen out of favor because of the risk of hepatotoxicity.

Bupropion, a norepinephrine-dopamine reuptake inhibitor (NDRI), comes in several formulations (immediate release, sustained release [SR], and extended release [XL]). In general, the immediate-release formulation has fallen out of favor. Bupropion is known to lower seizure threshold, especially with the immediate-release formulation and at higher doses. As such, the medication is relatively contraindicated in patients with increased risk of seizures (e.g., bulimia and anorexia nervosa, epilepsy, poorly controlled diabetes, acute alcohol withdrawal). Notable side effects include gastrointestinal symptoms, insomnia, headache, agitation, tinnitus, and hypertension. It has few, if any, anticholinergic effects and a relatively benign cardiovascular profile. Bupropion is also used in the treatment of sexual dysfunction caused by SSRI and SNRI medications.

Mirtazapine is a dual serotonin and norepinephrine agent which acts through a novel mechanism independent of norepinephrine and serotonin reuptake blockade. It is a commonly used treatment for depression, as well as anxiety disorders. Although rare, cases of agranulocytosis have been reported with mirtazapine. Mirtazapine is also known to cause weight gain. However, it may be useful to capitalize on some of the side effects of mirtazapine such as sedation and weight gain in, for example, cancer patients with insomnia, anorexia, and significant weight loss. Because of 5-HT_3 antagonism, mirtazapine may also have some antiemetic effects (Box 4.4).

Box 4.4   Clinical Pearls – Antidepressants

- Capitalize on "useful" side effects of some antidepressants to provide symptomatic benefit to patients in specific clinical contexts.
- Many non-psychotropic medications have serotonergic effects, sometimes acting as weak MAOIs (e.g., meperidine, linezolid, tramadol) increasing the potential for serotonin syndrome with the addition of an SSRI, SNRI, or other serotonergic psychotropic medication.

Key:
MAOIs = monoamine oxidase inhibitors
SNRI = serotonin-norephinephrine reuptake inhibitor
SSRI = selective serotonin reuptake inhibitor

Anxiolytics and sedatives

Benzodiazepines

Benzodiazepines bind to the "benzodiazepine"-GABA$_A$ ligand–gated chloride channel receptor complex, thereby facilitating the action of the neurotransmitter GABA, an inhibitory neurotransmitter. They are reported to have anxiolytic, hypnotic, anticonvulsant, and muscle relaxant effects. Benzodiazepines differ on the basis of various pharmacokinetic properties which can affect their use in medically ill patients. For example, diazepam has greater lipophilicity than lorazepam, resulting in a faster onset of action. However, diazepam has a longer elimination half-life than lorazepam; therefore it is washed out slowly, resulting in potentially less severe or intense rebound symptoms. Common side effects include sedation, dizziness, and impaired cognition, especially in the elderly. (See Table 4.1 for dose adjustments due to hepatic or renal disease.) These agents are also associated with tolerance and dependence with prolonged use, as well as uncomfortable (e.g., agitation, insomnia, anxiety) and potentially dangerous withdrawal symptoms (e.g., seizures) with abrupt withdrawal. In addition, in the context of more severe or end-stage lung disease, benzodiazepines can suppress respiratory drive and therefore should be used with caution.

Non-benzodiazepine sedative/hypnotic medications

Zolpidem, zopiclone, eszopiclone, and zaleplon exert their pharmacologic actions through selective binding to $GABA_{A1}$ (omega-1) receptors. These medications are used for insomnia and differ in their half-lives and effective duration of action. They are increasingly recommended as first-line medications for the treatment of insomnia rather than benzodiazepines. Although the evidence is limited, zopiclone is thought to result in less respiratory depression than the benzodiazepines. However, daytime sedation, anterograde amnesia, and rebound insomnia have all been reported with this group.

Ramelteon is a melatonin MT_1 and MT_2 receptor agonist that is thought to induce sleep by influencing homeostatic sleep signaling mediated by the suprachiasmic nucleus in the hypothalamus. Limited evidence suggests that ramelteon may not cause significant respiratory depression in individuals with mild to moderate chronic obstructive pulmonary disease (Kryger, Wang-Weigand, and Zhang, 2008).

Buspirone

Buspirone is a $5\text{-}HT_{1A}$ receptor agonist with anxiolytic properties. It has several potential advantages over the benzodiazepines: It reportedly lacks abuse potential (does not cause dependence or withdrawal); does not impair psychomotor performance; is less sedating than benzodiazepines; and is not associated with weight gain. A disadvantage versus the benzodiazepines in the management of acute anxiety symptoms is that buspirone may take up to 4 weeks to take effect. Side effects include dizziness, headache, nervousness, sedation, nausea, and restlessness (Box 4.5).

Box 4.5 Clinical Pearls – Anxiolytics and Sedatives

- Judicious use of anxiolytic medications can provide effective short-term relief to patients in the hospital who suffer from insomnia and anxiety. They can be used as monotherapy or as an adjunct to other therapies (e.g., antidepressants).
- Lorazepam, oxazepam, and temazepam are generally safe to use in the context of hepatic impairment; because of the variety of routes of administration available with lorazepam, it may be preferred in the case when parenteral (IV, IM) administration may be needed.
- Although the data are limited, non-benzodiazepine sedative/hypnotics may offer a relatively safer alternative to benzodiazepines in patients with more severe respiratory disease who may be sensitive to the respiratory depressant effects of benzodiazepines, or who are at higher risk of hypercarbic respiratory failure.
- Low-dose antipsychotics may be used for anxiolysis in patients unable to tolerate other anxiolytics or sedatives.

Antipsychotics

Antipsychotics are widely used in the C/L setting. They are used most commonly for "off label" indications, including delirium, insomnia, anxiolysis, adjuvant analgesia, and mood lability and regulation, and for the management of psychotic symptoms secondary to medications or medical conditions. They are also used at times as antinauseants and for the treatment of refractory hiccups. Although they are rare, the two side effects that engender the greatest concern with this group of medications are prolongation of the corrected QT interval (QTc) with torsades de pointes ventricular arrhythmia (Box 4.6) and neuroleptic malignant syndrome (Box 4.7).

Box 4.6 Neuroleptic Malignant Syndrome (NMS) (2, 47, 48)

- Uncommon but potentially fatal complication of antipsychotic therapy
- Typically occurs soon after an antipsychotic is started or dose is increased but may occur late
- Risk factors include depot antipsychotics, intramuscular administration, rapid increase in dose of antipsychotics, high doses of antipsychotics, dehydration, malnutrition, iron deficiency, underlying brain abnormalities, and agitation.
- Diagnostic triad – fever ≥38° C (100.4° F), muscle rigidity, mental status changes
- Autonomic instability and hyperthermia are the major causes of morbidity and mortality.
- Common lab abnormalities include ↑CPK or myoglobinuria, ↑WBC, metabolic acidosis
- Ensure other medical causes have been excluded.
- Management includes discontinuing antipsychotic(s), lithium, and dopamine blocking antiemetic agents and providing supportive care, most commonly in an ICU. Although older references recommend use of bromocriptine or dantrolene, more recent references show no advantage for these agents.
- NMS Info Service Hotline – www.nmsis.org, or in USA, 1-888-NMS-Temp – Calling from Outside USA 1-315-464-4001

Key:
CPK = creatine phosphokinase
WBC = white blood cell count

Box 4.7 QTc Prolongation and Torsades de Pointes (TdP) Ventricular Arrhythmia (17, 31)

- Uncommon but potentially fatal complication of antipsychotic therapy
- Monitor QTc via daily (or more frequent) ECGs when using antipsychotics in medically ill patients especially if using higher doses or if patient has other risk factors.
- Risk factors include female sex, cardiac conditions (bradyarrhythmia, congenital long QT syndrome, congestive heart failure, atrioventricular heart block, hypertension, ischemic heart disease, myocardial infarction, valvular disease, cardiomyopathy), medications prolonging QTc (Group Ia and III antiarrhythmics, anti-infectives, vasodilators, other psychotropics), electrolyte disturbances (low Mg, low K, low Ca), metabolic disturbances (hypothyroidism, renal or liver dysfunction).
- The QTc duration associated with increased risk of TdP is somewhat controversial: <440 ms is clearly normal. Borderline values are 440–460 ms in men and 440–470 ms in women. A QTc ≥500 ms is of concern and may warrant not starting an antipsychotic or changing dose or agent. An increase of 60 ms or ≥25% with initiation/dose increase is of concern.
- Weigh risks versus benefits in individuals with increased QTc. Uncontrolled agitation may have a much higher probability of serious negative events than the more remote risk of TdP.
- If the risk/benefit evaluation favors treatment, then mitigate risk of TdP as best as you can by running Mg high normal and K mid to high normal and by doing serial ECGs daily (or more frequently if high-dose antipsychotics are used or if patient is at higher risk).
- Dose may need to be held or the time between doses increased to allow QTc to come down within an acceptable range.

Box 4.7 *(cont.)*

- High-risk mediations include mesoridiazine, thioridazine, pimozide, high-dose IV haldol (>100 mg/24 hr)
- The University of Arizona (Arizona-CERT) maintains a database of QT prolonging drugs stratified by relative risk – www.torsades.org, www.qtdrugs.org

Key:
ECGs = electrocardiograms
QTc = corrected QT interval

Conventional/first-generation antipsychotics

Haloperidol is the most widely used conventional antipsychotic for the management of delirium in the medical setting, particularly in intensive care and step-down units, because of its minimal effects on hemodynamic and respiratory parameters and minimal EPS (17). Its mechanisms of action in delirium have not been fully explicated, but it is presumed to act through blockade of dopamine-2 receptors. Haloperidol may increase the effects of antihypertensive agents apart from guanethidine. Epinephrine may interact with haloperidol to lower blood pressure. Haloperidol may reduce the effects of anticoagulants. It should not be used in patients with parkinsonism, Lewy Body dementia, or HIV brain disease, unless an intravenous route of administration is the only possibility, in which case very careful dose titration and follow-up are required. It should not be used in patients with thyrotoxicosis because of potential neurotoxicity. Haloperidol is not particularly sedating and is often used in combination with lorazepam if sedation is required. Low-dose haloperidol administered subcutaneously is a popular palliative care intervention for nausea.

Chlorpromazine has FDA approval for use in refractory hiccups and nausea and vomiting. Patients who have been on conventional antipsychotics for long-term management of psychotic illnesses require special attention in the medical context. Caution must be exercised with patients on mesoridazine or thioridazine with respect to addition of other QTc-prolonging medications or drug-drug interactions that could increase their level and thus the risk of QTc prolongation.

Atypical/second-generation antipsychotics

Atypical/second-generation antipsychotics are used "off label" for the management of delirium, particularly in patients outside of the intensive care unit environment and when an oral route of administration is preferred.

All of these drugs have some potential for dysregulating glycemic control and increasing lipids, but typically these effects are not relevant with the short-term use that is common in the medical setting. Increased risk of stroke in the demented elderly receiving atypical antipsychotics has been an area of recent although controversial concern (18–20).

Risperidone is the preferred agent when sedation should be avoided. On initiation, it can be associated with orthostatic hypotension and syncope, presumably secondary to its alpha$_1$-receptor–blocking properties, and should be used with caution in patients with cardiac impairment. Elderly patients with atrial fibrillation are reportedly at increased risk of CVA.

Olanzapine is a widely used agent because of its sedating properties secondary to blockade of histamine 1, alpha$_1$-adrenergic, and muscarinic 1 receptors. It may be associated with orthostatic hypotension on initial dose titration, especially when used intramuscularly. It should be used with caution in medically unstable patients, particularly those with cardiac issues. It may enhance the effects of antihypertensives. Its actions on muscarinic 1 receptors contraindicate its use in patients with known narrow-angle closure glaucoma, and caution is recommended in patients with prostatic hyperplasia or paralytic ileus.

Quetiapine is the preferred agent in the context of delirium in patients with Parkinson's disease, Lewy Body dementia, or HIV dementia. Its most problematic side effects in medically ill populations include dizziness related to orthostatic hypotension and sedation. It should be started at low doses (e.g., 25 mg twice daily) in the medically ill and may be used in low dose (e.g., 12.5 to 25 mg) for the management of insomnia in the medically ill.

Clozapine typically is not initiated in a patient with a major medical illness because of its complexities. Sialorrhea may complicate GI surgical procedures but often can be managed without discontinuing the clozapine (e.g., ipratropium nasal inhalers) (21) (Box 4.8).

Box 4.8 Clinical Pearls – Antipsychotics

- Risk/benefit analyses need to done when patients with long-term antipsychotic therapy for psychotic illnesses are admitted with major medical illnesses. Their pharmacotherapy should be changed only if a significant medical risk is associated with their usual regimen in the context of their current medical problems. If a change is needed, then ensure that the patient is being adequately "covered" with the new antipsychotic regimen (e.g., compare antipsychotic dosage equivalencies of the new regimen and the former regimen).
- Antipsychotics may be useful in low doses for a variety of "off-label" indications, including anxiolysis when benzodiazepines are contraindicated and the need to attenuate steroid-induced mood lability.

Psychostimulants

Psychostimulants have shown utility in improving depression and fatigue in the medically ill and are used clinically to address apathy and amotivation. The two primary psychostimulants used in this patient population are methylphenidate and dextroamphetamine. Methylphenidate and dextroamphetamine both act as inhibitors of the norepinephrine transporter (NET) and the dopamine transporter (DAT). Adverse effects of psychostimulants include nervousness, insomnia, anorexia, and, rarely, psychosis. Furthermore, potential cardiac side effects include tachycardia, hypertension, and, rarely, arrhythmias.

Psychostimulants can improve appetite in depressed medically ill patients. Moreover, depression in hospitalized cancer patients can improve within two days of administration of psychostimulant treatment (22). Fatigue in the absence of depression has demonstrated significant improvement following treatment with methylphenidate in patients with HIV and advanced cancer (23, 24). Cancer patients with hypoactive delirium may benefit from methylphenidate treatment, although an exacerbation of sleep or restlessness should be monitored (25). Early studies suggest that methylphenidate may ameliorate apathy in Alzheimer's dementia or improve neurocognitive symptoms post traumatic brain injury (26, 27).

In medically ill patients, modafinil may be used "off-label" for treating fatigue, and for augmentation in depression. Modafinil has shown benefit in preliminary studies in treating fatigue in patients with multiple sclerosis, myotonic dystrophy, fibromyalgia, and hepatitis C

(35–38). However, these studies have been tempered by negative studies (28). Depression with fatigue or hypersomnia may also be responsive to modafinil augmentation of antidepressant treatment, although rigorous studies in medically ill patients are needed (29) (Box 4.9).

Box 4.9 Clinical Pearls – Psychostimulants

- Monitor potential abuse of psychostimulants in patients with an addiction history, and consider long-acting preparations if stimulants are required.
- If a second dose of a psychostimulant is needed, give second dose in the early afternoon to minimize insomnia.
- Psychostimulants have minimal cytochrome P450 (CYP450) drug-drug interactions.

References

1. Guengerich FP. Role of cytochrome P450 enzymes in the drug-drug interactions. Adv Pharmacol. 1997;43:7–35.

2. Bourgeois JA, Kike AK, Simmons JE, et al. Adjunctive valproic acid for delirium and/or agitation on a consultation-liaison service: a report of six cases. J Neuropsychiatry Clin Neurosci. 2005;17(2):232–8.

3. Reoux JP, Saxon AJ, Malte CA, et al. Divalproex sodium in alcohol withdrawal: a randomized double-blind placebo-controlled clinical trial. Alcohol Clin Exp Res. 2001;25(9):1324–9.

4. Raja M, Azzoni A. Valproate-induced hyperammonaemia. J Clin Psychopharmacol. 2002;22(6):631–3.

5. Joffe H, Cohen LS, Suppes T, et al. Valproate is associated with new-onset oligoamenorrhea with hyperandrogenism in women with bipolar disorder. Biol Psychiatry. 2006;59(11):1078–86.

6. Van Amelsvoort T, Bakshi R, Devaux CB, Schwabe S. Hyponatremia associated with carbamazepine and oxcarbazepine therapy: a review. Epilepsia. 1994;35(1):181–8.

7. Perry C, Mackay-Sim A, Feron F, McGrath J. Olfactory neural cells: an untapped diagnostic and therapeutic resource. The 2000 Ogura Lecture. Laryngoscope. 2002;112(4):603–7.

8. Astrup A, Toubro S. Topiramate: a new potential pharmacological treatment for obesity. Obes Res. 2004;12(Suppl): 167S–173S.

9. Meador KJ, Loring DW, Hulihan JF, et al. Differential cognitive and behavioral effects of topiramate and valproate. Neurology. 2003;60(9):1483–8.

10. Kirov G, Tredget J, John R, et al. A cross-sectional and prospective study of thyroid disorders in lithium-treated patients. J Affect Disord. 2005;87(2-3): 313–7.

11. Lombardi G, Panza N, Biondi B, et al. Effects of lithium treatment on hypothalamic-pituitary-thyroid axis: a longitudinal study. J Endocrinol Invest. 1993;16(4):259–63.

12. Boton R, Gaviria M, Batlle DC. Prevalence, pathogenesis, and treatment of renal dysfunction associated with chronic lithium therapy. Am J Kidney Dis. 1987;10(5):329–45.

13. Presne C, Fakhouri F, Noel NH, et al. Lithium-induced nephropathy: rate of progression and prognostic factors. Kidney Int. 2003;64(2):585–92.

14. Gitlin M. Lithium and the kidney: an updated review. Drug Saf. 1999;20(3): 231–43.

15. Evans DL, Charney DS, Lewis L, et al. Mood disorders in the medically ill: scientific review and recommendations. Biol Psychiatry. 2005;58(3):175–89.

16. de Abajo FJ, Rodriguez LA, Montero D. Association between selective serotonin reuptake inhibitors and upper gastrointestinal bleeding: population

based case-control study [comment]. BMJ. 1999;319(7217):1106–9.

17. Robinson MJ, Owen JA. Psychopharmacology. In: Levinson J, editor. The American Psychiatric Publishing textbook of psychosomatic medicine. Washington (DC): American Psychiatric Publishing Inc; 2005. p. 871–922.

18. Herrmann N, Lanctot KL. Atypical antipsychotics for neuropsychiatric symptoms of dementia: malignant or maligned? Drug Saf. 2006;29(10): 833–43.

19. Schneider LS, Dagerman KS, Insel P. Efficacy and adverse effects of atypical antipsychotics for dementia: meta-analysis of randomized, placebo-controlled trials. Am J Geriatr Psychiatry. 2006;14(3):191–210.

20. Trifuro G, Spina E, Gambassi G. Use of antipsychotics in elderly patients with dementia: do atypical and conventional agents have a similar safety profile. Pharmacol Res. 2009;59(1):1–12.

21. Robinson RG, Jorge RE, Clarence-Smith K. Double-blind randomized treatment of poststroke depression using nefiracetam. J Neuropsychiatry Clin Neurosci. 2008; 20(2):178–84.

22. Orengo CA, Kunik ME, Molinari V, Workman RH. The use and tolerability of fluoxetine in geropsychiatric inpatients. J Clin Psychiatry. 1996;57(1):12–6.

23. Breitbart W, Rosenfeld B, Pessin H, et al. Depression, hopelessness, and desire for hastened death in terminally ill patients with cancer. JAMA. 2000;284(22):2907–11.

24. Bruera E, Driver L, Barnes EA, et al. Patient-controlled methylphenidate for the management of fatigue in patients with advanced cancer: a preliminary report. J Clin Oncol. 2003;21(23):4439–43.

25. Barberger-Gateau P, Commenges D, Gagnon M, et al. Instrumental activities of daily living as a screening tool for cognitive impairment and dementia in elderly community dwellers. J Am Geriatr Soc. 1992;40(11):1129–34.

26. Herrmann N, Rothenburg LS, Black SE, et al. Methylphenidate for the treatment of apathy in Alzheimer disease: prediction of response using dextroamphetamine challenge. J Clin Psychopharmacol. 2008; 28(3):296–301.

27. Port A, Willmott C, Charlton J. Self-awareness following traumatic brain injury and implications for rehabilitation. Brain Inj. 2002;16(4):277–89.

28. Stankoff B, Waubant E, Confavreux C, et al. Modafinil for fatigue in MS: a randomized placebo-controlled double-blind study. Neurology. 2005;64(7):1139–43.

29. Fava M, Thase ME, DeBattista C. A multicenter, placebo-controlled study of modafinil augmentation in partial responders to selective serotonin reuptake inhibitors with persistent fatigue and sleepiness. J Clin Psychiatry. 2005;66(1): 85–93.

30. Birmes P, Coppin D, Schmitt L, Lague D. Serotonin syndrome: a brief review. CMAJ. 2003;168(11):1439–42.

31. Gupta A, Lawrence AT, Krishnan K, et al. Current concepts in the mechanisms and management of drug-induced QT prolongation and torsade de pointes. Am Heart J. 2007;153(6):891–9.

Suicide risk assessment

James J. Amos

Typical consult question

"Is the patient suicidal?"

This question often comes from intensive care units where patients are typically admitted after attempting suicide, and can make up about 15% or so of all psychiatric consultation requests. Staff members usually want a quick response, so you should get over there as soon as possible.

Background

It has been said that "there are only two kinds of psychiatrists – those who have had patients commit suicide, and those who will" (1). No task is more difficult for the psychiatrist or any other healthcare professional than suicide risk assessment. No treatment outcome is more devastating than suicide. Academic departments and private practice organizations are in many cases ill prepared to help their members or the families who are left behind cope with the devastating aftermath – shock, guilt and shame, isolation, grief, dissociation, crises of faith about psychotherapy and other treatments, and grandiosity associated with the suicide of a loved one (2).

Making suicide assessment a practical and routine part of psychiatric consultation will help the clinician become more proficient with this part of the examination, and may help prevent some suicides. Suicide is the 11th leading cause of death in the United States, with one person dying of suicide every 16 minutes (3). About 30,000 suicide attempts are reported annually in the United States alone. Some estimates indicate that 5% to 6% occur in hospitals (4). In Busch's study of 76 patients who committed suicide on an inpatient psychiatric unit, 78% denied suicide ideation or intent as their last communication. Severe agitation or anxiety was found in 79% of the patients during the week before their suicide. One other disheartening finding was that 9% of the patients who committed suicide somehow managed to kill themselves while under 1:1 observation (4). This study highlighted the need to pay closer attention to psychic and motoric anxiety as a risk factor for suicide, and to not rely on denials of suicidality from the patient.

In one study, after adjustment was made for the presence of other illnesses, several common medical conditions were found to be independent predictors for increased suicide risk, including severe pain, congestive heart failure, seizure disorder, and chronic lung disease. Bipolar disorder, depression, anxiety, and sleep disorders are the psychiatric disorders which had the highest likelihood of association with suicide (5).

Psychosomatic Medicine: An Introduction to Consultation-Liaison Psychiatry, eds. James J. Amos and Robert G. Robinson. Published by Cambridge University Press. © Cambridge University Press 2010.

The need to monitor and respond to complaints of severe anxiety as an acute risk factor for suicide was noted by Bostwick and Rackley regarding inpatients who commit suicide in general hospital medical/surgical units (6). A clear and urgent need has been identified for more detailed and prospective data collection on reported suicides in the general medical inpatient setting. When suicides do occur in the medical setting, they are devastating for families, medical personnel, and hospital administrators. The association between medical illness and suicide may be independent of two other major and well-established risk factors: substance abuse and depression. Although systematic data collection methods are limited, some findings are notable. Medical inpatients tend to commit suicide by jumping from heights, in contrast to patients on psychiatric units, who tend to hang themselves, and in contrast to community-based persons, who tend to shoot themselves (7). Medical inpatients tend to be older, married, and employed, in contrast to psychiatric inpatients, and tend to commit suicide on hospital grounds.

Conducting suicide risk assessment face to face is difficult enough, although guidelines have been put forth by the American Psychiatric Association (APA) (8). Conducting these assessments remotely by telemedicine may be considerably more challenging. However, the Department of the Veterans Administration (VA) has been a leader in this area since 2007, when the VA initiated a major suicide prevention campaign, in part in response to a study indicating that veterans were twice as likely to die of suicide when compared with non-veterans in the general population (3).

Work-up

The components of a suicide risk assessment, ideally, should (1) be easy to remember, (2) be based on empirically demonstrable essential features, (3) be readily transferable from emergency room or intensive care unit to consulting room, (4) foster a therapeutic alliance, (5) facilitate the gathering of valid information, and (6) guide treatment decisions.

One suggested example is the Chronological Assessment of Suicide Events (CASE) approach proposed by Shea (9). Four "regions" of inquiry are explored in order:

1. The presenting suicide ideation and behaviors
2. Recent suicide ideation and behavior over the preceding 8 weeks
3. Past suicide ideation and behaviors
4. Immediate suicide ideation and future suicide plans

While the progression from present to past to immediate suicide ideation may seem backwards, especially to time-pressured emergency room clinicians, Shea's rationale is that rapport and trust-building may be easier if one delays exploring the region of immediate suicidality until the patient learns that it's okay to talk about suicide.

Another somewhat more complicated component model of inquiry has been proposed by Bryan and Rudd (10):

1. Predisposition to suicidal behavior

   a. Previous psychiatric diagnoses, including depressive disorder, substance abuse, borderline personality disorder (BPD), and antisocial personality disorder (ASPD), all of which raise the risk for suicide
   b. Previous suicidal behavior
   c. History of abuse

    d. Recent discharge from inpatient psychiatric unit

    e. Demographics, including middle-aged or elderly white married or recently separated/ divorced or white homosexual male

2. Identifiable precipitants or stressors

    a. Acute or chronic medical illness, especially with increasing pain

    b. Family instability

    c. Significant losses of an interpersonal or financial nature

3. Symptomatic presentation

    a. Consider diagnoses such as those mentioned above (BPD, ASPD), as well as major depressive disorder (MDD).

    b. Low self-esteem especially when combined with substance dependence

    c. Psychotic illness, especially during periods of symptomatic improvement implying increased awareness of implications of the disorder and functional losses

    d. Instrumental suicide-related behavior designed to inflict pain on others, seek help, and get attention without intent to die; lethality of suicidal behavior may be underestimated

4. Presence of hopelessness

    a. Hopelessness and its duration and degree figure importantly in suicide attempters compared with non-attempters

5. Nature of suicidal thinking

    a. Estimate frequency and intensity on 1–10 scales.

    b. Ask about distant suicidal episodes before more recent episodes to reduce resistance.

    c. Ask about means, availability of means, steps to prepare, and deterrents to suicide.

6. Previous suicidal behavior

    a. Although it is recommended to get details about each and every episode, this may not be practical with some multiple attempters.

    b. Recalling the absence of previous attempts does not necessarily indicate reduced risk.

7. Impulsivity and self-control

    a. Ask directly about self-control, previous arrest, substance abuse, violent acting out, and methods for coping with stress.

8. Protective factors

    a. Suicide-related writing may serve a protective role (e.g., "journaling") through discharge of impulsive and maladaptive coping, although when it is used to communicate plans and preparation, it is obviously not protective.

    b. Interpersonal supports, young children in the home, religious faith, and spirituality may be important protective factors.

    c. Interventions that shore up protective factors may be more effective than focusing on risk factors alone.

Bryan and Rudd also recommend a hierarchical approach to questioning, but prefer starting from identification of the precipitant, to symptomatic presentation, to hopelessness, to the ultimate nature of the patient's suicidal thinking. The rationale is the same – to improve rapport, enhance the honesty of the report, and gradually reduce anxiety by normalizing the suicidal thinking. Trying to clarify the difference between explicit and implicit intent is emphasized. Confronting the patient with discrepancies between behavior and statements can be difficult. Besides asking at least twice about the suicide method, one can elicit patient ratings on a 1–10 scale regarding suicide ideation intensity, intent, and hopelessness (10).

Other interview techniques adapted from Shea and designed to facilitate getting valid information and reducing anxiety follow:

1. Behavioral incident

This consists of asking many detailed, directed questions to get a verbal walkthrough of a suicide event, such as an aborted or completed suicide attempt. It is time consuming, so should be used judiciously early in the interview, after sufficient rapport building has been done.

2. Denial of the specific

Often, asking simple, open-ended questions (sometimes called "gate" questions; e.g., "Have you ever had a suicide plan?") yields negative answers. If the examiner follows by asking a series of closed-ended questions (e.g., "Well, for example, have you ever thought of shooting yourself, hanging, overdosing?"), this may jog the patient's memory. This kind of sifting through a list may result in a surprising array of responses not obtainable with the use of simple open-ended questions. This is also potentially time consuming, because the examiner may then follow up with behavioral incident–type questions.

3. Shame attenuation

Sometimes, the examiner can break the taboo against talking about subjects typically freighted with shame and guilt, such as suicidal thoughts. This entails using openers designed to help de-stigmatize the subject (e.g., "With all this pressure, I would think that you might think things are pretty hopeless, even think about ending the pain once and for all"). This is based on patients' perception of the difficulties that triggered their thoughts and behaviors.

4. Normalization

Some people are very sensitive to being viewed as different, so they may be helped by pointing out that a lot of people under similar circumstances might feel the same way (e.g., "Many people I've talked to who have these stressors may sometimes begin to think about suicide. Does that ever happen to you?"). This is based on what other people sometimes think or do.

5. Gentle assumption

This technique can be used by experienced examiners when a good deal of information about the patient is gathered by observation, collateral history, and close listening, followed by application of a well-practiced algorithm-type assessment. One is playing the odds that this will permit an educated guess to be used in gently confronting a patient about an assumption that the examiner arrives at. For example, if the patient is brought to the ER by a relative who has told the nurse that she's concerned about the patient being "desperate," if the chart reveals a history of previous suicide attempts, and if the patient breaks eye contact and cries several times during general history taking about self-harm, the examiner might ask, "So, what are some ways that you've thought about killing yourself, if any?" This approach should be used sparingly, as patients can sometimes feel affronted by it.

6. Symptom amplification

This is another advanced technique that may offset the tendency of patients to minimize suicidality. The examiner strategically exaggerates in anticipation of this tendency. This technique may be more effective when used with patients who have a reputation for minimizing and have been confronted about it previously. For example, "So, what do you estimate the percentage of time is that you spend thinking about suicide in a given week, 75% or 95%?" The examiner might get a more accurate answer of, say, 50%, but without the technique, the patient may underestimate or deny altogether thinking about suicide. The exaggerated number should make sense; if it's fantastic, it may tip the patient off or put him off.

Clinical decision-making and treatment

The default plan for someone judged to be at high risk for suicide is hospitalization, either voluntary or involuntary. Serial suicide risk assessments are done while the patient is in the hospital, while modifiable risk factors are dealt with pharmacologically (e.g., global insomnia, major Axis I disorders) and psychologically with evidence-based interventions, including supportive and cognitive-behavioral therapies.

Often after a serious suicide attempt, the patient suffers from medical complications while at the same time needing intensive psychiatric evaluation and treatment. Most intensivists are reluctant to house such patients, who no longer need critical care, for very long because they believe that this is an inappropriate use of their service. Medical-psychiatry units (MPUs), when available, can fill this gap in care for those with combined, complex medical and psychiatric illness. These units often help prevent the practice of restraining patients on 1:1 observation through 24-hour shifts by non–psychiatrically trained sitters. When MPUs are appropriately designed and built, they contain both medical and psychiatric safety features, and are staffed by nurses and physicians with combined medical and psychiatric training (11).

The first priority in preventing suicide in the medically ill is to search for and treat underlying psychiatric illness. It is very important to "restrain other physicians from automatically prescribing antidepressants for every medically ill patient who expresses a wish to die," which tends to pathologize normal grieving and leads to the overuse of psychotropic drugs (12).

It is recommended to assign and document specific risk categories (10):

Baseline: absence of acute overlay without significant stressors, appropriate only for ideators and single attempters

Acute: presence of acute overlay and significant stressors and/or symptoms, appropriate only for ideators and single attempters

Chronic high risk: baseline risk for multiple attempters, absence of acute overlay, no significant stressors or symptoms

Chronic high risk with acute exacerbation: acute risk for multiple attempters, presence of acute overlay, significant stressors and/or prominent symptoms

No empirical evidence has been found to support no-suicide or no-harm contracts; these contracts do not prevent suicides, nor do they protect one against malpractice lawsuits. The use of no-suicide contracts is currently not recommended as a tool for suicide risk assessment (10, 13).

Rudd proposes an alternative to no-suicide contracts, called the "commitment to treatment statement" (14). This is defined as an agreement between the patient and the clinician in which the patient agrees to commit to the treatment process and to living by doing the following:

1. Identifying the roles and expectations of both treater and patient
2. Communicating candidly about all aspects of treatment, including suicide
3. Accessing emergency services during crises that could hinder honoring the agreement (crisis plan)

Rudd recommends not making these agreements on a preprinted form and placing a time restriction on them. They can include statements about taking medications, keeping appointments with therapists, and using a crisis plan when necessary. Both patient and treater sign it, and it also can be signed by a family member or support person, as well as by a witness.

The crisis plan could be placed on the back of a business card, a 3 × 5-in. index card, or, probably, in the case of a busy consultation service in a large hospital, a preprinted form. It provides specific instructions for what the patient is to do during crises when suicidal thinking or behavior is imminent. It can include crisis line and support person phone numbers, activities to comfort oneself, reasons for living, and contingencies for going to the emergency room if preliminary efforts fail (14).

A great deal more information can be conveyed through body language than through words. It is estimated that we communicate only 7% of what we intend through words (15). This is a reciprocal interaction. How we ask questions is at least as important as what we ask. Important behaviors to note in ourselves and in our patients include eye contact, conviction in the voice, approach versus withdrawal gestures, and the nuances of laughter that can indicate anxiety or genuine humor. "Don't just do something, sit there" comes close to what a clinician should do first on entering the room. More important, in a noisy, crowded hospital room, where suicide risk assessments are often conducted, it's best to find a place to sit down.

None of the aforementioned interview techniques will matter if you're not prepared to do more listening than talking. Try to remember that the suicide risk assessment is more like a "difficult conversation" than an interrogation (16).

References

1. Simon RI. Assessing and managing suicide risk: guidelines for clinically based risk management. Washington (DC): American Psychiatric Publishing; 2003.

2. Hausmann K, Psychiatrists Often Overwhelmed By a Patient's Suicide. Psychiatr News. 2003;38(13):6–43.

3. Godleski L, Nieves JE, Darkins A, Lehmann L. VA telemental health: suicide assessment. Behav Sci Law. 2008;26(3): 271–86.

4. Busch K, Fawcett J, and Jacobs D. Clinical correlates of inpatient suicide. J Clin Psychiatry. 2003;64(1):14–9.

5. Juurlink DN, Herrmann N, Szalai JP, et al. Medical illness and the risk of suicide in the elderly. Arch Intern Med. 2004;64(11): 1179–84.

6. Bostwick JM, Rackley SJ. Completed suicide in medical/surgical patients: who is at risk? Curr Psychiatry Rep. 2007;9(3): 242–6.

7. Ballard ED, Pao M, Henderson D, et al. Suicide in the medical setting. Jt Comm J Qual Patient Saf. 2008;34:474–81.

8. American Psychiatric Association. Practice guideline for the assessment and treatment of patients with suicidal behaviors. Washington (DC): American Psychiatric Association; 2003.

9. Shea SC. The practical art of suicide assessment: a guide for mental health professionals and substance abuse counselors. 2nd ed. Hoboken (NJ): John Wiley and Sons; 2002.

10. Bryan CJ, Rudd MD. Advances in the assessment of suicide risk. J Clin Psychol. 2006;62(2):185–200.

11. Amos JJ, Kijewski V, and Kathol R. The Medically Ill or Pregnant Psychiatric Inpatient, in Principles of Inpatient Psychiatry, Ovsiew F, and Munich RL, Editors. 2009, Wolters Kluwer: Lippincott Williams & Wilkins: Philadelphia; 333–343.

12. Bostwick JM, Levenson JL. Suicidality. In: Levenson JL, editor. Textbook of psychosomatic medicine. Washington (DC): American Psychiatric Publishing, Inc; 2005. p. 219–34.

13. Lewis LM. No-harm contracts: a review of what we know. Suicide Life Threat Behav. 2007;37(1):50–7.

14. Rudd MD, Mandrusiak M, and Joiner TE Jr. The case against no-suicide contracts: the commitment to treatment statement as a practice alternative. J Clin Psychol. 2006;62(2):243–51.

15. Mehrabian A. Silent messages. Belmont (CA): Wadsworth Publishing Co; 1971.

16. Stone D, Patton B, Heen S. Difficult conversations: how to discuss what matters most. New York (NY): Penguin Books; 2000.

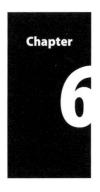

Assessment and management of the violent patient

James J. Amos

Typical consult question

"Can you help us manage this patient who threatened us on rounds?"

Most of the time in the general hospital or in clinics, this question is preceded by an alarm of some kind, notifying pertinent staff members who may be part of a team of people designated to manage situations in which a patient is likely to become or has already become violent. In any case, this is a situation for which there is an immediate need to saddle up and get up to the floor.

Background

Nothing gets the adrenaline rushing like the panic button call from one of the med/surg units requesting immediate help in managing the patient who is violent or is about to become violent. Some hospitals have rapid response teams that are available by special page or overhead speaker announcement. They often include the consultation psychiatrist.

Recognizing the gut feeling that a threat exists is imperative in maintaining a safe environment for you, the patient, and others in the evaluation area. Denial, freezing, and bravado are some of the symptoms of unacknowledged fear of a threat. They can contribute to rapid escalation of agitation in the patient, who will almost certainly be more ready to obey gut impulses than you will be. It's important to acknowledge fear when you sense danger; some experts believe that this is intuitive and that judgment interferes in the heat of the moment (1). However, sizing up a volatile patient quickly, which could be called thin-slicing, is fraught with peril if it's done on the basis of stereotypes (2).

There are many ways to conceptualize algorithms for managing the acutely agitated and potentially violent patient. Here is a suggested mnemonic:

Containment before
Assessment before
Non-violent
Intervention before
Take down

Frequently the consultant is called to intensive care units and emergency rooms to assist in the management of patients who are rapidly getting out of control or are already out of control.

Psychosomatic Medicine: An Introduction to Consultation-Liaison Psychiatry, eds. James J. Amos and Robert G. Robinson. Published by Cambridge University Press. © Cambridge University Press 2010.

The idea behind CAN IT is to facilitate recall of basic principles of assessment and management of acute agitation. Containment refers to ensuring that you and the patient both feel relatively safe in the assessment area. Preferably, both of you should have easy access to the door for escape if necessary. At first, it may seem odd to recommend letting the patient escape from the room, but the point is not to force the patient to run over you to get to the door.

Another issue of containment is to ensure that the patient gives up any weapons before you agree to do the evaluation. Sometimes, offering food or drink (not hot enough to injure if hurled in your face) will help set a non-threatening atmosphere. It's helpful to avoid making intense or prolonged eye contact with the patient, because this may be viewed as threatening. Always make sure that plenty of other people are available to help you if a take-down situation develops.

Containment under these conditions sometimes is achievable by simply being honest with the patient who is still able to hear you by admitting that he/she is saying or doing things that make you afraid. This may seem counterintuitive. But, provided it's delivered calmly as a statement followed by reassurance that you and everyone else involved are committed to maintaining the safety of all persons present (including the patient), this may capitalize on the patient's own fear of losing control by assuring that you'll do everything in your power to keep the lid on the situation. Now it won't contain the occasional sadistic psychopathic personality who enjoys making people afraid. In this case, it has to be abundantly clear to this individual that many people are around who could physically control him if absolutely necessary.

Work-up

Assessment is vital, but it can be adequately carried out only if safety issues have been addressed first. To manage the agitated patient, it's critical to understand the origin of the behavior. And that doesn't mean theorizing about the neurobiological underpinnings. The following list presents some of the most commonly associated disorders in agitated patients:

1. Primary Psychiatric Disorders

   a. Psychotic disorders

      i. Schizophrenia
      ii. Affective illness
         1. Bipolar affective disorder, manic with psychosis
         2. Major depression can be accompanied by anger attacks and psychosis

   b. Cognitive disorders

      i. Dementia with psychosis and behavior disturbance
      ii. Mental retardation

   c. Personality disorders

      i. Antisocial and borderline

   d. Substance abuse disorders

      i. Intoxications

2. Medical Disorders

    a. Delirium due to a general medical condition

        i. Seizure disorder
        ii. CNS malignancy, trauma, or infection
        iii. Medications
        iv. Cerebrovascular disease
        v. Systemic disorders
            1. Toxic, metabolic
            2. Infectious
            3. Environmental

Thinking "both/and" rather than "either/or" about etiologies is prudent. Treatment of the underlying cause is always advisable, but is not feasible in some situations. The underlying illness may be chronic, for example, or the patient may be too agitated initially to allow a full medical examination.

Many authors agree that the best predictor of future violence in psychiatric patients is past violence, especially recent past violence. High arousal states including fear, anger, confusion, or humiliation may underlie aggression.

Clinical decision-making and treatment

Attempts to de-escalate agitation with non-violent means constitute the next step. Offering to inject the patient with an antipsychotic would not usually be welcomed as a first intervention. Paying attention to your own body language is important. Crossed arms or hands held behind the back can be seen as threatening. Stay out of arms reach. Avoid challenging the patient by "correcting" faulty reality testing. Open-ended questions may invite excessive, non-productive scapegoating, overinclusive rumination, and suspicion (e.g., "you trying to crawl inside my head – what do you mean by that?").

Try to keep questions to the point, obtaining as much information as possible about such things as triggering social crises. If a therapeutic alliance is achieved, capitalize by giving the patient a sense of control by offering choices regarding requests for urine drug screens or blood tests.

Only if non-violent means fail should the take-down be considered. This is when seclusion and restraints, and involuntary administration of medications, happen. It's unfortunate when this occurs because it wrests freedom and control away from the patient. At all times an effort should be made to utilize the least restrictive alternative doctrine. If the patient will accept an oral formulation of a sedative rather than an injection, this choice should be respected, along as there is no medical reason not to do so.

Sometimes a show of force is all that is required to convince someone that it would be too costly to fight. This entails gathering at least five people to non-violently simply confront the patient with an overwhelming number of potential opponents.

Psychopharmacologic management of the agitated, violent patient

No specific medication is approved by the FDA for control of agitation and combative behavior. Medications of choice are haloperidol and lorazepam, used singly or in combination.

Droperidol is another very effective agent, although recent FDA black box warnings about the risk for cardiac arrhythmias and case reports of sudden death reported with its use have led to greater caution. Of course, the first questions you should ask before administering any sedatives are the following:

- Does the patient have any known general medical relative or absolute contraindications to specific agents (e.g., cardiac, pulmonary, renal, or liver disease)?
- Does the patient have any known specific drug allergies or potentially life-threatening idiosyncratic drug sensitivities?

Antipsychotics often provide non-specific but effective control of violent behavior regardless of its cause. Haloperidol is the most studied agent. Some clinicians prefer IM chlorpromazine, especially if patients report intolerance of haloperidol. However, it's debatable whether management of agitation with haloperidol alone is optimally beneficial in someone who is violent primarily because of antisocial personality traits. An angry sociopathic individual may require one or more (rarely requiring >3) doses of oral or injectable lorazepam. Sedation is achieved often in minutes, with an amnestic effect as well. The efficacy of these agents for violence associated with borderline personality disorder is unknown. It is possible that benzodiazepines at lower doses may disinhibit the behavior of patients with personality disorders.

Comparative studies in patients with schizophrenia, mania, or schizoaffective disorder suggest that the combination of haloperidol and lorazepam is more effective than the use of either drug alone.

Rapid tranquilization is referred to in the medical literature with variable recommendations about dosing schedules. One suggested regimen is haloperidol 5 mg IM/concentrate q 30 minutes until calm but awake. Other regimens call for increasing (usually doubling) doses of haloperidol every 20 to 30 minutes until the patient is calm or until a set total dose is reached, after which alternative combination regimens of haloperidol and lorazepam are recommended. Another regimen administered haloperidol 5 mg and lorazepam 2 mg IM/concentrate q 1 hour to endpoint.

Regardless of the dosing interval, haloperidol up to 40 mg IM (equivalent to 80 mg PO) in 7 hours and lorazepam 24 mg/day have been safely administered in studies. It is important to note that dose-ranging studies do not consistently demonstrate that giving doses of haloperidol >10 mg IM (20 mg PO) per day significantly increases the response rate. However, these doses do increase the risk (percentage) that patients may experience extrapyramidal side effects (e.g., dystonia). Extrapyramidal adverse effects (e.g., dystonia) may be managed with benztropine 2 mg IM (onset 20–40 minutes) or IV (onset 1–2 minutes). Cogentin can be made available for management of extrapyramidal adverse effects at 2 mg IM/oral q 4 hours prn.

Agitation of delirium is generally responsive to monotherapy with antipsychotics, and haloperidol is the agent with which physicians have the most experience and for which efficacy is best supported by the medical literature. Attempting to treat this condition with benzodiazepines alone usually leads to worsening delirium, except in the special case of alcohol or benzodiazepine withdrawal delirium.

In delirious patients, one regimen suggests increasing (usually doubling) doses of haloperidol every 20 to 30 minutes until the patient is calm or until a set total dose is reached. In medically ill patients, a safe starting dose might be 1 to 2 mg. However, this strategy may also increase the risk for side effects, including extrapyramidal effects and neuroleptic malignant syndrome.

Recently, the FDA required a black box warning suggesting that unexpected cardiovascular death could occur when normal therapeutic doses of droperidol are used. This has had consequences for use of the agent in emergency rooms and on hospital wards lacking the capacity for cardiac monitoring. Mullins et al. reviewed this topic in the January 2004 issue of *American Journal of Emergency Medicine*, as did Shale et al. in the May 2003 issue of *Journal of Clinical Psychiatry*. They concluded that cardiovascular deaths are rare with doses at or below 2.5 mg, that mandatory electrocardiographic screening appears unnecessary, and that it's an extremely effective and safe method for treating severely agitated or violent patients, provided that the drug is administered in 5 mg intramuscular doses (with or without lorazepam). Because it is absorbed almost as quickly with intramuscular injection as with intravenous administration, the latter method offers no great advantage (3, 4).

Based on the FDA's black box warning for droperidol, the policy of the University of Iowa Health Care Hospitals and Clinics (UIHC) Pharmacy and Therapeutics (P & T) Subcommittee is that an EKG must be obtained before droperidol is administered and for 2 to 3 hours after the dose is administered. Its use is restricted to units that have developed a protocol for its use (usually intensive care units with cardiac monitoring available).

In most cases, the practical effect of this is to sharply limit the use of droperidol. It has also been associated with postural hypotension (due to alpha-adrenergic blockade) and corrected QT interval (QTc interval) prolongation, which could potentially progress to torsades de pointe and malignant ventricular arrhythmias. The latter problem has also been known to occur with large doses of intravenous haloperidol (although it has no black box warning), and thioridazine, (which has a black box warning). Ziprasidone has no black box warning (although there is a warning about possible QTc prolongation), and the trials using IM injections have not been notable for QTc prolongation. It may be more likely to occur if the baseline corrected QTc interval is in excess of 450 milliseconds in length, so a baseline EKG should be reviewed if it's available.

Intramuscular ziprasidone has been approved to treat acute agitation associated with schizophrenia and IM olanzapine to treat acute agitation associated with schizophrenia and bipolar mania. Although potentially efficacious, the use of IM **olanzapine** and **ziprasidone** in an emergent situation may be problematic because of the extra time required to reconstitute the product. This would become less of an issue if ward personnel would request pharmacy staff to demonstrate the reconstitution protocol so that nurses on the inpatient psychiatric units can perform this themselves rather than waiting for assistance from the pharmacy. Olanzapine is obtainable as the intramuscular injectable form.

Clinical trials with intramuscular ziprasidone and olanzapine have shown these agents to be more efficacious than placebo in treating acute agitation associated with schizophrenia or bipolar mania, and efficacy was achieved fairly quickly (5–7). It has been suggested that these agents may be more effective or may have a faster onset of action than IM haloperidol. Acutely agitated patients with schizophrenia treated with IM ziprasidone for 3 days had a significantly greater reduction in agitation than those treated with IM haloperidol in a double-blind, controlled trial (8). Likewise, patients with acute agitation associated with schizophrenia or bipolar mania treated with IM olanzapine had a significantly greater reduction in agitation at 15, 30, and 45 minutes compared with those treated with IM haloperidol in a double-blind, controlled trial, but no difference was noted between the two medications at the end of 2 hours (7).

The very low rates of dystonia and other extrapyramidal side effects and the lack of QTc interval prolongation in clinical studies with intramuscular ziprasidone and olanzapine have been reassuring (5–7).

Following is recommended dosing for IM ziprasidone and olanzapine:

- Ziprasidone 20 mg IM (preferred dose) every 4 hours as needed; maximum dose 40 mg per 24 hours. In the elderly, one should start with 10 mg IM.
- Olanzapine 10 mg IM every 2 hours as needed; maximum dose 30 mg per 24 hours.

References

1. De Becker G. The gift of fear: survival signals that protect us from violence. 1st ed. Boston: Little, Brown; 1997. p. viii, 334.

2. Gladwell M. Blink: the power of thinking without thinking. 1st ed. New York: Little, Brown and Co; 2005. p. viii, 277.

3. Mullins M, Van Zwieten K, Blunt JR. Unexpected cardiovascular deaths are rare with therapeutic doses of droperidol. Am J Emerg Med. 2004;22(1):27–8.

4. Shale JH, Shale CM, Mastin WD. A review of the safety and efficacy of droperidol for the rapid sedation of severely agitated and violent patients. J Clin Psychiatry. 2003; 64(5):500–5.

5. Daniel DG, Zimbroff DL, Swift RH, Harrigan EP. The tolerability of intramuscular ziprasidone and haloperidol treatment and the transition to oral therapy. Int Clin Psychopharmacol. 2004;19(1):9–15.

6. Meehan K, Zhang F, David S, et al. A double-blind, randomized comparison of the efficacy and safety of intramuscular injections of olanzapine, lorazepam, or placebo in treating acutely agitated patients diagnosed with bipolar mania. J Clin Psychopharmacol. 2001;21(4):389–97.

7. Wright P, Birkett M, David SR, et al. Double-blind, placebo-controlled comparison of intramuscular olanzapine and intramuscular haloperidol in the treatment of acute agitation in schizophrenia. Am J Psychiatry. 2001;158(7):1149–51.

8. Brookes G, Ahmed AG. Pharmacological treatments for psychosis-related polydipsia. Cochrane Database of Syst Rev. 2002(3):CD003544.

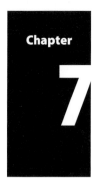

Chapter

7

Evaluation and management of delirium

John Querques, Carlos Fernandez-Robles, Davin Quinn, Megan Moore Brennan, and Gregory Fricchione

Typical consult questions

Consultation requests in patients with delirium rarely include the word *delirium*. Rather, they frequently contain one or more of the following: altered mental status, disoriented, confused, agitated, out of it, not making sense, manic, psychotic, depressed, withdrawn.

Examples of typical scenarios that raise concern for delirium include the following:

- A man with a history of heavy alcohol use becomes agitated and combative two days after undergoing a surgical procedure.
- An elderly woman with coronary artery disease and hypertension is brought in from a nursing home for psychosis; she is found to have a urinary tract infection.
- A woman with bipolar disorder and hepatitis C becomes confused and psychotic after starting interferon.

Although the sensitivity and specificity of recognizing delirium vary widely among clinicians, most recognize when patients are behaving, emoting, or thinking strangely or differently. Non-psychiatric clinicians often attribute disturbances in behavior, affect, or cognition to major mental illness, whether or not the patient has a psychiatric diagnosis. For example, clinicians are likely to attribute hallucinations and erratic behavior to schizophrenia; social withdrawal and low mood in elderly or severely ill patients to depression; or impulsive hyperactivity to bipolar disorder.

Background

The essence of delirium is captured in the *Diagnostic and Statistical Manual of Mental Disorders* definition (1):

- A perturbation in consciousness manifested in a reduced ability to focus, maintain, or shift attention
- A change in cognition or the development of hallucinations or illusions not caused by dementia
- Development over hours to days
- Fluctuation during the day
- A direct consequence of a general medical or surgical condition or its treatment

Although delirium is an acute derangement primarily in cognition, affect and behavior also become dysregulated. Affect varies from lability and emotional incontinence to affective

Psychosomatic Medicine: An Introduction to Consultation-Liaison Psychiatry, eds. James J. Amos and Robert G. Robinson. Published by Cambridge University Press. © Cambridge University Press 2010.

Table 7.1 Risk factors for delirium

- Advanced age
- Vision impairment
- Hearing impairment
- Baseline cognitive impairment
- Dehydration
- Malnutrition
- Sleep deprivation
- Social isolation
- Restraints
- Bladder catheters
- Polypharmacy
- Some psychoactive medications (e.g., benzodiazepines, those with prominent anticholinergic effects)

Data from references 14 and 15

constriction and blunting, behavior from docility to fulminant agitation. Therefore, just as we speak of heart, kidney, and liver failure, delirium should be thought of as *acute brain failure* (2).

Delirium affects 10% to 30% of hospitalized patients (3, 4) and is more common in patients of advanced age or in intensive care units (5–7). Delirium correlates with greater morbidity and mortality (8), longer hospital stays (9), and cognitive deterioration (10).

The pathophysiology of delirium may be explained by two neurotransmitter states: high dopaminergic tone and low cholinergic tone. Dopamine increase in mesolimbic and meso-cortical tracts may cause agitation and delusions, whereas acetylcholine decrease in hippocampal and basal forebrain regions may lead to disorientation, hallucinations, and memory impairment (11). Thus there is a hypothetical inverse relationship between dopamine and acetylcholine that tips in the direction of more dopamine and less acetylcholine (12). Inflammatory mediators that lead to neuronal oxidative stress may also play a role (13).

Risk factors for delirium are listed in Table 7.1 (14, 15). These same factors also retard the resolution of delirium once its reversible causes are treated.

Assessment and work-up

The work-up for delirium includes a detailed history, a methodical physical examination, and laboratory studies that help make the diagnosis, identify the cause(s) of the delirium, and establish an appropriate treatment plan (16).

The timing of events is key and often provides the best clues to the cause of the delirium. In a majority of cases, the patient will be unable to provide valid or reliable information. A review of physicians' and nurses' notes, vital signs, anesthesia reports, and medication administration records – correlating this information with behavioral changes – will help in constructing a time line. Exploring episodes of delirium reported during previous admissions may uncover useful data.

Consideration of substance intoxication and withdrawal is essential. A thorough alcohol and drug use history, as well as blood alcohol levels and blood and urine toxicology results, should be obtained in the emergency department and at the time of your examination.

Dementia can be difficult to distinguish from delirium. Abrupt onset, a waxing and waning course, and significantly disturbed or fluctuating attention characterize delirium, whereas late-stage dementia can lead to confusion, agitation, and psychosis (17). Any type of

Table 7.2 Glasgow Coma Scale

Eye Opening	
Spontaneous	4
To verbal command	3
To pain	2
No response	1
Motor	
Obeys verbal command	6
Localizes pain	5
Withdraws limb	4
Abnormal flexion (decortication)	3
Extension (decerebration)	2
No response	1
Verbal	
Oriented, converses	5
Disoriented, converses	4
Inappropriate words	3
Incomprehensible sound	2
No response	1
Score = total of 3 domains	Range 3 to 15

Adapted from reference 19

cognitive impairment can predispose to delirium (17). History obtained from family members and primary care physicians can help establish the patient's baseline cognitive status.

The formal mental status examination begins with an assessment of the level of consciousness. Alteration in consciousness is the *sine qua non* of delirium and is best measured by testing attention (18). Tests of attention include digit span; the number tapping test; recitation of the months of the year or the days of the week backward; and alternating alphabet recitation and counting (a verbal form of the Trails B test). If the patient does not speak, a handy test is to ask yourself this question: Do the patient's eyes look back at me? It is useful to examine the patient two or three times during the day to document waxing and waning symptoms and fluctuation in the level of consciousness.

The Glasgow Coma Scale, as modified for the Acute Physiology and Chronic Health Evaluation (APACHE) III study (Table 7.2), formally rates consciousness (19). It is particularly useful because it yields a number that can be tracked over time and that can be used in discussions with non-psychiatric clinicians, to whom "hard numbers" often mean more than abstract ideas. The Folstein Mini-Mental State Examination (MMSE) is a helpful tool that tests orientation, attention, memory, language, comprehension, and construction (20). Specific deficits are more important than the score, and it can be repeated serially to gauge a patient's progress. Mild confusion can be detected by asking the patient to draw a clock (21).

The neurological examination is as important as the mental status evaluation. Myoclonus, asterixis, and hyperreflexia are usual findings. Abnormalities of the eyes and pupils, nuchal rigidity, unilateral weakness, hyporeflexia, Babinski reflexes, abnormal gait, and absent vibratory or position sense can all point to specific causes of delirium. Frontal release signs (grasp,

Table 7.3 Life-threatening causes of delirium: WHHHIMP

- **W**ernicke's encephalopathy
- **H**ypoxia
- **H**ypoglycemia
- **H**ypertensive encephalopathy
- **I**ntracerebral hemorrhage
- **M**eningitis/encephalitis
- **P**oisoning

Data from reference 17

Table 7.4 A more comprehensive list of causes of delirium: I WATCH DEATH

Infection	Encephalitis, meningitis, syphilis, HIV infection, sepsis
Withdrawal	Alcohol, benzodiazepines, barbiturates
Acute metabolic	Acidosis, alkalosis, electrolyte derangements, liver failure, kidney failure
Trauma	Closed head injury, postoperative states, burns
CNS pathology	Abscess, hemorrhage, hydrocephalus, subdural hematoma, infection, seizures, stroke, tumors (primary or metastatic), vasculitis
Hypoxia	Anemia, carbon monoxide poisoning, hypotension, respiratory failure, heart failure
Deficiencies	Vitamins B1 (thiamine), B3 (niacin), B9 (folate), and B12 (cyanocobalamin)
Endocrinopathies	Overactivity or underactivity of thyroid, parathyroid, and adrenal glands, hyperglycemia or hypoglycemia
Acute vascular	Severe hypertension, stroke, arrhythmia, shock
Toxins or drugs	Medications, illicit drugs, pesticides, solvents
Heavy metals	Lead, manganese, mercury

Adapted from reference 21

snout, palmomental, suck, and glabellar), normally present only during the neonatal period, may emerge during an episode of delirium (17).

Several rating scales serve different purposes when delirium is assessed. The Confusion Assessment Method (CAM) aids in formal diagnosis, whereas the Delirium Rating Scale and the Memorial Delirium Assessment Scale rate the severity of the delirium and track its course (22).

Delirium is merely an epiphenomenon of an underlying problem; therefore, once delirium is identified, the principal task is to identify its cause – often more than one. Clinically it is helpful to divide possible culprits into two groups: those that are immediately life threatening (Table 7.3) and those that form a more comprehensive differential (Table 7.4) (17, 21).

A panel of basic laboratory tests (Table 7.5) aimed at identifying the most frequent underlying causes of delirium should be considered in every patient with delirium.

If the evaluation suggests a specific pathology, additional work-up to confirm or to exclude this diagnosis should be ordered. Cerebrospinal fluid analysis, brain computed tomography or magnetic resonance imaging, and additional blood tests (e.g., rapid plasma reagin, heavy metals, antinuclear antibodies, urine porphyrins, human immunodeficiency virus antibodies) are some examples.

Table 7.5 Laboratory evaluation of delirium

- Complete blood count
- Serum chemistries
- Serum and urine toxicology
- Urinalysis and urine culture
- Electrocardiogram
- Chest X-ray
- Arterial blood gases or oxygen saturation
- Serum drug levels (e.g., digoxin, amitriptyline)
- Thyroid-stimulating hormone
- Serum B12 and folate levels

Changes in the electroencephalogram (EEG) virtually always accompany delirium (16). An EEG can be helpful when the diagnosis of delirium is obscured by cognitive or psychiatric co-morbidities. In most non–alcohol-withdrawal deliria, the EEG shows generalized slowing and increased amplitude (23). The presence of triphasic waves may be helpful in identifying certain specific metabolic deliria (e.g., hepatic encephalopathy) (21).

Clinical decision-making and treatment

The primary, definitive treatment of delirium is reversal of its underlying cause(s), while dopamine blockade is adjunctive. The physician must evaluate the risk/benefit ratio of employing a dopamine antagonist. We favor using a dopamine blocker on a standing basis if the patient is continuously agitated or is clearly suffering from his confusion (even if not agitated). Whenever standing medication is used, we suggest that as-needed doses also be available for breakthrough agitation. Some, although not consistent, evidence suggests that dopamine blockade may be beneficial even in hypoactive patients, although use in this situation is elective and more speculative (24, 25).

Haloperidol administered IV is the mainstay in the dopamine-blocking management of delirious agitation. This route of administration is not approved by the FDA, and haloperidol now carries a black box warning (concerning its use in elderly patients with dementia-related psychosis) because of the potential for lethal ventricular arrhythmias, including torsades des pointes (TdP) (26, 27). However, its strong D_2 receptor binding affinity affords the safest and quickest way to calm the patient, in whom the risk of insufficiently treated, severe agitation often outweighs the risk of side effects. Although drug-induced prolongation of the QT interval corrected for heart rate (QTc) is relatively common in clinical practice, QTc intervals >500 ms are uncommon and TdP is rare. Secondary risk factors include high doses, rapid administration, inhibition of cytochrome P450 liver enzymes (e.g., paroxetine and ketoconazole inhibit the oxidative metabolism of haloperidol), impaired drug elimination, bradycardia, hypokalemia, hypomagnesemia, left ventricular hypertrophy, heart failure, recent conversion of atrial fibrillation, hypothyroidism, older age, female gender, concomitant use of other potassium channel blockers, undetected ion channel polymorphisms, and congenital long QT syndrome.

After reviewing in detail the QTc risk factor profile, we minimize these risks as best we can (e.g., we supplement potassium to 4 mmol/L and magnesium to 2 mEq/L) before giving haloperidol IV. We monitor the EKG closely. When the QTc increases to 450 to 500 ms, there is reason for caution; when it surpasses 500 ms, risk of TdP is increased (27). We concur with American Psychiatric Association (APA) guidelines (28): a QTc interval >450 msec, or more than 25% over baseline, may warrant consultation with a cardiologist and reduction or discontinuation of the antipsychotic medication. We regularly re-evaluate the risk/benefit ratio to determine whether haloperidol administration continues to make sense.

Haloperidol has little anticholinergic liability and few active metabolites. The effects of haloperidol on blood pressure, pulmonary artery pressure, heart rate, and respiration are milder than those of other antipsychotics and of intravenous benzodiazepines, and it is less sedating (28–30). Haloperidol may lower seizure threshold, although it is one of the safest neuroleptics in this regard. Haloperidol administered IV is less likely to produce extrapyramidal syndromes than is intramuscular or oral haloperidol (31).

We generally use haloperidol 2 to 2.5 mg IV for mild agitation, 5 mg for moderate agitation, and 7.5 to 10 mg for severe agitation. In the elderly, doses should be approximately one-third of the usual prescribed dose. APA guidelines recommend 0.25 to 0.5 mg every 4 hours as needed for elderly delirious patients (28, 30).

Doses can be repeated every 30 minutes until the patient is calm yet arousable to normal voice. When serious agitation persists, the previous dose can be doubled 30 minutes later; this approach of successive doubling can be repeated. The goal is to break the agitation rapidly, as partial control sometimes prolongs the delirious state. For agitation re-emerging after a calm period, the last effective dose can be administered. For persistent agitation, a continuous infusion of 5 to 10 mg/hr can be instituted, although we have very rarely needed this approach. More than 1000 mg of intravenous haloperidol has been used with safety (32).

A common problem in the general hospital is the urgency to discharge patients quickly to rehabilitation or nursing facilities. Often these facilities are not permitted to administer haloperidol IV, and so an oral agent is sought. The danger here is that an oral agent may be insufficient to keep the delirium under control and the patient may become floridly delirious once again, thus counterproductively prolonging the hospitalization. It is worth the investment of time to administer the haloperidol IV until the delirium is lysed, and only then taper it and perhaps replace it with an oral agent. When the delirium has resolved, the dopamine blocker should not be stopped at the first instance the patient is lucid. Because delirium waxes and wanes, you simply may have caught the patient when the mental state was clear. As a practical rule of thumb, two consecutive instances of lucidity should be observed before the dopamine blocker is altered; the first step then is to decrease it, not stop it outright.

Other parenteral neuroleptic drugs that have occasionally been used for treatment of agitation include perphenazine and chlorpromazine. These phenothiazines are relatively anticholinergic, can lower the seizure threshold and blood pressure, and can prolong the QTc interval. However, in smaller doses, they can be both safe and effective.

Adding lorazepam (1–2 mg IV every 2–4 hr) to haloperidol in the management of severely agitated patients can be helpful because lorazepam may reduce the extrapyramidal side effects of haloperidol, especially akathisia and catatonic features (33, 34).

Atypical antipsychotics given orally or intramuscularly may be useful for mild and perhaps moderate delirious agitation. These agents are now known to run the same dose-related risk of QTc prolongation and sudden cardiac death as haloperidol (35).

The addition of IV valproate (Depacon) may help in management of severe agitation when conventional therapy is inadequate or when problematic side effects emerge (36). Fentanyl or hydromorphone can also be added in severely agitated patients who are being mechanically ventilated, or when pain is an aggravating factor. Meperidine is to be avoided because of the deliriogenic effects of its active metabolite, normeperidine. If the patient is not sufficiently calmed with these usual measures, sedation with ventilator support can be achieved with propofol or dexmedetomidine (37–39).

Other methods of management include limb restraints, either soft or leather; torso restraints (e.g., Posey vests); soft hand mitts (to prevent removal of intravenous lines, Foley catheters, and the like); 1:1 observation; Vail beds; and orienting cues (e.g., calendars, clocks). In our view, the emphasis in the delirium literature on provision of orienting cues and on other, similar nonpharmacologic approaches is overstated (40). Although such maneuvers may be helpful in mild delirious states, they are ineffective in the floridly hyperactive delirious patient and may actually be harmful if they are used in place of pharmacologic agents.

Resolution of the delirious state frequently lags behind improvement in infectious, metabolic, hemodynamic, and toxic parameters. For example, a urinary tract infection may be successfully eradicated with antibiotics, but the patient may still be confused and at times agitated. This time lag is underappreciated by many physicians, and thus it is not uncommon for general physicians to declare that a patient is better and ready to be discharged while his mental state is still grossly deranged. Normal laboratory values do not guarantee normal mental states.

Conclusion

As a disturbance of consciousness with cognitive, affective, and behavioral manifestations, delirium – put simply – is acute brain failure. Although its pathophysiology is not known with certainty, its causes are legion, the determination and treatment of which are the first and second steps in management. Use of dopamine antagonists is adjunctive; haloperidol remains the treatment of choice for fulminant delirium with agitation. Resolution of the delirious state often lags behind reversal of the causative medical or surgical problem.

References

1. American Psychiatric Association. Diagnostic and statistical manual of mental disorders. 4th ed. Text Revision. Washington (DC): American Psychiatric Association; 2000.

2. Lipowski ZJ. Delirium: acute brain failure in man. Springfield (IL): Charles C Thomas Publisher; 1980.

3. Levkoff S, Cleary P, Liptzin B, Evans DA. Epidemiology of delirium: an overview of research issues and findings. Int Psychogeriatr. 1991;3(2):149–67.

4. Trzepacz PT. Delirium: advances in diagnosis, pathophysiology, and treatment. Psychiatr Clin North Am. 1996;19(3):429–48.

5. Francis J, Kapoor WN. Delirium in hospitalized elderly. J Gen Intern Med. 1990;5(1):65–79.

6. Roberts B. Screening for delirium in an adult intensive care unit. Intensive Crit Care Nurs. 2004;20(4):206–13.

7. Demeure MJ, Fain MJ. The elderly surgical patient and postoperative delirium. J Am Coll Surg. 2006;203(5):752–7.

8. McCusker J, Cole M, Abrahamowicz M, Primeau F, et al. Delirium predicts 12-month mortality. Arch Intern Med. 2002;162(4):457–63.

9. McCusker J, Cole M, Dendukuri N, Belzile E, et al. Delirium in older medical inpatients and subsequent cognitive and functional status: a prospective study. Can Med Assoc J. 2001;165(5):575–83.

10. McCusker J, Cole MG, Dendukuri N, Belzile E. Does delirium increase hospital stay? J Am Geriatr Soc. 2003;51(11):1539–46.

11. Murray GB. Excess endogenous dopamine and decreased endogenous acetylcholine responsible for acute delirium: an hypothesis. J Neuropsychiatr. 1993;5(4):456.

12. Coffman JA, Dilsaver SC. Cholinergic mechanisms in delirium. Am J Psychiatry. 1988;145(3):382–3.

13. Fricchione GL, Nejad SH, Esses JA, et al. Postoperative delirium. Am J Psychiatry. 2008;165(7):803–12.

14. Inouye SK. Delirium in hospitalized older patients: recognition and risk factors. J Geriatr Psychiatry Neurol. 1998;11(3):118–25.

15. Inouye SK. Predisposing and precipitating factors for delirium in hospitalized older patients. Dement Geriatr Cogn Disord. 1999;106(5):565–73.

16. Wise MG, Rundell JR. Clinical manual of psychosomatic medicine: a guide to consultation-liaison psychiatry. Arlington (VA): American Psychiatric Publishing; 2005. p. 29–47.

17. Cassem NH, Murray GB, Lafayette JM, A Stern T. Delirious patients. In: Stern TA, Fricchione GL, Cassem NH, Jellinek MS, Rosenbaum JF, editors. The MGH handbook of general hospital psychiatry. 5th ed. Philadelphia: Mosby; 2004. p. 119–34.

18. Macleod AD. Delirium: the clinical concept. Palliat Support Care. 2006;4(3):305–12.

19. Bastos PG. Sun X. Wagner DP, et al. Glasgow Coma Scale score in the evaluation of outcome in the intensive care unit: findings from the Acute Physiology and Chronic Health Evaluation III study. Crit Care Med. 1993;21(10):1459–65.

20. Folstein MF, Folstein SE, McHugh PR. "Mini-mental state": a practical method for grading the cognitive state of patients for the clinician. J Psychiatr Res. 1975;12(3):189–98.

21. Wise MG, Trzepacz PT. Delirium (confusional states). In: Rundell JR, Wise MG, editors. The American Psychiatric Press textbook of consultation-liaison psychiatry. Washington (DC): American Psychiatric Press; 1996. p. 268.

22. Trzepacz PT, Mulsant BH, Dew MA, et al. Is delirium different when it occurs in dementia? A study using the Delirium Rating Scale. J Neuropsychiatry Clin Neurosci. 1998;10(2):199–204.

23. Engel GL, Romano J. Delirium, a syndrome of cerebral insufficiency. J Chronic Dis. 1959;9(3):260–77.

24. Platt MM, Breitbart W, Smith M, et al. Efficacy of neuroleptics for hypoactive delirium. J Neuropsychiatry Clin Neurosci. 1994;6(1):66–7.

25. Breitbart W, Tremblay A, Gibson C. An open trial of olanzapine for the treatment of delirium in hospitalized cancer patients. Psychosomatics. 2002;43(3):175–82.

26. Shapiro BA, Warren, J, Egol AB, et al. Practice parameters for intravenous analgesia and sedation for adult patients in the intensive care unit: an executive summary. Crit Care Med. 1995;23(9):1596–1600.

27. Heist EK, Ruskin JN. Drug-induced proarrhythmia and use of QTc-prolonging agents: clues for clinicians. Heart Rhythm. 2005;2(2 Suppl):S1–S8.

28. American Psychiatric Association. Practice guideline for the treatment of patients with delirium. Am J Psychiatry. 1999;156(5 Suppl):1–20.

29. Sos J, Cassem NH. The intravenous use of haloperidol for acute delirium in intensive care settings. In: Speidel H, Rodewald G, editors. Psychic and neurological dysfunctions after open heart surgery. Stuttgart: Thieme; 1980.

30. Cook IA. Guideline watch: practice guideline for the treatment of patients with delirium. Arlington (VA): American Psychiatric Association; 2004. Available from: http://www.psych.org/psych_pract/treatg/pg/prac_guide.cfm.

31. Menza MA, Murray GB, Holmes VF, Rafuls WA. Decreased extrapyramidal symptoms with intravenous haloperidol. J Clin Psychiatry. 1987;48(7):278–80.

32. Tesar GE, Murray GB, Cassem NH. Use of high-dose intravenous haloperidol in the treatment of agitated cardiac patients. J Clin Psychopharmacol. 1985;5(6): 344–7.

33. Menza MA, Murray GB, Holmes VF, Rafuls WA. Controlled study of extrapyramidal reactions in the management of delirious, medically ill patients: intravenous haloperidol versus intravenous haloperidol plus benzodiazepines. Heart Lung. 1988;17(3): 238–41.

34. Adams F, Fernandez F, Andersson BS. Emergency pharmacotherapy of delirium in the critically ill cancer patient. Psychosomatics. 1986;27(1 Suppl):33–8.

35. Ray WA, Chung, CP, Murray KT, et al. Atypical antipsychotic drugs and the risk of sudden cardiac death. N Engl J Med. 2009;360(3):225–325.

36. Bourgeois JA, Koike AK, Simmons JE, et al. Adjunctive valproic acid for delirium and/or agitation on a consultation-liaison service: a report of six cases. J Neuropsychiatry Clin Neurosci. 2005;17(2):232–8.

37. Smith I, White PF, Nathanson M, Gouldson R. Propofol: an update on its clinical use. Anesthesiology. 1994;81(4): 1005–43.

38. Currier DS, Bevacqua BK. Acute tachyphylaxis to propofol sedation during ethanol withdrawal. J Clin Anesth. 1997;9(5):420–3.

39. Szumita PM, Baroletti SA, Anger KE, Wechsler ME. Sedation and analgesia in the intensive care unit: evaluating the role of dexmedetomidine. Am J Health Syst Pharm. 2007;64(1):37–44.

40. Inouye S. Delirium in older persons. N Engl J Med. 2006;354(11):1157–65.

Chapter 8

Management of somatoform disorders

Kathy Coffman

Typical consult question

"Please see this thirty-two year old male coroner with many baseless somatic complaints of chest pain, shortness of breath, back pain, and difficulty urinating without catheterization, who requires a bowel regimen for defecation and has bone pain in the joints of both legs."

Background

Medically unexplained symptoms (MUSs) have been estimated at about 10% (1). Estimates are that 27% of patients present to outpatient clinics with unexplained conditions (2). These conditions are seen frequently by the various medical specialties, including chronic fatigue syndrome, fibromyalgia, multiple chemical sensitivity, non-cardiac chest pain, and non-epileptiform seizures (NESs) (3, 4).

Recent proposals made to change classification of somatoform disorders include the following:

i. Relocating hypochondriasis, disease phobia, persistent somatization, conversion symptoms, illness denial, demoralization, and irritability to factors influencing medical illness in the *Diagnostic and Statistical Manual of Mental Disorders (DSM) V* (5).
ii. Placing hypochondriasis (renamed "health anxiety disorder") and body dysmorphic disorder with the anxiety disorders.
iii. Somatization disorder would be considered a combination of Axis II personality disorder and Axis I mood or anxiety disorder. Pain disorder and other somatic symptoms and syndromes would be placed under Axis III (6).
iv. Reclassifying hypochondriasis under anxiety disorders along a spectrum of obsessive-compulsive disorders (7).
v. Reclassifying conversion disorder as a dissociative disorder in *DSM V*, as in the International Statistical Classification of Diseases and Health-Related Problems, 10th revision (ICD-10). To support the re-classification, one group cites the high correlations between conversion symptoms and dissociative symptoms and shared features such as the role of trauma and similar underlying psychodynamics (8, 9).

Psychosomatic Medicine: An Introduction to Consultation-Liaison Psychiatry, eds. James J. Amos and Robert G. Robinson. Published by Cambridge University Press. © Cambridge University Press 2010.

Somatization disorder

Background

Some familial preponderance with somatization disorder has been found in 10% to 20% of first-degree female relatives (10). An increased incidence of alcohol abuse, antisocial personality disorder, and depression has been reported in first-degree male relatives (11).

Psychiatric co-morbidity includes 75% with Axis I diagnoses such as dysthymia, major depression, panic disorder, simple phobia, and substance abuse (12, 13). Women with somatization disorder have a higher likelihood of having a history of sexual abuse than those with primary mood disorders (14). Outcomes are unknown, but complete remission is thought to be rare.

Work-up

As defined by the *DSM IV*, somatization disorder requires onset of unexplained multi-system physical symptoms before age 30 years that last for several years and include two gastrointestinal symptoms, four pain symptoms, one pseudoneurological symptom, and one sexual symptom. Lifetime prevalence of this disorder is estimated at 0.2% to 2% in women, and less than 0.2% in men (15).

The differential diagnosis includes anxiety disorders, factitious disorder, malingering, mood disorders, multi-system medical disorders, schizophrenia with somatic delusions, and other somatoform disorders (16). Undifferentiated somatoform disorder is used when the cluster of symptoms do not meet the criteria for somatization disorder or another somatoform disorder. A majority of patients with somatoform disorder are diagnosed with somatoform disorder NOS or undifferentiated somatoform disorder.

Clinical decision-making and treatment

Cognitive-behavioral therapy (CBT) reduces disability, physical symptoms, and psychological distress for both somatoform disorders and medically unexplained physical symptoms (17). A consultation letter to the primary care physician has been shown to be effective, outlining the disorder, suggesting frequent office visits and conservative work-up only as indicated by physical findings, limiting medications, and addressing underlying factors affecting the symptoms (18). Although duloxetine has been touted in company publications as approaching significance for general somatic symptoms (19), and even though it has been marketed for depression with painful physical symptoms, a meta-analysis showed a very small statistically insignificant analgesic effect for duloxetine (20).

Conversion disorder

Background

Hysterical symptoms were first treated as religious phenomena (21). Sydenham noted that the symptoms followed strong emotion (22). By the 19th century, hysterical symptoms were thought to be caused and cured by psychosocial factors. Charcot's students differed on the mechanisms involved. Janet favored dissociation, whereas Freud viewed conversion as arising from repressed conflicts or fantasy expressed through somatic and behavioral symptoms with unconscious meanings (23). Although some may relegate conversion to history, a recent survey of 22 neurologists revealed that conversion was seen in up to 20% of patients in their clinical workload (24).

The prevalence of conversion disorder in the general population is around 0.3%, with a female predominance. Onset can range from ages 3 to 98 years. Prevalence of conversion disorder among inpatient neurological consultations in the United States is estimated at between 5% and 16%.

Confirming Charcot's idea that one day technology would find the "lesion" for conversion disorders, Kanaan et al. (25) used functional MRI with cued recall of a repressed event and found activation of brain regions associated with emotion, as well as decreased motor activity in the area matching the paralyzed limb.

Work-up

Caution is prudent in making this diagnosis as many organic disorders may present in a similar fashion to conversion disorders. Reportedly, 13% to 35% of patients with conversion disorder diagnoses are later found to have a medical diagnosis (26, 27).

Conversion symptoms are thought to occur at times of stress, are sensory-motor, provide secondary gain, are modeled on a significant other, and have symbolic meaning. With non-epileptic seizures (NESs), the nature of the movements, whether combative or sexual, may express anger or sexual conflict. Many patients with NESs may also have epileptic seizures. Prognosis is reportedly better with acute onset in the setting of major stressors, with short duration of symptoms, in patients with or without pre-morbid medical or psychiatric problems (28). Some syndromes such as amnesia, NES, and tremor (29) are thought to carry a poor prognosis.

Motor symptoms include aphonia, gait disturbance, globus hystericus, NESs, paralysis, tremor, and urinary retention. Sensory symptoms may include anesthesia, blindness, deafness, and paresthesias.

Clinical decision-making and treatment

Ruddy and House found only three randomized controlled studies comparing psychosocial interventions with standard care, all of poor methodologic quality (30).

Generally if symptoms are sensory-motor, physical therapy may provide a face-saving milieu to allow the patient to gradually relinquish the symptoms. Occasionally, the patient may recall the angry conflict that led to paralysis of a limb when the urge was to strike someone. With NESs, if movements are combative or sexual in nature, the patient or spouse may be aware of the underlying conflict, which then may be amenable to marital therapy.

Anniversary reactions may provide the underlying dynamic for some conversion symptoms. Many times the author has seen patients using identification as a defense who professed to have the symptoms of the deceased, usually within two weeks before the anniversary. For example, two patients presented with thrashing movements on the anniversary of having witnessed a drowning. These patients are not consciously aware of the connection between their symptoms and bereavement, and may not recall the anniversary unless questioned. Grief therapy exploring feelings towards the deceased and any remaining guilt or anger may relieve the symptoms within days to weeks. In Freud's day, sexuality was the big taboo, but in the present day, death is the major taboo in our society. However, the author has seen a case of globus hystericus wherein the patient was "choked up" about an impending divorce, and another in which the patient had been forced to perform fellatio. Both were amenable to supportive therapy once the underlying dynamic was revealed by inquiry about significant life events surrounding the onset of the symptom.

Hypochondriasis
Background
Hypochondriasis (HC) is the misinterpretation of benign symptoms resulting in preoccupation with having a serious disease, which does not respond to appropriate medical evaluation and reassurance, and disrupts family, occupation, and social functioning. Prevalence is 14% in primary care settings in the United States (31–33). The ratio of females to males is equal in HC. Onset is most often seen in early adulthood, but can be seen at any age (7). Stressful life events, such as diagnosis or death of a close friend or relative with a serious illness, or recuperation of the patient from an illness, may result in the appearance of symptoms (34). Co-morbidity includes major depressive disorder, dysthymic disorder, generalized anxiety disorder, and panic disorder (35, 36).

Work-up; clinical decision-making and treatment
Differential diagnosis includes generalized anxiety disorder, obsessive-compulsive disorder (OCD), and panic disorder. Cognitive-behavioral therapy approaches HC as the result of excessive anxiety resulting from learned sensitivity to normal bodily functioning, resulting in repeated checking behavior through doctor's visits in response to a perceived threat to one's health. Patients with HC disregard information suggesting good health in favor of body checking during times of stress, resulting in catastrophic rumination. A treatment approach suggested by Abramowitz and Braddock includes the following:

1) Medical evaluation with physical examination and review of records to rule out any medical condition contradicting the diagnosis of HC.
2) Functional assessment to collect patient-specific health-anxiety triggers and a list of safety behaviors used in response to the triggers. Ask what the patient considers to be evidence of serious illness, and why medical evidence fails to reduce health-related anxiety. A 0–10 scale can be used to rate symptom severity and the urge to perform safety behaviors.
3) Pharmacologic treatment for HC with antidepressants may be useful even in the absence of depression to decrease anxiety, dysfunctional beliefs, fear of disease, reassurance behavior, and somatic complaints.

    Medications that have been effective include clomipramine, fluoxetine, fluvoxamine, imipramine, paroxetine, and nefazodone.

    The author has successfully used desipramine in HC, along with exercise, relaxation tapes, and other behavioral methods, to encourage healthy behaviors and avoid reinforcing symptoms. Some patients with HC may become alarmed about side effects of the antidepressants, so may do better taking those with a low side effect profile, such as escitalopram. The rationale for use of these agents is to decrease anxiety about bodily symptoms.
4) Cognitive-behavioral therapy may help to educate patients about the pernicious cycle of negative perceptions of normal bodily sensations, which leads to health anxiety and use of maladaptive strategies to reduce anxiety, such as doctor shopping and repeated

testing, which carries risk of iatrogenic injury. Recognizing dysfunctional beliefs will help patients refrain from reassurance seeking and will remove barriers to correction of faulty beliefs (7).

Body dysmorphic disorder

Background

This disorder is defined as having a preoccupation with appearance because of a real or imagined defect in the body. A random sample national telephone survey in the United States indicated a point prevalence of body dysmorphic disorder (BDD) of 2.4% (2.5% in women, 2.2% in men) (37). In cosmetic surgery settings the prevalence is around 10%, and up to 20% is reported in those seeking rhinoplasty. These patients were more likely to attempt do-it-yourself surgery and believed that rhinoplasty would bring dramatic changes in their lives (39). However, in patients with BDD, surgery generally only leads to shifting of symptoms to another area (40).

Because onset generally occurs in adolescence, the differential diagnosis includes somatic delusions seen in schizophrenia. This condition may be chronic and may carry the risk of iatrogenic problems due to repeated surgical interventions (41).

Co-morbidity includes social phobia in 34.4%, which usually begins before BDD, and depression and substance abuse disorders that develop after onset of BDD (42, 43); eating disorders are seen in 32.5% (44) and OCD in 70% (45). Phillips et al. estimated a lifetime prevalence of major depression of 74.2% and a current diagnosis of major depression in 38.2% of patients with BDD (46).

The prevalence of BDD in patients with OCD was 15.3%, with worse depression and increased checking, hoarding, symmetry, and seeking reassurance. Patients with BDD have high rates of suicide ideation (19%) and high rates of suicide attempts related to concerns about appearance (7%). About half of patients with BDD were delusional, but the clinical features and course were similar (47, 48). Attempted suicide in patients with BDD was associated with childhood abuse and neglect, as well as high lifetime rates of substance abuse (49).

Work-up

Diagnosis is often delayed because of reluctance to disclose these symptoms to a physician. Prevalence in an inpatient psychiatric setting was 13% but the condition was not diagnosed, as patients would not mention symptoms unless specifically asked, because of shame (50).

Patients with BDD may engage in compulsive behaviors, including camouflaging, checking behavior, do-it-yourself surgeries, excessive use of make-up, mirror gazing, pathological skin picking, measuring body parts, repetitive questioning of others to seek reassurance about their appearance, tanning, and trichotillomania (45, 48, 51).

Clinical decision-making and treatment

Treatment has not been well studied. However, patients with BDD are thought to be fearful of negative appraisals from others, because of a bias for misinterpreting facial expressions as negative, which may lead to ideas of reference and thinking that others pay special attention to their "defect" (52). In one case study, a combination of exposure and response prevention of

BDD-associated rituals plus doxepin 125 mg daily was effective (53). Cognitive restructuring and graded social exposure with recording a log of verbal responses of others to greetings, plus escitalopram, were effective in reducing BDD symptoms in another case. The expectation of rejection was refuted by the responses of others in public settings (54).

Two randomized controlled pharmacotherapy trials (RCTs) suggested that fluoxetine and clomipramine were superior to placebo. Three RCT psychotherapy trials indicated a reduction in symptom severity, and a low relapse rate (4/22) was seen in another trial (55). Some have reported poor responses to treatment (25% favorable response), but others have stated that patients with BDD may require higher doses of selective serotonin reuptake inhibitors (SSRIs) and longer trials than in major depressive disorder (45, 56).

Pain disorder

Background

Pain disorder consists of pain symptoms in excess of the medical findings. A recent study of 4181 participants in a community sample in Germany showed a 12-month prevalence of *DSM IV* pain disorder of 8.1%, with the majority having co-morbid anxiety and mood disorders. Most had more than one type of pain, with headache the most commonly reported type of pain (57).

Higher rates of alcohol dependence, chronic pain, and depressive disorder have been reported in first-degree relatives of patients with pain disorder versus the general population (15). Psychiatric co-morbidity in patients with pain disorder includes benzodiazepine and opioid dependence, as well as depression in 8% to 80% (58). Outcomes are poor in those on compensation, with long duration of untreated pain, and in patients who are unemployed or involved in litigation, and with somatization (59).

Rubin (60) has noted that 40% to 60% of women and 20% of men with chronic pain disorders have a history of emotional, physical, or sexual abuse in childhood or adulthood, a two to four times higher incidence than the general population, associated with chronic pelvic pain, facial pain, fibromyalgia, and other pain disorders. For women, more perpetrators correlated with more somatic symptoms.

Work-up; clinical decision-making and treatment

An approach outlined for diagnosis and treatment included (1) inquiring about current or past history of abuse, (2) using an empathic approach with validation of suffering, (3) recognizing dysfunctional pain behaviors, (4) documenting anatomic and non-anatomic pain features found on examination, (5) using a multi-disciplinary approach with psychotherapy when indicated, and (6) avoiding invasive procedures and addictive medications such as benzodiazepines and opioids when possible (60).

References

1. Ford CV. The somatizing disorders. Psychosomatics. 1986;27:327–31, 335–7.

2. Reid S, Wessely S, Crayford T, et al. Medically unexplained symptoms in frequent attenders of secondary health care: retrospective cohort study. Br Med J. 2001;322:767.

3. Bailer J, Witthoft M, Paul C, et al. Evidence for overlap between idiopathic environmental intolerance and somatoform disorders. Psychosom Med. 2005;67:921–9.

4. Richardson RD, Engel CC Jr. Evaluation and management of medically unexplained physical symptoms. Neurologist. 2004;10: 18–30.

5. Fava GA, Fabbri S, Sirri L, et al. Psychological factors affecting medical condition: a new proposal for DSM-V. Psychosomatics. 2007;48:103–11.

6. Mayou R, Kirmayer LJ, Simon G, et al. Somatoform disorders: time for a new approach in DSM-V. Am J Psychiatry. 2005;162:847–55.

7. Abramowitz JS, Braddock AE. Hypochondriasis: conceptualization, treatment, and relationship to obsessive-compulsive disorder. Psychiatr Clin North Am. 2006;29:503–19.

8. Brown RJ, Cardena E, Nijenhuis E, et al. Should conversion disorder be reclassified as a dissociative disorder in DSM-V? Psychosomatics. 2007;48:369–78.

9. Espirito-Santo H, Pio-Abreu JL. Psychiatric symptoms and dissociation in conversion, somatization and dissociative disorders. Aust N Z J Psychiatry. 2009;43:270–6.

10. American Psychiatric Association. Diagnostic and statistical manual of mental disorders, DSM-IV-TR. Washington (DC): American Psychiatric Association; 2000.

11. Golding JM, Rost K, Kashner TM: Does somatization disorder occur in men? Clinical characteristics of women and men with multiple unexplained somatic symptoms. Arch Gen Psychiatry. 1991;48: 231–5.

12. Katon W, Lin E, Von Korff M, et al: Somatization: a spectrum of severity. Am J Psychiatry. 1991;148:34–40.

13. Swartz M, Blazer D, George L, et al: Somatization disorder in a community population. Am J Psychiatry. 1986;143: 1403–8.

14. Morrison J. Childhood sexual histories of women with somatization disorder. Am J Psychiatry. 1989;146:239–41.

15. American Psychiatric Association. Diagnostic and statistical manual of mental disorder (DSM-IV). Washington (DC): American Psychiatric Association Press; 1994.

16. Abbey SE. Somatization and somatoform disorders. In: Rundell JR, Wise MG, editors. Essentials of consultation-liaison psychiatry. Washington (DC): American Press Association Press; 2005. p. 156–87.

17. Sumathipala A. What is the evidence for the efficacy of treatments for somatoform disorders? A critical review of previous intervention studies. Psychosom Med. 2007;69:889–900.

18. Kroenke K. Efficacy of treatment for somatoform disorders: a review of randomized controlled trial. Psychosom Med. 2007;69:881–8.

19. Mallinckrodt CH, Prakash A, Houston JP, et al. Differential antidepressant symptom efficacy: placebo-controlled comparisons of duloxetine and SSRIs (fluoxetine, paroxetine, escitalopram). Neuropsycho-biology. 2007;56:73–85.

20. Spielmans GI. Duloxetine does not relieve painful physical symptoms in depression: a meta-analysis. Psychother Psychosom. 2008;77:12–6.

21. Micale MS. Approaching hysteria: disease and its interpretations. Princeton (NJ), Chichester: Princeton University Press; 1995.

22. Veith I. Hysteria: the history of a disease. 1st soft cover ed. Northvale (NJ): Jason Aronson; 1993.

23. Erreich A. The anatomy of a symptom: concept development and symptoms formation in a four-year-old boy. J Am Psychoanal Assoc. 2007;55: 899–922.

24. Kanaan R, Armstrong D, Barnes P, et al. In the psychiatrist's chair: how neurologists understand conversion disorder. Brain Advance Access. March 24, 2009. Brain. Brain Advance Access. Published on April 16, 2009. DOI: 10.1093/brain/awp060.

25. Kanaan RA, Craig TK, Wessely SC, David AS. Imaging repressed memories in motor conversion disorder. Psychosom Med. 2007;69:202–5.

26. Slater E, Glithero E: A follow-up of patients diagnosed of suffering from "hysteria." J Psychosom Res. 1965;9:9–14.

27. Stefansson JG, Messina JA, Meyerowitz S: Hysterical neurosis, conversion type: clinical and epidemiological considerations. Acta Psychiatr Scand. 1976;53: 119–38.

28. Lazare A. Current concepts in psychiatry: conversion symptoms. N Engl J Med. 1981; 305:745–8.

29. Toone BK. Disorders of hysterical conversion. In: Oxford BC, editor. Somatization: physical symptoms and psychological illness. Oxford (UK): Blackwell Scientific; 1990. p. 207–34.

30. Ruddy R, House A. Psychosocial interventions for conversion disorder. Cochrane Database Syst Rev. 2005 Oct 19;(4):CD005331.

31. Bearber RJ, Rodney WM. Underdiagnosis of hypochondriasis in family practice. Psychosomatics. 1984;25:39–46.

32. Kellner R. Functional somatic symptoms and hypochondriasis: a survey of empirical studies. Arch Gen Psychiatry. 1985;42: 821–33.

33. Barsky AJ, Wyshak G, Lerman GI, et al. The prevalence of hypochondriasis in medical outpatients. Soc Psychiatry Psychiatr Epidemiol. 1990;25:89–94.

34. Barsky AJ, Klerman GL. Overview: hypochondriasis, bodily complaints, and somatic styles. Am J Psychiatry. 1983;140: 273–83.

35. Hiller W, Leibbrand R, Rief W, et al. Differentiation hypochondriasis from panic disorder. J Anxiety Disord. 2005;19:29–49.

36. Barsky AJ, Fama JM, Bailey E, et al. A prospective 4- to 5-year study of DSM-III-R hypochondriasis. Arch Gen Psychiatry. 1998;55:737–44.

37. Koran LM, Abujaoude E, Large MD, et al. The prevalence of body dysmorphic disorder in the United States adult population. CNS Spectr. 2008;13: 316–22.

38. Pavan C, Simonato P, Marini M, et al. Psychopathologic aspects of body dysmorphic disorder: a literature review. Aesthet Plast Surg. 2008;32:473–84.

39. Veale D, De Haro L, Lambrou C. Cosmetic rhinoplasty in body dysmorphic disorder. Br J Plast Surg. 2003;56:546–51.

40. Mehler-Wex C, Warnke A. Dysmorphophobia. MMW Fortschr Med. 2006;148: 37–9.

41. Phillips KA, McElroy SL, Keck PE, et al. Body dysmorphic disorder: 30 cases of imagined ugliness. Am J Psychiatry. 1993; 150:302–8.

42. Coles ME, Phillips KA, Menard W, et al. Body dysmorphic disorder and social phobia: cross-sectional and prospective data. Depress Anxiety. 2006;23:26–33.

43. Gunstad J, Phillips KA. Axis I comorbidity in body dysmorphic disorder. Compr Psychiatry. 2003;44:270–6.

44. Ruffolo JS, Phillips KA, Menard W, et al. Comorbidity of body dysmorphic disorder and eating disorders: severity of psychopathology and body image disturbance. Int J Eat Disod. 2006;39:11–9.

45. Fontenelle LF, Telles LL, Nazar BP, et al. A sociodemographic, phenomenological, and long- term follow-up study of patients with body dysmorphic disorder in Brazil. Int J Psychiatry Med. 2006;36: 243–59.

46. Phillips KA, Didie ER, Menard W. Clinical features and correlates of major depressive disorder in individuals with body dysmorphic disorder. Affect Disord. 2007;97:129–35. Epub 2006 Aug 7.

47. Rief W, Buhlmann U, Wilhelm S, et al. The prevalence of body dysmorphic disorder: a population-based survey. Psychol Med. 2006;36:877–85.

48. Phillips KA, Conroy M, Dufresne RG, et al. Tanning in body dysmorphic disorder. Psychiatr Q. 2006;77:129–38.

49. Didie ER, Tortolani CC, Pope CG, et al. Childhood abuse and neglect in body dysmorphic disorder. Child Abuse Negl. 2006;30:1105–15. Epub 2006 Sep 26.

50. Grant JE, Kim SW, Crow SJ. Prevalence and clinical features of body dysmorphic disorder in adolescent and adult psychiatric inpatients. J Clin Psychiatry. 2001;62:517–22.

51. Grant JE, Menard W, Phillips KA. Pathological skin picking in individuals with body dysmorphic disorder. Gen Hosp Psychiatry. 2006;28:487–93.

52. Buhlmann U, Etcoff NL, Wilhelm S. Emotion recognition for contempt and anger in body dysmorphic disorder. J Psychiatr Res. 2006;40:105–11.

53. Sobanski E, Schmidt MH. 'Everybody looks at my pubic bone' – a case report of an adolescent patient with body dysmorphic disorder. Acta Psychiatr Scand. 2000;101:80–2.

54. Coffman KL. Treatment of a case of body dysmorphic disorder, unpublished.

55. Ipser JC, Sander C, Stein DJ. Pharmacotherapy and psychotherapy for body dysmorphic disorder. Cochrane Database Syst Rev. 2009; (1):CD005332.

56. Grant JE, Phillips KA. Recognizing and treating body dysmorphic disorder. Ann Clin Psychiatry. 2005;17:205–10.

57. Frohlich C, Jacobi F, Wittchen HU. DSM-IV pain disorder in the general population: an exploration of the structure and threshold of medically unexplained symptoms. Eur Arch Psychiatry Clin Neurosci. 2006;256: 187–96.

58. Smith GR. The epidemiology and treatment of depression when it coexists with somatoform disorders, somatization, or pain. Gen Hosp Psychiatry. 1992;14: 265–72.

59. Tyrer S. Psychiatric assessment of chronic pain. Br J Psychiatry. 1992;160:733–41.

60. Rubin JJ. Psychosomatic pain: new insights and management strategies. South Med J. 2005;98:1099–110.

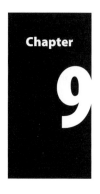

Managing factitious disorder and malingering

James J. Amos

Typical consult question

"Please transfer to psych this patient, who has no real physical disorder and who may be malingering."

The history of one of the first reported patients diagnosed with Munchausen's syndrome, a man known as The Indiana Cyclone, was recorded in a very long poem by William H. Bean, M.D., entitled "The Munchausen Saga":

The Munchausen Saga

> *In the summer of nineteen and fifty-four*
> *At Iowa City, to our hospital door –*
> *Mecca for hundreds every day –*
> *A merchant seaman found his way,*
> *A part-time wrestler, in denim jacket,*
> *He crashed through the door with a horrible racket,*
> *Two hundred and sixty pounds at least,*
> *And covered with blood like a wounded beast…* (1)

It goes on for many pages about his colorful stories, many of which were not true, and his astonishing ability to feign impressive bouts of bleeding that were medically unexplained. His motives for producing medical symptoms and signs, including external incentives for financial gain from insurance fraud, were obviously mixed. He also underwent excruciatingly painful procedures which malingerers usually avoid (2). Important clinical and conceptual differences between factitious disorder and malingering have been noted. However, the boundary between them tends to blur because of the difficulty clinicians have in determining intentions and incentives that are driving these abnormal illness behaviors.

Background

Factitious disorder was first described most compellingly by Asher in his article, "Munchausen's Syndrome" (3). He described patients who faked medical illnesses. He also told tall tales in a manner ascribed falsely to the eighteenth century German raconteur Baron von Münchausen. Asher gave colorful, Latinized names to some of the patients, including *hemorrhagica histrionica*, *laparotomophilia migrans*, and *neurologica diabolica*. Chapman, who

Psychosomatic Medicine: An Introduction to Consultation-Liaison Psychiatry, eds. James J. Amos and Robert G. Robinson. Published by Cambridge University Press. © Cambridge University Press 2010.

wrote the case report on The Indiana Cyclone, thought these were whimsical appellations that Asher coined with tongue in cheek. The gist of the definition of this disorder is that patients lie about medical or psychiatric symptoms to healthcare providers to adopt the sick role, presumably because they crave attention, especially from doctors. It is distinguished from malingering by not defining malingering as a disorder and by identifying external incentives as the major reason to fake medical or psychiatric illness (e.g., escaping penalties or obligations such as incarceration or military service, obtaining entitlements). The *Diagnostic and Statistical Manual of Mental Disorders (DSM)-IV-TR* criteria for factitious disorder follow:

A. Intentional production or feigning of physical/psychological signs/symptoms
B. Motivation for the behavior is to assume the patient role.
C. External incentives for the behavior (such as economic gain, avoiding legal responsibility, or improving physical well-being, as in malingering) are absent (4).

The *DSM-IV-TR* classifies malingering as "V" code, meaning "Other conditions that may be the focus of clinical attention" – but it's not considered a mental disorder. It is defined as "the intentional production of false or grossly exaggerated physical or psychological symptoms motivated by external incentives" (4).

The place of factitious disorder in *DSM-V* is being debated, as are all of the somatoform disorders themselves. Factitious disorder, in the opinion of some experts, is more about lying than about somatizing (5). Turner's proposal to emphasize pseudologia fantastica or pathological lying as the major feature was based on the idea that it is central to the disorder. Although no epidemiologic data on the phenomenon of pseudologia fantastica are available, the general characteristics are as follows:

1. The fluent answering of questions with elaborate falsehoods, often casting the teller in the role of victim and/or hero, who often looks as though she/he believes the tale
2. The story often contains a kernel of truth.
3. Imaginary adventures manifest in a variety of circumstances and are durable.
4. Evokes a complex subjective response from the listener (e.g., intriguing) (6)

Others believe that it should be a subtype of somatoform disorders, conceptualized and perhaps managed in similar ways (e.g., "somatoform disorder with factitious behavior") (7). Bass and Halligan carry the underlying criticism of the primacy of deception as a defining feature even further, claiming that the disorder is "conceptually flawed, diagnostically impractical and clinically unhelpful and should be dropped from existing nosologies" (8).

Despite the preference of some experts who prefer that the categories of factitious disorder and malingering be mutually exclusive, evidence indicates that both behavior patterns can coexist, just as they appeared to in the case of The Indiana Cyclone (9).

The conceptualization of the disorder has been complexified by the false report of a case of alleged "Factitious Munchausen's Syndrome." The authors, Gurwith and Langston, reported seeing a patient in the emergency room who claimed to have Munchausen's syndrome and demanded to be admitted for treatment of the disorder itself. He was described as confessing to having undergone many unnecessary surgeries resulting in gridiron abdomen – which washed off with soap and water. The authors later confessed to the fiction, which Marc Feldman, a published expert on the disorder, suggested should be retitled "Fictitious Factitious Munchausen's Syndrome" (10, 11). The tipoff that it was a hoax was within the article itself. The name of the patient was revealed as "Norman U. Senchbau," an anagram of Baron Munchausen. However, the paper was cited by other authors in apparent belief of its authenticity.

One author proposed that it was an elaborate and clever joke that played on the paradoxes inherent in the disorder:

"…Clearly, Gurwith and Langston intend the word factitious to signify in two opposite directions. In the first sense, factitious describes the patient's false enactment of a known malady. His symptoms would be true enough if he was suffering from a real disorder but, given that the patient is faking, the symptoms are considered merely made up. In this sense, factitious signifies that the disorder is not real: none of the symptoms that the patient described are thus true indicators of Munchausen syndrome. Instead of producing the symptoms and signs of an affliction such as epilepsy or AIDS, as is usually the case, the patient simulated the syndrome itself. By choosing to imitate Munchausen syndrome, the patient cannily provided the sign that indicates authentic Munchausen syndrome. Epilepsy can't be faked with tales of seizures; AIDS can't be imitated with handwritten notes about low t-cell counts. Unlike patients simulating physical afflictions, a patient can simulate the psychiatric disorder of Munchausen syndrome by telling tall tales, for, when they are revealed to be factitious, those symptomatic tall tales themselves signify as pseudologica fantastica, as real signs of Munchausen syndrome. Paradoxically, by choosing to fake Munchausen syndrome, the patient proves that he or she suffers from it. As a result, the term factitious, which initially signifies that the patient does not really suffer from Munchausen syndrome, now signifies that the patient really does" (12).

The epidemiology of both factitious disorder and malingering with respect to estimating prevalence is hindered by the obvious problems with ascertainment. One of the more recent estimates of the frequency of factitious disorder hovers around 1% (13). It may be more frequent on psychiatric inpatient units than was hitherto suspected. One case series report put the prevalence at about 6% of 100 admissions, with overdose being one of the initial reasons for some admissions and with more than half of those with physical illness having multiple psychiatric diagnoses as well (14).

Estimates of the frequency of malingering are less certain, although specific complaints, such as mild head injury followed by fibromyalgia or chronic pain syndrome, pain, neurotoxic disorders, electrical injury, seizure disorders, and moderated or severe head injury, are thought to be more likely to be malingered (9). Malingered mental illness is believed to occur more often in the context of criminal charges, but in medical illness the incentive may be primarily financial gain.

The cause of factitious disorder is a matter of speculation. Risk factors are thought to include histories of child abuse, childhood hospitalizations that may have been attempts to escape abusive and chaotic families and households, and parental rejection or over-reaction to illness. Dynamic themes may include masochism, counterphobia, mastery and control, and attempts to establish relationships (15). A disturbed sense of self and of reality has been hypothesized as well (16). It is often co-morbid with antisocial and borderline personality disorders. A diathesis-stress model follows (17):

1. Early trauma creating psychological vulnerability (e.g., unbearable stress with the need to escape)
2. Leads to reporting of physical symptoms; support from hospitals which reinforces the behavior
3. Subsequent stressors dealt with similarly

Patients with factitious disorder can self-induce illness in ways that result in severe disfigurement or death, often from unnecessary medical interventions. And they have successfully sued physicians who unwittingly caused iatrogenic harm for failing to recognize their disorder – despite denying the true nature of their feigned illnesses in the first place early on. The cost of their excessive health utilization has been estimated to run in the millions of dollars. Their subterfuge can also result in the physician's ignoring genuine disease.

Work-up

Presentations of factitious disorder and its most severe variant, often called Munchausen's syndrome, can range from completely fabricating a medical (or psychiatric) illness, to aggravating or exaggerating symptoms, to simulating an illness, such as by mimicking a generalized seizure episode or by inducing one (e.g., injecting a wound with fecal bacteria). Often patients take flight by leaving the hospital against medical advice when their impostorship is uncovered. Factitious psychiatric disorders are often co-morbid with factitious medical disorders. The prognosis of the faked mental disorders is viewed not infrequently to be worse than that of the genuine disorder. Polysymptomatic psychiatric disorders and multiple syndromes with inconsistent presentations are not uncommon. General features include the following:

- Non-response to usually effective treatment
- Massive medical care histories
- Accurate forecast of waxing/waning disease
- Lack of appropriate worry in families
- Aliases and impostorship
- Pseudologia fantastica

The clinical course often is marked by the following:

- Usually chronic, although remissions occur
- Morbidity high
- Mortality data lacking, but deaths occur as the result of disease simulation/suicide

The clinician should maintain a high degree of suspicion in the face of long and complex histories, histrionic symptom presentations, and an uncanny ability to predict when the course of a disease will wax or wane.

Clues to malingering include claiming to have a large number of drug allergies when pursuing drugs. Patients also may insist on a specific drug, such as Demerol. Malingers may feign an acute problem to avoid an immediate predicament, or may feign a subacute problem when seeking permanent disability.

No objective laboratory tests can confirm malingering. Detecting malingered pain is extremely difficult because the experience is subjective. The role of neuropsychology is important in establishing malingering with greater certainty than simple clinical suspicion. The Minnesota Multi-Phasic Personality Inventory, 2nd edition (MMPI-2), can be helpful for identifying malingered mental illness, although it is less useful in evaluating malingered medical illness. The Test of Malingered Memory (TOMM) can show prolonged reaction times on correct responses in simulators. In one study, the Modified Somatic Perception Questionnaire distinguished malingerers from non-malingerers with a sensitivity and specificity of 0.90 (9). Attempts to evaluate facial expressions and physical examination findings are less reliable. The hallmark of malingering has been said to be "the inconsistency between reported symptoms and collateral reports, observed behaviors, and physical and psychological assessments" (9).

Clinical decision-making and treatment

Most authors do not discuss treatment for malingering because it is not considered a mental illness. However, some authors emphasize the importance of letting the malingerer save face while giving up the sick role. Recovery, not confession, is often the most realistic goal. It's important to recognize the treatable and treatment-refractory disorders that contribute to the self-perceived need to malinger. Treatment of underlying depression, anxiety, and personality disorders, specifically antisocial personality disorder (ASPD), is appropriate, although many would regard ASPD as one of the refractory disorders.

No evidence-based literature talks about factitious disorder in terms of controlled trials from 1998 to 2005, although about 1900 papers have been published from 1985 to the present: two meta-analyses, eight reviews, and case reports. A few comments on the reviews follow (18):

- Early detection will likely prevent future chronic illness.
- Therapeutic approach is emphasized with psychiatrist and primary care physician collaborating, the latter adopting a conservative medical management approach.
- The development of a therapeutic alliance is essential for treatment.
- Demographics show overwhelmingly that patients tend to be young, educated, white female healthcare workers.

The consultant will do well to consult early with the hospital attorney to develop a plan for risk management regarding any patient suspected of factitious disorder or malingering, given the propensity to litigate that often is attributed to patients in both categories.

Whether to confront or not to confront the patient with factitious disorder is a matter of some debate, with proponents in support of both depending on the situation. Patients who are in serious danger of accidental death or severe bodily injury often may need transfer to a locked medical-psychiatry unit (MPU), if one is available. One may have to confront the patient who is infecting a wound or poisoning himself, and who may refuse rescue from his own dangerous behavior. In many jurisdictions, it is impossible to certify a patient to a judge or a judicial magistrate to obtain a court order to involuntarily hospitalize him, unless one tells the patient why this is being done.

If an MPU is not available or if the patient's self-harm behavior does not put him at risk for imminent danger, then non-confrontational methods are preferred. One of these might be the therapeutic double-bind. Rather than telling the patient that one believes he is harming himself and lying about it, one poses a dilemma that is ironically a form of deception about what one really suspects. In the case of a feigned medical problem, one tells the patient that either a medical problem or a psychiatric problem exists – it's just not clear which. If the problem is medical, then the next proposed conservative, safe, noninvasive treatment will result in complete and sustained resolution of the problem. If the problem continues, then a psychiatric disorder is the explanation for lack of resolution.

In some cases, the double-bind produces what the name of the technique implies. The patient must choose either to identify himself as a psychiatric patient (which is often the last thing he wants) or to give up the abnormal illness behavior. It's simply not clear how often this strategy is employed and how successful it is. The intervention is based on strategic-behavioral treatment guided by a specific script and presented to patients with chronic non-organic motor disorders, as described by Shapiro and Teasell (19):

1. The core element involves telling the patient that full recovery is proof of a physical cause, while failure to recover provides conclusive evidence of a psychiatric cause.
2. Slower than expected recovery is due to only one of two factors: either the disorder is not physical but is a psychiatric problem, or a modification to the treatment is needed, and once that is made, rapid and complete recovery would ensue – if the problem is physical. If the modification is made and recovery is still incomplete, then the problem is psychiatric.
3. Incomplete recovery includes resumption of symptoms after discharge, retention of some symptoms, development of new symptoms despite resolution of others for which there's no organic basis, or request for discharge before full resolution of symptoms.
4. Full recovery would be possible with long-term psychiatric treatment.
5. A key factor is presentation of this script to family and other support persons in a family conference (scheduled just before discharge if symptoms have resolved, or earlier if insufficient improvement occurred). This is designed to overcome resistance and prevent relapse. The physician emphasizes that even when patients recover fully, there's always a small chance that the problem was psychiatric. Accordingly, the only way to know for certain that the problem was not psychiatric is to see whether the patient remains asymptomatic after discharge. If old symptoms re-emerge or new non-organic symptoms appear, the patient and his family are advised to seek psychiatric treatment.

Shapiro and Teasell reported a 71% improvement rate in the small case series upon which the above protocol is based. However, unless one can lie and do it well, one is probably better off avoiding the double-bind, except in extreme cases when no other alternative is available. That said, the literature otherwise does not contain much guidance about treatment, although case reports that claim success can be found. No robust research has been done to determine effectiveness of any management technique for factitious disorder, whether confrontational or non-confrontational. According to a recent review, most are not engaged in treatment and are lost to follow-up (20). There is little to recommend drug treatment for the behavior itself, although if the patient suffers from mood, anxiety, or psychotic disorders, the indicated pharmacotherapy should be applied. Psychotherapy is the treatment of choice, although the patient is often difficult to engage.

One can be sure that the conclusion of the above mentioned review will not prevent medical and surgical colleagues from calling psychiatric consultants for help when faced with what looks like factitious behavior. Hamilton and Feldman propose three new working assumptions about factitious disorder (21):

1. Factitious disorder is neither rare nor is it always severe.
2. Factitious disorder is not categorically distinct from somatoform disorders.
3. Factitious disorder develops gradually.

What can develop from re-framing like this is the deployment of cognitive-behavioral therapy and contingency management strategies (such as regular follow-up regardless of the existence of an active medical complaint). Encouraging early consultation when factitious disorder is suspected can reduce the number of unnecessary medical interventions that carry risk for iatrogenic harm. Pediatricians and primary care physicians can try to prevent chronic patterns of illness behavior from developing by educating families about the importance of minimizing sick role behavior and by encouraging growth-promoting activities at home, school, and work.

A key role for psychiatric consultants is to facilitate the consulting physicians' decision-making about when enough medical evaluation has been done, so as to avoid iatrogenic harm. It's also important to help them recognize and prevent the strong emotional reactions that such patients engender and which can split the care team into opposing camps.

References

1. Bean WB. The Munchausen syndrome. Perspect Biol Med. 1959;2(3):347–53.

2. Chapman JS. Peregrinating problem patients: Munchausen's syndrome. JAMA. 1957;165(8):927–33.

3. Asher R. Munchausen's syndrome. Lancet. 1951;1(6650):339–41.

4. American Psychiatric Association, American Psychiatric Association Task Force on DSM-IV. Diagnostic and statistical manual of mental disorders: DSM-IV-TR. Washington (DC): American Psychiatric Association; 2000.

5. Turner MA. Factitious disorders: reformulating the DSM-IV criteria. Psychosomatics. 2006;47(1):23–32.

6. Newmark N, Adityanjee, Kay J. Pseudologia fantastica and factitious disorder: review of the literature and a case report. Compr Psychiatry. 1999;40(2): 89–95.

7. Krahn LE, Bostwick JM, Stonnington CM. Looking toward DSM-V: should factitious disorder become a subtype of somatoform disorder? Psychosomatics. 2008;49(4): 277–82.

8. Bass C, Halligan PW. Illness related deception: social or psychiatric problem? J R Soc Med. 2007;100(2):81–4.

9. McDermott BE, Feldman MD. Malingering in the medical setting. Psychiatr Clin North Am. 2007;30(4):645–62.

10. Feldman MD. Factitious Munchausen's syndrome – a confession. N Engl J Med. 1992;327(6):438–9.

11. Gurwith M, Langston C. Factitious Munchausen's syndrome. N Engl J Med. 1980;302(26):1483–4.

12. Amirault C. Pseudologica fantastica and other tall tales: the contagious literature of Munchausen syndrome. Lit Med. 1995; 14(2):169–90.

13. Fliege H, Grimm A, Eckhardt-Henn A, et al. Frequency of ICD-10 factitious disorder: survey of senior hospital consultants and physicians in private practice. Psychosomatics. 2007;48(1): 60–4.

14. Gregory RJ, Jindal S. Factitious disorder on an inpatient psychiatry ward. Am J Orthopsychiatry. 2006;76(1):31–6.

15. Klonoff EA, et al. Chronic factitious illness: a behavioral approach. Int J Psychiatry Med. 1983;13(3):173–83.

16. Spivak H, Rodin G, Sutherland A. The psychology of factitious disorders: a reconsideration. Psychosomatics. 1994;35(1):25–34.

17. Feldman MD, Eisendrath SJ. The spectrum of factitious disorders. 1st ed. Washington (DC): American Psychiatric Press; 1996.

18. Straker D, Hyler S. Factitious disorders. In: Blumenfield MJ, Strain JJ, editors. Psychosomatic medicine. New York: Lippincott Williams & Wilkins; 2006. p. 571–8.

19. Shapiro AP, Teasell RW. Behavioural interventions in the rehabilitation of acute v. chronic non-organic (conversion/ factitious) motor disorders. Br J Psychiatry. 2004;185(2):140–6.

20. Eastwood MR, Rifat SL, Nobbs H, et al. Mood disorder following cerebrovascular accident. Br J Psychiatry. 1989;154: 195–200.

21. Hamilton JC, Feldman MD. Factitious disorder and malingering. In: Gabbard GO, editor. Gabbard's treatments of psychiatric disorders. Washington (DC): American Psychiatric Publishing, Inc; 2007. p. 629–35.

10

Agitation in patients with dementia

Debra R. Kahn, Raheel A. Khan, and James A. Bourgeois

Typical consult question

"A seventy-two year old man with a history of Parkinson's disease is admitted to the hospital for placement because his family 'can't handle him anymore.' The patient has been paranoid and frequently refuses medications. Please help us with management."

Background

Dementia is an increasingly frequent and costly disease of our aging population. An estimated 5% to 15% of the U.S. population over the age of 65 has dementia. Worldwide estimates are 25 million with an expected doubling by 2020 (1, 2). Neuropsychiatric symptoms occur in more than 80% of those with Alzheimer's disease (AD) (1, 3). Symptoms may include mood disorders, sleep disturbance, irritability, aggression, psychosis, and agitation. Behavioral and mood disturbances in patients with dementia are associated with patient and caregiver distress, greater impairment in activities of daily living (ADLs), decreased cognition, increased care costs, and nursing home placement (2, 4).

Among the most troubling neuropsychiatric symptoms is agitation, found in 40% to 60% of nursing home patients with AD (1, 5). Similar rates of agitation and psychosis have been found in patients with vascular dementia (1, 6, 7). Cohen-Mansfield (2001) delineated several categories of "inappropriate behavior" associated with dementia, summarized as follows (8):

1. Physically aggressive behaviors (e.g., hitting, kicking, biting)
2. Motoric restlessness that is not aggressive (e.g., pacing, repetitive mannerisms)
3. Verbalizations (e.g., perseverations, cursing, screaming)

Agitation in patients with dementia may present acutely, follow a "waxing and waning" course, or develop slowly over months to years. Patients may experience a pattern of nightly increases in confusion and agitation, referred to as "sundowning." Demented patients also may become agitated when they are unable to verbalize physical discomfort, or when they become medically ill.

Examples of causes of dementia can be seen in Table 10.1. Dementias are also frequently described in terms of patterns of deficits (cortical, subcortical, or mixed) (Table 10.2). Identifying a specific cause of dementia can help clinicians predict the course of illness and the pattern of neuropsychiatric symptoms. Accurate diagnosis is also essential for selecting the

Psychosomatic Medicine: An Introduction to Consultation-Liaison Psychiatry, eds. James J. Amos and Robert G. Robinson. Published by Cambridge University Press. © Cambridge University Press 2010.

89

Table 10.1 Causes of dementia

Degenerative	Infectious
Cortical	HIV
Alzheimer's disease	CJD
Dementia with Lewy Bodies	Syphilis
Fronto-temporal dementia	PML
Subcortical	**Metabolic**
Parkinson's disease	Vitamin deficiencies (e.g., thiamine)
Huntington's disease	Anoxia/hypoxia
Wilson's disease	Recurrent hypoglycemia
	Porphyrias
Vascular	**Traumatic/structural**
Binswanger's disease	Subdural hematoma
Post-CVA dementia	Subarachnoid hemorrhage
	Normal pressure hydrocephalus
	Traumatic brain injury
Inflammatory	**Other**
Systemic lupus erythematosus	Multiple sclerosis

Adapted from Lobo A, Saz P. Dementia. In: Levenson JL, eds: Textbook of Psychosomatic Medicine. Arlington, VA; APPI: 2005:131–169.
Key:
CJD = Creutzfeldt-Jakob disease
CVA = cerebrovascular disease
HIV = human immunodeficiency virus
PML = progressive multifocal leukoencephalopathy

Table 10.2 Cortical vs. subcortical dementia

Cortical	Subcortical
Agnosia	Abnormalities of movement (extrapyramidal symptoms/gait changes)
Aphasia	Apathy
Apraxia	Bradyphrenia
Executive dysfunction	Early personality changes
Memory impairment that is not helped by cues	Memory impairment that is responsive to cues

safest and most effective treatments for dementia and its associated neuropsychiatric symptoms. The following paragraphs outline several of the most common types of dementia and their associated symptoms.

Cortical dementias

Alzheimer's disease

Alzheimer's disease (AD) is the most common type of dementia in Western cultures, representing 55% to 75% of all cases (9). Symptoms typically begin after age 65, and median time between diagnosis and death varies from 3.4 to 8.3 years, depending on age at diagnosis (9, 10). AD is associated with a relentless progression of symptoms and impairment of ADLs. Early findings include mild impairments in recent memory, language, and planning. Mood and personality changes may also occur. Disturbances in middle stages may include psychosis, aggression, gait impairment, and frontal release signs. End stages are associated with severe impairment in all activities, incontinence, mutism, and lack of responsiveness to the environment (9).

Fronto-temporal dementia

Fronto-temporal dementia (FTD) is marked by an insidious onset of personality changes, mood disorders, and impulsivity, which frequently cause disability before memory impairment is observed. Mild deficiencies in social conduct or grossly inappropriate behavior, such as violence and sexual disinhibition, may result in social isolation.

Dementia with Lewy bodies

Findings of Dementia with Lewy bodies (DLB) may include the early onset of psychotic symptoms, motor symptoms characteristic of Parkinson's disease (PD), and fluctuations in cognition/mental status. Visual hallucinations and delusions are very common in DLB, occurring in 60% to 70% of patients (1, 11, 12). These represent great treatment challenges, because patients are exquisitely sensitive to adverse effects of antipsychotic medications.

Subcortical dementias

Parkinson's disease

Patients with Parkinson's disease (PD) may experience neuropsychiatric symptoms at any time, although psychosis tends to occur later in the course of the illness or in relation to PD medications (dopamine agonists, anticholinergics, monoamine oxidase inhibitors [MAOIs]) (13). Dementia also tends to present late in the course of PD, occurring in about one-third of patients (9, 14). Similar to patients with DLB, those with PD show marked sensitivity to the motoric side effects of antipsychotic medications and should be treated cautiously with medications that have antidopaminergic activity.

Huntington's disease

Huntington's disease (HD) is an autosomal dominant degenerative disease primarily affecting the basal ganglia. Characteristic findings include motor disturbances, decreased cognition, and neuropsychiatric symptoms. The prevalence of neuropsychiatric symptoms in HD has been estimated at between 33% and 76%, with disturbances including irritability, depression, apathy, paranoia, hallucinations, impulsivity, and suicidality (15–18).

Mixed dementias

Vascular dementia

Vascular dementia (VaD) is the second most common type of dementia in Western cultures. Deficits characteristic of both cortical and subcortical dementias, depending on the location and extent of cerebrovascular lesions, may occur (9). Although agitation and psychosis are equally common in AD and VaD, mood and anxiety disorders are considered more common in patients with vascular dementia (6, 19). Risk factors for VaD greatly overlap with risk factors for cardiovascular disease (hypertension, smoking, diabetes mellitus, dyslipidemia). Patients who have cerebrovascular, cardiovascular, or diabetic vascular complications are at particularly high risk for VaD. Therefore, exercise caution using medications which may influence underlying cardiovascular disease.

Traumatic brain injury

Numerous neuropsychiatric sequelae are associated with traumatic brain injury (TBI), making it difficult to identify a well-defined syndrome. Aggression after TBI has been linked with pre-morbid aggression, arrest, and substance abuse (20). Yudofsky et al. (1990) characterized aggression after TBI as non-reflective, non-purposeful, reactive, periodic, explosive, and ego-dystonic (20, 21).

Work-up

It is critical to diagnose before treating. The treating clinician must ask, "Why is the patient behaving this way?" Vigorously search for acute treatable causes of behavioral disturbances. An initial evaluation for dementia is also an evaluation for delirium. Acute mental status changes must be thoroughly worked up before they can be attributed to "dementia-related agitation." A useful metaphor is that the "smoke" of delirium may clear to reveal the "fire" of underlying dementia. Remember that patients with dementia are subject to other psychiatric disorders associated with agitated or psychotic behavior (e.g., bipolar disorder, schizophrenia, personality disorder).

History

Thorough psychiatric and medical histories are critical in diagnosing patients who present with agitation and cognitive changes. Important aspects include prior mood, anxiety, psychosis, substance abuse, and cognitive disorders. When patients are unable to supply a history because of memory impairment, agitation, or other barriers to communication, gather collateral history from family members, the patient's chart, and previous care providers.

Relevant questions about symptoms include the following:

- Time of onset?
- Gradual or acute onset?
- Getting better or getting worse?
- Fluctuating since onset?
- Diurnal variations?
- Recent medication changes?
- Recent trauma (especially head injury) and other recent illnesses?
- Similar past episodes?
- Family/patient theories about symptom causes?
- Family history of dementia/neuropsychiatric illness?
- Substance abuse history?

Physical exam/neuropsychiatric testing/labs/studies

A complete physical and neurological exam will help identify "focal findings" suggestive of particular neurological pathology or indicators of other medical disease. Note the presence or absence of tremor, diaphoresis, abnormalities in tone, asymmetry of movement, respiratory abnormalities, gait abnormalities, and speech/language abnormalities. A Folstein Mini-Mental State Examination (MMSE) or other standardized bedside cognitive testing is essential for identifying abnormalities of orientation, attention, memory, and calculation (22). Additional neuropsychiatric testing can be invaluable in making a diagnosis and following the progress of a dementing illness.

Laboratory and neuroimaging studies are of variable utility in evaluating for "reversible causes of altered mental status," which may include normal pressure hydrocephalus, subdural hematoma, nutritional deficiencies, metabolic and toxic dementias, and CNS tumors. Given an aging patient with a history of slow and gradual cognitive decline, the likelihood of finding something truly reversible on testing is low (9). Although the likelihood of finding a treatable cause of acute changes in cognition and attention in a patient without a history of prior cognitive decline is probably much higher, persistent cognitive impairments may be observed following the delirium episode (23).

Laboratory tests that should be considered include the following:
- Urinalysis/urine culture
- CBC with differential
- Complete metabolic panel
- Liver-associated enzymes, or "LFTs"
- Serum ammonia (NH3)
- RPR, HIV, hepatitis panel
- TSH
- ESR, rheumatologic panel
- Blood alcohol level
- Urine toxicology screen

Studies that should be considered include the following:
- Head imaging (CT or MRI)
- Chest X-ray
- ABG
- EEG
- Lumbar puncture

Relevant laboratory tests should also be ordered for porphyrias, heavy metal toxicity, and Wilson's disease, if the history or physical exam is suggestive.

Clinical decision-making and treatment

The diagnosis typically will determine the appropriate course of treatment. If the patient's symptoms are due to delirium, substance intoxication/withdrawal/adverse effects, primary psychotic or mood disorder, or underlying personality pathology, then treat the underlying disorder.

Primary treatment principles for patients with dementia and agitation include the following:
- Immediately treat symptoms due to reversible causes such as a urinary tract infection, pain, constipation, or medications.
- Immediately treat agitation that may cause harm to the patient, family, or staff. This may mean using chemical or physical restraints.
- Assess environmental triggers and minimize agitating factors while maximizing cues for orientation.

Acute, non-pharmacologic management of agitation in demented patients frequently involves the use of physical restraints. This may paradoxically increase distress and agitation.

Restraints should be used only for as long as needed to ensure the safety of patient and staff, and these patients should be continuously monitored while restrained. Minimize environmental triggers of agitation and frequently reorient the patient. Interventions may include the use of eyeglasses, hearing aids, circadian rhythm lighting, and clocks, as well as verbal reorientation and the presence of family members and friends. Environmental interventions known to minimize delirium-related agitation can likewise be helpful for dementia-related agitation.

In a 2001 review of non-pharmacologic interventions for dementia-related inappropriate behavior, Cohen-Mansfield identified a variety of promising treatment modalities, including sensory interventions, social contact, behavior therapy, staff training, activities, environmental interventions, medical/nursing interventions, and combination therapy (8). Many of the interventions described make "common sense" in terms of identifying and targeting particular patients' needs (e.g., more contact for isolated individuals, increased activity for bored individuals).

Sensory interventions include massage and touch, white noise, and music therapies. On the basis of data from a limited number of randomized-controlled trials (RCTs), reviewers concluded that hand massage was useful in reducing immediate and short-term agitation (24). Several trials looking at music and relaxation during meals and bathing found positive associations for the time of listening (8).

Social contact therapies such as pet therapy, individual interaction, and simulated interaction have led to some improvements in behavior.

Medications for agitation in dementia

A number of medications have been studied for their effects on dementia-related agitation. The most common categories include antipsychotics, antiepileptic medications, antidepressants, and cognitive enhancers.

Antipsychotics

Antipsychotics are frequently prescribed for agitation and psychosis in dementia, although this use is not supported by an official FDA indication in the United States. Evidence for the utility of antipsychotics in treating dementia-related agitation and psychosis is sparse, but is still greater than evidence for many other medications used for this indication. A 2006 Cochrane review of randomized, placebo-controlled trials of atypical antipsychotics used for psychosis and agitation in dementia found the following (29):

- Compared with placebo, risperidone and olanzapine significantly improved aggression.
- Risperidone significantly improved psychosis.
- The review by Schneider et al. of RCTs of atypical antipsychotics used to treat agitation and psychosis in demented patients (most with AD) found the following (2, 30, 31):

  ○ Risperidone was associated with improvements in psychosis.
  ○ General neuropsychiatric functioning improved with "pooled analysis of aripiprazole and risperidone."

The Clinical Antipsychotic Trials of Intervention Effectiveness – Alzheimer's Disease (CATIE–AD) trial compared the atypical antipsychotics olanzapine, quetiapine, and risperidone with placebo for the treatment of psychosis and/or agitation in subjects with dementia (32). Outcomes were measured primarily by time to medication discontinuation and secondarily by Clinical Global Impression of Change (CGIC). Olanzapine and risperidone were found to have benefits in terms of longer times to discontinuation compared with other antipsychotics. However, they also were found to have shorter times to discontinuation because of intolerability compared with placebo.

Data for the utility of typical antipsychotics in neuropsychiatric symptoms of dementia are even more limited. A 2005 review of medications used for neuropsychiatric symptoms in dementia found little evidence that typical antipsychotics were useful, but a 2004 Cochrane review found some evidence that haloperidol may help treat aggression (33, 34). Studies comparing typical and atypical antipsychotics generally have found little difference in efficacy, but increased extrapyramidal symptoms (EPS) with haloperidol (2).

Any positive findings must be balanced against a growing body of evidence that both typical and atypical antipsychotics may cause significant increases in morbidity and mortality in patients with dementia (35). Multiple studies have verified the increased risk of obesity, metabolic disturbance, hypotension, and sedation with atypical antipsychotics. U.S. FDA "black box" warnings of increased rates of cerebrovascular accident and death with atypical antipsychotics in demented patients have been in place for a number of years, but more recent reports suggest that this increased risk extends to typical antipsychotics (36, 37). Additional risks of antipsychotics include parkinsonism, sedation, edema, chest infection, and cognitive decline (1).

As mentioned earlier, special caution must be taken for patients with DLB or PD. In PD, antipsychotics are known to cause significant worsening of underlying movement disorders; in DLB, antipsychotics have been associated with rigidity, falls, sedation, and increased confusion. These phenomena are likely mediated by dopaminergic and cholinergic blockade in patients with dopamine and acetycholin imbalances (13). Antipsychotics with less D_2 affinity and more serotonergic receptor activity, such as clozapine and quetiapine, would theoretically provide greater efficacy and decreased side effect burden in patients with both DLB and PD. Clozapine has been shown to be beneficial in PD with psychosis, although use of this medication is limited by concerns for multiple serious toxicities such as orthostatic hypotension, seizures, and agranulocytosis. Although quetiapine has yet to be proven efficacious for psychosis in PD, this medication is typically considered first line because of its lower potential toxicity. In DLB psychosis, quetiapine proved helpful in an open-label study, but several patients discontinued it because of side effects (13).

Despite the published risks of atypical antipsychotics in dementia, they have a greater quantity of efficacy data than other medications. The clinician must carefully weigh the risks/benefits of their use. Consideration of medication interactions, side effects, and co-morbidities may help in choosing the safest antipsychotic for a particular patient. Frequent monitoring of clinical status and continuous reassessment of the need for medication may help reduce the morbidity and mortality associated with atypical antipsychotics in patients with dementia.

Anticonvulsants

In a literature review of anticonvulsants used for neuropsychiatric symptoms of dementia, Konovalov et al. identified very few placebo-controlled trials (two RCTs for carbamazepine and five for valproate) (38). This group concluded that these medications did not have sufficient data for clinicians to recommend them routinely. Additionally, adverse effects occurred with significant frequency (most commonly falls, ataxia, drowsiness, GI disturbances).

Cholinesterase inhibitors and memantine

Data on the effectiveness of cholinesterase inhibitors in treating neuropsychiatric symptoms of dementia have been mixed (39). Although some controlled studies have reported behavioral and psychiatric benefits in demented subjects taking cholinesterase inhibitors, a 2007 RCT specifically looking at agitation found no benefit with donepezil in patients with AD (1, 40, 41).

Open-label studies in patients with PD have found donepezil and rivastigmine helpful for psychosis (42), although only rivastigmine was found to have significant effects on neuropsychiatric symptoms in a placebo-controlled study (13). In patients with DLB, rivastigmine was found helpful in neuropsychiatric symptoms in "observed cases," but significance was lost when intention-to-treat analyses were conducted.

Studies of memantine for agitation in patients with dementia are more promising. A recent Cochrane review noted a small but consistent finding of a decreased incidence of agitation in patients with moderate to severe dementia taking memantine. This medication was also noted to be well tolerated (43).

Antidepressants

Several controlled trials have found citalopram to be more effective than placebo for neuropsychiatric symptoms in dementia, but a review of controlled studies of trazodone did not find enough data to support its effectiveness for agitation in demented subjects (1, 44, 45).

Medications for agitation in Huntington's disease and traumatic brain injury

Controlled studies on pharmacologic treatment for agitation in HD are rare. In case reports and open-label trials, olanzapine was found to have some benefit for a variety of neuropsychiatric symptoms (15). Despite the lack of published data, practitioners frequently use antipsychotics, mood stabilizers, and antidepressants for these patients. Beta-blockers may also be useful for aggression related to HD (46).

Data from high-quality studies regarding pharmacologic treatment for agitation following TBI have been limited. The best evidence appears to be related to beta-blockers (20, 47). Buspirone, selective serotonin reuptake inhibitors (SSRIs), carbamazepine, and valproic acid also have shown some efficacy for agitation in patients with TBI. Although commonly recommended by psychiatrists, patients with TBI are particularly sensitive to the side effects of antipsychotics, and these medications should be used cautiously. Of special concern is the association in animal models of haloperidol with impaired neuronal recovery (20).

References

1. Ballard C, Day S, Sharp S, et al. Neuropsychiatric symptoms in dementia: importance and treatment considerations. Int Rev Psychiatry. 2008;204:396–404.

2. Jeste DV, Blazer D, Casey D, et al. ACNP white paper: update on use of antipsychotic drugs in elderly persons with dementia. Neuropsychopharmacology. 2008;33: 957–70.

3. Howard R, Ballard C, O'Brien J, et al, UK and Ireland Group for Optimization of

Management in Dementia. Guidelines for the management of agitation in dementia. Int J Geriatr Psychiatry. 2001;357: 1382–92.

4. Yaffe K. Treatment of neuropsychiatric symptoms in patients with dementia. N Engl J Med. 2007;357:1441–3.

5. Margallo-Lana M, Swann A, O'Brien J, et al. Prevalence and pharmacological management of behavioral and psychological symptoms amongst dementia

sufferers living in care environments. Int J Geriatr Psychiatry. 2001;16:39–44.

6. Lyketsos CG, Steinberg M, Tschanz JT, et al. Mental and behavioral disturbances in dementia: findings from the Cache County Study on Memory in Aging. Am J Psychiatry. 2000;157:708–14.

7. Sultzer DL, Levin HS, Mahler ME, et al. A comparison of psychiatric symptoms in vascular dementia and Alzheimer's disease. Am J Psychiatry. 1993;150:1806–12.

8. Cohen-Mansfield J. Non pharmacologic interventions for inappropriate behaviors in dementia: a review, summary, and critique. Am J Geriatr Psychiatry. 2001; 9:361–81.

9. Lobo A, Saz P. Dementia. In: Levenson JL, editor. Textbook of psychosomatic medicine. Arlington (VA): American Psychiatric Publishing, Inc; 2005. p. 131–69.

10. Brookmeyer R, Corrada MM, Curriero FC, et al. Survival following a diagnosis of Alzheimer disease. Arch Neurol. 2002;59: 1764–7.

11. Ballard C, Ayre G, Gray A. Psychotic symptoms and behavioural disturbances in dementia: a review. Rev Neurol. 1999;155: 44–52.

12. Klatka L, Louis E, Schiffer RB. Psychiatric features in diffuse Lewy body disease: a clinicopathologic study using Alzheimer's disease and Parkinson's disease control groups. Neurology. 1996;47:1148–52.

13. Weintraub D, Hurtig HI. Presentation and management of psychosis in Parkinson's disease and dementia with Lewy Bodies. Am J Psychiatry. 2007;164:1491–8.

14. Breteler MM, DeGroot RR, Van Romunde LK, et al. Risk of dementia in patients with Parkinson's disease, epilepsy and severe head trauma: a register-based follow-up study. Am J Epidemiol. 1995;142:1300–5.

15. Adam OR, Jankovic J. Symptomatic treatment of Huntington disease. Neurotherapeutics. 2008;5:181–97.

16. van Duijn E, Kingma EM, Van Der Mast RC. Psychopathology in verified Huntington's disease gene carriers.

J Neuropsychiatry Clin Neurosci. 2007;19:441–8.

17. Cummings JL: Behavioral and psychiatric symptoms associated with Huntington's disease. In: Weiner WJ, Lang AE, editors. Behavioral neurology of movement disorders. New York (NY): Raven Press; 1995. p. 179–86.

18. Watt DC, Seller A. A clinico-genetic study of psychiatric disorders in Huntington's chorea. Psychol Med. 1993;Suppl 23;1–46.

19. Ballard CG, Eastwood C, Gahir M, et al. A follow up study of depression in the carers of dementia sufferers. Br Med J. 1996;312: 947.

20. Fann JR, Kennedy R, Bombardier CH. Physical medicine and rehabilitation. In: Levenson JL, editor. Textbook of psychosomatic medicine. Arlington (VA): American Psychiatric Publishing, Inc; 2005. p. 787–825.

21. Yudofsky SC, Silver JM, Hales RE. Pharmacologic management of aggression in the elderly. J Clin Psychiatry. 1990;51: 22–8.

22. Folstein MF, Folstein SE, McHugh PR. "Mini-mental state": a practical method of grading the cognitive state of patients for the clinician. J Psychiatr Res. 1975;12: 189–98.

23. Trzepacz PT, Meagher DJ. Delirium. In: Levenson JL, editor. Textbook of psychosomatic medicine. Arlington (VA): American Psychiatric Association, Inc; 2005. p. 91–130.

24. Viggo Hansen N, Jorgensen T, Ortenblad L. Massage and touch for dementia. Cochrane Database Syst Rev. 2006(4):CD004989. DOI:10.1002/14651858,CD004989.pub2.

25. Livingston G, Johnston K, Katona C, et al. Old Age Task Force of the World Federation of Biological Psychiatry. Systematic review of psychological approaches to the management of neuropsychiatric symptoms of dementia. Am J Psychiatry. 2005; 62:1996–2021.

26. Holt FE, Birks TPH, Thogrimsen LM, et al. Arometherapy for dementia. Cochrane

Database Syst Rev. 2003;(3):CD003150. DOI:10.1002/14651858.CD003150.

27. Ballard CG, O'Brien JT, Reichelt K, et al. Aromatherapy as a safe and effective treatment for the management of agitation in severe dementia: the results of a double-blind placebo-controlled trial with Melissa. J Clin Psychiatry. 2002;63:553–8.

28. Forbes D, Morgan DG, Bangma J, et al. Light therapy for managing sleep, behaviour, and mood disturbances in dementia. Cochrane Database Syst Rev. 2004;(2):CD003946. DOI:10.1002/14651858.CD003946.pub2.

29. Ballard CG, Waite J, Birks J. Atypical antipsychotics for aggression and psychosis in Alzheimer's disease. Cochrane Database Syst Rev. 2006;(1):CD003476. DOI:10.1002/14651858.CD003476.pub2.

30. Schneider LS, Dagerman K, Insel PS. Efficacy and adverse effects of atypical antipsychotics for dementia: meta-analysis of randomized, placebo-controlled trials. Am J Geriatr Psychiatry. 2006;14:191–210.

31. Schneider LS, Tariot PN, Dagerman KS, et al. Effectiveness of atypical antipsychotic drugs in patients with Alzheimer's disease. N Engl J Med. 2006;355:1525–38.

32. Sultzer DL, Davis SM, Tariot PN, et al. CATIE-AD Study Group. Clinical symptom responses to atypical antipsychotic medications in Alzheimer's disease: Phase 1 outcomes from the CATE-AD effectiveness trial. Am J Psychiatry. 2008;165:844–54.

33. Sink KM, Holden KF, Yaffe K. Pharmaco-logical treatment of neuropsychiatric symptoms of dementia: a review of the evidence. JAMA. 2005;293:596–608.

34. Lonergan E, Luxemberg J. Valproate preparations for agitation in dementia. Cochrane Database Syst Rev. 2004;(2):CD003945. DOI:10.1002/14651858.CD003945.pub2.

35. Schneider LS, Dagerman KS, Insel P. Risk of death with atypical antipsychotic drug treatment for dementia: meta-analysis of randomized placebo-controlled trials. JAMA. 2005;294:1934–43.

36. Kales HC, Valenstein M, Kim HM, et al. Mortality risk in patients with dementia treated with antipsychotics versus other psychiatric medications. Am J Psychiatry. 2007;164:1568–76.

37. Rochon PA, Normand S-L, Gomes T, et al. Antipsychotic therapy and short-term serious events in older adults with dementia. Arch Intern Med. 2008;168:1090–6.

38. Konovalov S, Muralee S, Tampi RR. Anticonvulsants for the treatment of behavioral and psychological symptoms of dementia: a literature review. Int Psychogeriatr. 2008;20:293–308.

39. Rossi P, Serrao M, Pozzessere G. Gabapentin-induced worsening of neuropsychiatric symptoms in dementia with Lewy bodies: case reports. Eur Neurol. 2002;47:56–7.

40. Howard RJ, Juszczak E, Ballard CG, et al. Donepezil for the treatment of agitation in Alzheimer's disease. N Engl J Med. 2007;357:1382–92.

41. Wild R, Petit TACL, Burns A. Cholinesterase inhibitors for dementia with Lewy Bodies. Cochrane Database Syst Rev. 2003;(3):CD003672. DOI:10.1002/14651858.CD003672.

42. McKeith I, Del Ser T, Spano P, et al. Efficacy of rivastigmine in dementia with Lewy bodies: a randomized, double-blind, placebo-controlled international study. Lancet. 2000;356:2031–6.

43. McShane R, Arosa Sastre A, Makaran N. Memantine for dementia. Cochrane Database Syst Rev. 2006(2):CD003154. DOI:10.1002/14651858.CD003154.pub5.

44. Martinon-Torres G, Fioravanti M, Grimley Evans J. Trazodone for agitation in dementia. Cochrane Database Syst Rev. 2004(3):CD004990. DOI:10.1002/14651858.CD004990.

45. Pollock BG, Mulsant BH, Rosen J, et al. Comparison of citalopram, perphenazine, and placebo for the acute treatment of psychosis and behavioral disturbances in

hospitalized, demented patients. Am J Psychiatry. 2002;159:460–5.

46. Rosenblatt A, Leroi I. Neuropsychiatry of Huntington's disease and other basal ganglia disorders. Psychosomatics. 2000;41: 24–30.

47. Fleminger S, Greenwood RRJ, Oliver DL. Pharmacological management for agitation and aggression in people with acquired brain injury. Cochrane Database Syst Rev. 2006(4):CD003299. DOI:10.1002/ 14651858.CD003299.pub2.

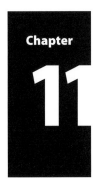

Depression and heart disease

Jess G. Fiedorowicz

Typical consult question

"Could you please see this patient who is refusing to take his medications for heart disease because he doesn't care and doesn't want to live anymore?"

Despite its potential clinical significance, major depression often may be missed in patients hospitalized for cardiovascular conditions unless the manifestation is overt or interferes with treatment.

Background

Bidirectional links exist between mood disorders and cardiovascular disease. Individuals with mood disorders bear a greater burden of cardiovascular morbidity and mortality than would be expected from general population estimates. Those with depression have approximately double the risk of developing cardiovascular disease (CVD). Similar elevations in risk have been documented for patients with bipolar disorder (1). Further, individuals with CVD are at greater risk of developing major depression – a development that may pose important prognostic implications. Approximately 20% of patients with cardiovascular disease meet criteria for major depressive disorder (2, 3). A variety of mechanisms have been hypothesized to mediate this relationship between depression and CVD, as outlined in Table 11.1. Proposed biological links include autonomic nervous system dysfunction, hypothalamic-pituitary-adrenal axis dysfunction, pro-coagulant states, vascular dysfunction, altered immune function, and inflammation. Behavioral and psychosocial links may include poor diet, physical inactivity, treatment non-adherence, smoking, and social isolation. Individuals with major depression are also more likely to have established risk factors for heart disease such as diabetes mellitus, hyperlipidemia, hypertension, obesity, and smoking (4). Further, a number of medical conditions may convey increased risk of depression and CVD, such as arthritis, hyperlipidemia, hypothyroidism, obesity, and obstructive sleep apnea.

The presence of depression has been independently associated with a number of cardiovascular outcomes, several of which are illustrated in Table 11.2. Some studies have suggested that depression with onset after an acute coronary syndrome or myocardial infarction conveys particularly negative prognostic significance (5). Treatment-resistant depression may be associated with a particularly high risk (6). Beyond impact on cardiovascular outcomes, depression may have other adverse effects, including impaired function, reduced quality of life, increased resource utilization, and general suffering. Thus, recognition of treatment of depression in general is clinically relevant, although it assumes particular importance in

Psychosomatic Medicine: An Introduction to Consultation-Liaison Psychiatry, eds. James J. Amos and Robert G. Robinson. Published by Cambridge University Press. © Cambridge University Press 2010.

Table 11.1 Proposed mechanisms linking depression to CVD

Biological	Behavioral
Autonomic nervous system dysfunction	Poor diet
Hypothalamic-pituitary-adrenal axis dysfunction	Physical inactivity
Procoagulant states	Smoking
Enhanced platelet activation	Social isolation
Impaired immune function	Medication non-adherence
Vascular dysfunction	Non-adherence to treatment programs
Inflammation	Stress

Table 11.2 Adverse cardiovascular outcomes associated with depression

Sample	Outcome
Suspected MI	Death or cardiovascular events
Acute MI	Cardiovascular complications
Patients receiving CABG	Death
Patients with ACS	Cardiovascular events
Unstable angina	Death

Key:
ACS = acute coronary syndrome
CABG = coronary artery bypass grafting
MI = myocardial infarction

individuals with CVD. Unfortunately, among those with CVD, depression is often under-recognized and undertreated. Screening for depression subsequently has been recommended for individuals with CVD. Because of the bidirectional associations between depression and heart disease, individuals with depression should be closely monitored and treated for risk factors for cardiovascular disease.

Depression and cardiovascular disease are common conditions, are risk factors for each other, and consequently commonly co-occur. Depression negatively influences prognosis in heart disease and is associated with a myriad of adverse outcomes. Patients with CVD should be screened for depression and appropriate treatments delivered following identification. The selective serotonin reuptake inhibitors (SSRIs) clearly represent first-line pharmacologic therapy for major depression in CVD because of their demonstrated effectiveness for the depressive syndrome and an established safety profile. Although all SSRIs may be considered, sertraline, citalopram, and escitalopram have the lowest risk for drug interactions with commonly prescribed medications for patients with CVD. Non-pharmacologic therapies including psychotherapy, exercise, relaxation, and stress management may be considered as alternatives or adjuncts. Exercise and cardiovascular rehabilitation are particularly noteworthy for their potential cardiovascular and mood benefits. Further research is warranted to conclusively determine whether specific or general treatments for depression may reduce the risk of subsequent cardiovascular events. Non-adherence to treatment is common and should be anticipated, heeded, and addressed when identified.

Screening and assessment

The American Heart Association and others have recommended screening for depression among those with CVD (7). It has been further suggested that this screening should occur at least quarterly (3). Screening can be accomplished by asking about the presence of depressed mood, anhedonia, and suicide ideation. In response to a positive screen, other symptoms suggestive of a depressive syndrome can be explored in the context of a medical and psychiatric history. Clinicians and patients alike may attribute symptoms of depression to manifestations of CVD, particularly the somatic symptoms. Depressive symptoms should not be assumed to be related to symptoms of CVD. For instance, if a patient with congestive heart failure presents with fatigue or even weight gain, these signs and symptoms should not be simply attributed to the heart failure. Accurate diagnosis can be made by including symptoms such as fatigue or weight gain towards a diagnosis of depression, regardless of presumed origin (8).

Work-up

In addition to an appropriate and targeted work-up for CVD, patients should be screened for conditions related to depression and heart disease, such as sleep apnea. Individuals with depression and heart disease should receive a comprehensive psychiatric evaluation. This evaluation can help to distinguish major depression from demoralization, as detailed in the chapter by Wellen and Wise entitled "Demoralization in the Medical Setting." The evaluation can be augmented with depression rating scales if desired. Because vascular disease may also be associated with impaired cognition, particular attention should be paid to the assessment of cognitive function on mental status exam. Any subjective concerns or objective findings on exam related to cognition may be followed up with neuropsychological testing. Patients should be evaluated for substance abuse, which may potentially impact both mood and cardiovascular prognosis. Tobacco use should be assessed. Hypothyroidism may adversely affect mood and cardiac function, so a thyroid-stimulating hormone (TSH) level should be checked. The medications used to treat CVD, especially when heart failure is present, may result in electrolyte abnormalities that may adversely affect mood and sensorium. Many antidepressants may worsen orthostatic hypotension, and orthostatic vital signs should be assessed and monitored as indicated. Orthostatic hypotension may be particularly problematic in elderly patients or in those at risk of falls.

Clinical decision-making and treatment

Once the diagnosis of depression has been made, a variety of treatment options are available. These include antidepressants, psychotherapy, and exercise. Relaxation and stress management approaches also may be of benefit. Any eligible patient should be referred to cardiac rehabilitation (9). Treatments generally can be expected to have at least modest effects on depression and uncertain effects on cardiovascular events.

The selective serotonin reuptake inhibitors (SSRIs) are considered first line in the management of depression in CVD, including in the setting of heart failure. Sertraline, citalopram, or escitalopram are often selected because of the low risk of drug interactions. SSRIs are preferable for patients with CVD because they are unlikely to alter heart rate or blood pressure. SSRIs may also reduce platelet aggregation and may have favorable effects on sympathetic and vasomotor tone (10).

Although these biological effects of SSRIs have been purported as a potential mechanism to reduce cardiovascular risk, current evidence does not convincingly support a reduction in cardiovascular events with SSRIs. Treatment with SSRIs for depression in CVD has been demonstrated effective in treating depression, improving quality of life, and improving adherence to medications. Treatment has not convincingly demonstrated any reduction in cardiovascular morbidity or mortality. The Enhancing Recovery in Coronary Heart Disease (ENRICHD) trial comparing cognitive-behavioral therapy (CBT) versus usual care demonstrated improved depression but no improvement in survival for the CBT group. Although not randomized to antidepressants and subsequently susceptible to confounding, those receiving antidepressants in the ENRICHD trial had a 42% reduction in death or nonfatal myocardial infarction (11). In the Sertraline Antidepressant Heart Attack Randomized Trial (SADHART) study, sertraline was demonstrated effective for major depression in patients with acute MI or unstable angina, although it did not result in a statistically significant reduction in adverse cardiovascular events (12); however, the study was underpowered to assess this outcome (13). In the Myocardial INfarction and Depression Intervention Trial (MIND-IT), mirtazapine demonstrated no improvement in depression or cardiac events (14), although a follow-up secondary analysis found greater mortality among non-responders to mirtazapine or citalopram (15). Despite some encouraging findings from secondary analyses of the aforementioned studies, randomized, controlled trials of SSRIs in cardiovascular disease have not demonstrated significant reductions in cardiovascular mortality. However, given the difficulty in powering treatment trials of depression to assess this outcome, the issue remains unsettled.

Beyond SSRIs, other antidepressants have also been studied for major depression with heart disease. Nefazodone and mirtazapine have been used safely in patients with congestive heart failure (3). Bupropion and mirtazapine have been studied post myocardial infarction and appear generally safe (16). In one small study of patients with CVD, bupropion resulted in a small but significant increase in supine blood pressures (17). Mirtazapine may cause orthostatic hypotension.

The serotonin-norepinephrine reuptake inhibitors (SNRIs), duloxetine and venlafaxine, may increase heart rate and blood pressure, which may be problematic for patients with CVD. Venlafaxine may also result in QTc prolongation. The norepinephrine reuptake inhibitor, reboxetine, may also increase blood pressure. These medications, however, do not appear to share the pro-arrhythmic properties of the tricyclic antidepressants (TCAs). SNRIs may be considered in patients, particularly given a compelling indication such as prior response. However, because SNRIs are not well studied in CVD and may cause some undesirable side effects for patients with CVD, they generally should not be considered first- or even second-line options.

TCAs and monoamine oxidase inhibitors (MAOIs) should be avoided in patients with CVD and are even considered contraindicated by some. TCAs may increase heart rate, blood pressure, and risk of orthostatic hypotension. TCAs may antagonize sodium and potassium channels, resulting in intraventricular conduction delays and a prolonged QT interval (16). These type 1A antiarrhythmic effects may be problematic in patients with ischemic heart disease (18). Nortriptyline also may reduce heart rate variability (19), which may adversely affect cardiovascular prognosis. MAOIs may increase risk of orthostatic hypotension and may cause transient but clinically significant increases in blood pressure shortly after ingestion (20). MAOIs further have the potential for life-threatening drug interactions secondary to serotonin syndrome. Meperidine and narcotic analgesics at anesthetic doses may

Table 11.3 Potential drug interactions associated with antidepressants for commonly prescribed cardiovascular medications

Enzyme	Inhibitor	Substrate
1A2	Fluvoxamine	Propranolol, Warfarin
2C19	Fluoxetine, Fluvoxamine, Paroxetine	Digoxin, Propranolol, Warfarin
2D6	Bupropion, Fluoxetine, Paroxetine	Captopril, Carvedilol, Encainide, Flecainide, Metoprolol, Propranolol, Timolol
3A4	Fluoxetine, Fluvoxamine, Nefazodone	Amiodarone, calcium channel blockers, Digoxin, Disopyramide, Dofetilide, Lidocaine, Quinidine, Statins

precipitate such reactions. Given the demand for narcotic adjuncts with cardiopulmonary bypass and up to a 14-day period required to wash out the pharmacodynamic effects of MAOIs (20), MAOIs generally should be avoided in patients with CVD.

Patients with CVD may be reluctant to take yet another medication for depression. Further, patients with depression and CVD may be at greater risk of non-compliance for cardiovascular and antidepressants alike (21, 22). Upfront efforts to facilitate communication, establish a therapeutic alliance, and engage the patient's family or other supports may be effective towards the aim of preventing non-adherence. Physicians should monitor adherence and explore any reasons for non-adherence or barriers to adherence. For patients concerned about the risk/benefit ratio of medications, psychoeducational strategies may help mitigate the risk of non-compliance. Medication monitoring by family or other supports, case managers, or visiting nurses may prove valuable. Given the complex medication regimens often involved, such assistance may be of considerable value.

Monitoring for adverse events and drug-drug interactions is important, as polypharmacy is common in patients with CVD. A number of antidepressants may interact with medications used to treat CVD. Fluvoxamine may inhibit cytochrome P450 (CYP450) 1A2. Fluoxetine, fluvoxamine, and paroxetine inhibit CYP 2C19. The antidepressants bupropion, fluoxetine, and paroxetine inhibit CYP 2D6. Sertraline may exhibit mild inhibition of CYP 2D6. Individual patients may be poor metabolizers at CYP 2D6 and particularly sensitive to any such effects. Fluoxetine, fluvoxamine, and nefazodone inhibit CYP 3A4. Inhibition of CYP 1A2 and 2D6 may increase levels of beta-blockers. Inhibition of CYP 3A4 may increase levels of amiodarone, calcium channel blockers, antiarrhythmics, digoxin, and statins. Fluoxetine, fluvoxamine, and paroxetine may inhibit CYP 2C19, which may increase risk of bleeding for patients on warfarin. Potential drug interactions between antidepressants and commonly prescribed medications for patients with cardiovascular disease are highlighted in Table 11.3.

Although not shown to reduce cardiovascular events, psychotherapy has demonstrated effectiveness for major depression in CVD and should be considered in addition to pharmacologic management. Psychotherapeutic approaches studied in patients with depression and CVD include cognitive-behavioral therapy, mindfulness-based psychoeducation, and interpersonal psychotherapy. In the Cardiovascular Risk reduction by Early Anemia Treatment with Epoetin Beta (CREATE) trial, citalopram but not interpersonal therapy produced better results than clinical management alone for the treatment of depressive symptoms (23). Other therapeutic approaches useful for major depression but not studied for cardiovascular disease may also be considered.

Relaxation therapy and exercise training have also been studied, may benefit mood, and produce physical health benefits. The exercise obtained in cardiac rehabilitation has been demonstrated to improve depressive symptoms and mortality (24). Depression may also impede adherence to cardiac rehabilitation, especially if hopelessness is present (25). Efforts to promote adherence to behavioral recommendations, non-pharmacologic therapies, and cardiac rehabilitation are worthwhile. Depressed patients may be less likely to follow behavioral recommendations such as diet modification, exercise, and smoking cessation (26). These important efforts may subsequently require extra attention and emphasis.

Suggestions of adverse psychiatric effects of commonly prescribed cardiovascular medications generally have not been substantiated. Beta-blockers do not cause depression and should not be avoided in patients with depression and CVD. The initial concern that beta-blockers may induce depression was based on case reports and is no longer supported by current best evidence (27, 28). There has also been concern about potential psychiatric side effects of lipid-lowering therapies. Although low cholesterol has been associated with suicide, this association is neither strong nor robust (29). Although case reports have documented a number of psychiatric adverse effects of hydroxymethylglutaryl-coenzyme A (HMG-CoA) reductase inhibitors or statins, such effects have not been reported in systematic studies. Use of statins does not appear to increase risk of suicide (30). It is thus important to not withhold these potentially life-saving interventions from those with major depression and heart disease. Monitoring for changes in mental status is nonetheless worthwhile during treatment of patients with depression and heart disease, although caution should be exercised before any changes are attributed to cardiovascular medications.

References

1. Weiner M, Warren L, Fiedorowicz JG. Cardiovascular morbidity and mortality in bipolar disorder. Ann Clin Psychiatry. In press.

2. Thombs BD, de Jonge P, Coyne JC, et al. Depression screening and patient outcomes in cardiovascular care: a systematic review. JAMA. 2008;300(18):2161–71.

3. Watson K, Summers KM. Depression in patients with heart failure: clinical implications and management. Pharmacotherapy. 2009;29(1):49–63.

4. Joynt KE, Whellan DJ, O'Connor CM. Depression and cardiovascular disease: mechanisms of interaction. Biol Psychiatry. 2003;54(3):248–61.

5. Parker GB, Hilton TM, Walsh WF, et al. Timing is everything: the onset of depression and acute coronary syndrome outcome. Biol Psychiatry. 2008;64(8): 660–6.

6. Carney RM, Freedland KE. Treatment-resistant depression and mortality after acute coronary syndrome. Am J Psychiatry. 2009;166(4):410–7.

7. Lichtman JH, Bigger JT Jr, Blumenthal JA, et al. Depression and coronary heart disease: recommendations for screening, referral, and treatment: a science advisory from the American Heart Association Prevention Committee of the Council on Cardiovascular Nursing, Council on Clinical Cardiology, Council on Epidemiology and Prevention, and Interdisciplinary Council on Quality of Care and Outcomes Research: endorsed by the American Psychiatric Association. Circulation. 2008;118(17):1768–75.

8. Williams JW Jr, Noel PH, Cordes JA, et al. Is this patient clinically depressed? JAMA. 2002;287(9):1160–70.

9. Pozuelo L, Tesar G, Zhang J, et al. Depression and heart disease: what do we know, and where are we headed? Cleve Clin J Med. 2009;76(1):59–70.

10. van Melle JP, de Jonge P, Van Den Berg MP, et al. Treatment of depression in acute

coronary syndromes with selective serotonin reuptake inhibitors. Drugs. 2006;66(16):2095–107.

11. Berkman LF, Blumenthal J, Burg M, et al. Effects of treating depression and low perceived social support on clinical events after myocardial infarction: the Enhancing Recovery in Coronary Heart Disease Patients (ENRICHD) Randomized Trial. JAMA. 2003;289(23):3106–16.

12. Glassman AH, O'Connor CM, Califf RM, et al. Sertraline treatment of major depression in patients with acute MI or unstable angina. JAMA. 2002;288(6):701–9.

13. Joynt KE, O'Connor CM. Lessons from SADHART, ENRICHD, and other trials. Psychosom Med. 2005;67(Suppl 1):S63–S66.

14. van Melle JP, de Jonge P, Honig A, et al. Effects of antidepressant treatment following myocardial infarction. Br J Psychiatry. 2007;190:460–6.

15. de Jonge P, Honig A, van Melle JP, et al. Nonresponse to treatment for depression following myocardial infarction: association with subsequent cardiac events. Am J Psychiatry. 2007;164(9):1371–8.

16. Taylor D. Antidepressant drugs and cardiovascular pathology: a clinical overview of effectiveness and safety. Acta Psychiatr Scand. 2008;118(6):434–42.

17. Roose SP, Dalack GW, Glassman AH, et al. Cardiovascular effects of bupropion in depressed patients with heart disease. Am J Psychiatry. 1991;148(4):512–6.

18. Jiang W, Davidson JR. Antidepressant therapy in patients with ischemic heart disease. Am Heart J. 2005;150(5):871–81.

19. Yeragani VK, Pesce V. Jayaraman A. et al. Major depression with ischemic heart disease: effects of paroxetine and nortriptyline on long-term heart rate variability measures. Biol Psychiatry. 2002;52(5):418–29.

20. Fiedorowicz JG, Swartz KL. The role of monoamine oxidase inhibitors in current

psychiatric practice. J Psychiatr Pract. 2004;10(4):239–48.

21. Gehi A, Haas D, Pipkin S, et al. Depression and medication adherence in outpatients with coronary heart disease: findings from the Heart and Soul Study. Arch Intern Med. 2005;165(21):2508–13.

22. Rieckmann N, Kronish IM, Haas D, et al. Persistent depressive symptoms lower aspirin adherence after acute coronary syndromes. Am Heart J. 2006;152(5):922–7.

23. Lesperance F, Frasure-Smith N, Koszycki D, et al. Effects of citalopram and interpersonal psychotherapy on depression in patients with coronary artery disease: the Canadian Cardiac Randomized Evaluation of Antidepressant and Psychotherapy Efficacy (CREATE) trial. JAMA. 2007;297(4):367–79.

24. Milani RV, Lavie CJ. Impact of cardiac rehabilitation on depression and its associated mortality. Am J Med. 2007;120(9):799–806.

25. Dunn SL, Stommel M, Corser WD, et al. Hopelessness and its effect on cardiac rehabilitation exercise participation following hospitalization for acute coronary syndrome. J Cardiopulm Rehabil Prev. 2009;29(1):32–9.

26. Kronish IM, Rieckmann N, Halm EA, et al. Persistent depression affects adherence to secondary prevention behaviors after acute coronary syndromes. J Gen Intern Med. 2006;21(11):1178–83.

27. Bright RA, Everitt DE. Beta-blockers and depression: evidence against an association. JAMA. 1992;267(13):1783–7.

28. Ko DT, Hebert PR, Coffey CS, et al. Beta-blocker therapy and symptoms of depression, fatigue, and sexual dysfunction. JAMA. 2002;288(3):351–7.

29. Fiedorowicz JG, Haynes WG. Circulating cholesterol, depression, and suicide: chicken or egg? Curr Psychiatr. In press.

30. Lester D. Serum cholesterol levels and suicide: a meta-analysis. Suicide Life Threat Behav. 2002;32(3):333–46.

Chapter

12

Management of post-stroke depression

Robert G. Robinson, Sergio E. Starkstein, and Romina Mizrahi

Typical consult question

"Mr. S. is a fifty-seven year old married male hospitalized following an acute stroke. He appears uninterested and lethargic most of the time, but periodically he is observed to be crying. Please evaluate for post-stroke depression."

Background

Post-stroke depression (PSD) is generally considered to be the most frequent and important neuropsychiatric consequence of stroke. According to pooled data from studies of patients hospitalized with acute stroke or rehabilitation therapy involving more than 2700 patients, 21.6% meet the *Diagnostic and Statistical Manual of Mental Disorders (DSM-IV)* criteria for mood disorder due to a general medical condition (i.e., stroke) with major depressive-like episodes, and 20.0% meet *DSM-IV* criteria for minor depression (i.e., a sub-syndromal form of major depression in which at least two, but fewer than five, symptoms are present, the symptoms include depressed mood or loss of interest and pleasure) (1).

Prevalence varies over time with a slight peak noted 3 to 6 months after stroke, but prevalence rates remain steady at about 30% to 35% during the first two years after stroke. Robinson and colleagues characterized the natural course of major depression after stroke, with spontaneous remission typically occurring between 6 months and 1 year (1). Morris et al. reported a mean duration of 39±31 (SD) weeks for major depression (2). However, it was also noted by Astrom et al. that 24% of episodes of acute major depression persisted for longer than 3 years following the stroke (3). Longitudinal studies have also shown that approximately 40% of post-stroke patients who are non-depressed during acute stroke treatment will develop a depression at some time during the first 2 years after stroke (1). Thus, post-stroke depression may present at any time over the first few years following stroke.

Numerous risk factors for depression after stroke have been identified, including left frontal or left basal ganglia lesions (4), subcortical atrophy (5), female gender (6–8), family or previous history of mood disorder (9), neuroticism trait (10), greater impairment in activities of daily living (11), impaired social support, and negative life events (10). Morris et al. showed that these risk factors are cumulative, so patients with acute left frontal lesions, prior history of depression, severe impairment of activities of daily living (ADLs), and poor social support are at very high risk for post-stroke major depression (10).

Of six studies which examined the effects of PSD on recovery in ADLs, five found that patients with PSD within the first three months after stroke have significantly poorer

Psychosomatic Medicine: An Introduction to Consultation-Liaison Psychiatry, eds. James J. Amos and Robert G. Robinson. Published by Cambridge University Press. © Cambridge University Press 2010.

Table 12.1 Differential diagnosis for post-stroke depression

Syndrome	Prevalence	Clinical symptoms	Associated lesion location
Major depression	22%	Depressed mood, diurnal mood variation, loss of energy, anxiety, restlessness, worry, weight loss, decreased appetite, early morning awakening, delayed sleep onset, social withdrawal, and irritability	Left frontal lobe, left basal ganglia
Minor depression	20%	Depressed mood, anxiety, restlessness, worry, diurnal mood variation, hopelessness, loss of energy, delayed sleep onset, early morning awakening, social withdrawal, weight loss, decreased appetite	Right or left posterior parietal and occipital regions
Anxiety disorder	18%	Symptoms of major depression, intense worry, and anxious foreboding, in addition to depression, associated light-headedness or palpitations, and muscle tension or restlessness, and difficulty concentrating or falling asleep	Left cortical lesions, usually dorsal lateral frontal lobe
Apathy			
Without depression	11%	Loss of drive, motivation, and interest, as well as low energy, slowed thought processes	Posterior internal capsule
With depression	11%		
Pathological crying	15%	Frequent, usually brief crying; crying not caused by sadness or that is out of proportion to it; social withdrawal occurs secondary to emotional outbursts	Frequently bilateral hemispheric Can occur with almost any location
Anosognosia	24%	Denial of impairment related to motor function, sensory perception; may include denial of sadness, but with other symptoms of depression (e.g.. sleep, appetite, energy, concentration disturbance)	Right hemisphere and enlarged ventricles
Catastrophic reaction	19%	Anxiety reaction, tears, aggressive behavior, swearing, displacement, refusal, renouncement, and compensatory boasting lasting a few minutes with return to baseline	Left anterior-subcortical
Aprosodia			
Motor	Unkn	Poor expression of emotional prosody and gesturing; may include denial of feelings of depression, but with symptoms of depression (e.g., sleep, appetite, energy and concentration disturbance)	Right hemisphere posterior inferior frontal lobe and basal ganglia
Sensory	32%	Good expression of emotional prosody and gesturing, poor understanding of the emotional state of others, and difficulty empathizing with others	Right hemisphere posterior inferior parietal lobe and posterior superior temporal lobe

recovery in ADLs up to two years after stroke compared with similar patients without PSD (1). In addition, PSD has been found to lead to greater cognitive impairment than is seen in comparable non-depressed patients, but only among patients with major depression following left hemisphere stroke (12). Moreover, patients with PSD have significantly more hospitalizations and outpatient visits, and longer lengths of hospital stay 12 months after the stroke, compared with patients without PSD (13); higher stress among caregivers (14) and increased risk of suicide (15) have also been noted. Finally, six studies now have shown that patients with PSD have significantly higher rates of short-term (twelve and twenty-four months) and long-term (six and ten years) mortality (3).

Work-up

Diagnosis

Practice guidelines for the care of post-stroke patients (16, p. 6–7) clearly state that all patients must be assessed for the presence of depression. However, several factors can complicate the diagnosis of depression following stroke: first, language disorders due to decreased level of consciousness or fluent (Wernicke's) aphasia with comprehension deficit. Patients with even moderate impairment in comprehension cannot be reliably diagnosed with depression. Another complication is anosognosia, or lack of insight or awareness of impairment, which sometimes may include depressive symptoms. Furthermore, depressive symptoms may overlap with symptoms of stroke. For example, a study examining the specificity of depressive symptoms found that during the first year post stroke, weight loss and early awakening were not significantly more frequent in depressed than in non-depressed elderly patients (17). In spite of the fact that some symptoms of depression may be due to the physical illness, the use of standard *DSM-IV* symptoms for major and minor depression was found to have 100% sensitivity and 97% specificity during the first year post stroke. On the other hand, if patients cannot be verbally examined, or if their awareness of their impairment appears to be altered and they cannot undergo the usual mental state examination to determine a diagnosis, you can only make an educated guess based on nursing observations, nursing reports, and family member information. These patients are often given a trial of antidepressants, even without a firm diagnosis of depression, to see if their behavior or affective state will change.

If the patient's comprehension is intact, a careful psychiatric interview of the patient with formal mental status exam and *DSM* criteria, corroborated by outside sources, serves as the basis for establishing a diagnosis. Table 12.1 shows the differential diagnosis for post-stroke depression.

Clinical decision-making and treatment of post-stroke depression

Although the pathogenesis of PSD remains unknown, a biopsychosocial approach to treatment is probably the most appropriate (18). It is important to keep in mind, however, that many patients with PSD do not receive effective treatment for their mood disorder. This may be related to failure of the treating physician to examine patients for depression or the inability of patients and their families to recognize symptoms of depression (19). A protocol for assessment and treatment is shown on Table 12.2.

Table 12.2 Assessment and treatment protocol for post-stroke depression

- Assess patient for symptoms of depression and other disorders using differential diagnoses in Table 12.1.
- If depression is diagnosed or is just suspected (e.g., in patients with comprehension impairment), assess for contraindications to treatment (e.g., medication allergies, heart conduction abnormalities, risk of bleeding) and assess for co-morbid conditions (e.g., generalized anxiety and apathy often accompany depression).
- Decide on the most appropriate treatment based on diagnosis, contraindications, and empirical data.
  - Depression with or without generalized anxiety – citalopram 20 mg or escitalopram 10 mg – if no response, nortriptyline with slow increase to 75–100 mg – if no response, ECT
  - Depression with pathological crying – citalopram 20 mg or escitalopram 10 mg or sertraline 50 mg. If no response, nortriptyline with slow increase to 75–100 mg.
  - Depression with apathy – citalopram 20 mg or escitalopram 10 mg. If no response, methylphenidate with slow increase to 30 mg.
- Assess drug side effects and tolerability in 1 week.
- Increase doses slowly in 1- to 2-week intervals and don't assume treatment failure until after 8 to 12 weeks of therapeutic doses.
- Continue treatment for 12 months or longer. If drug is stopped, be prepared for recurrence.
- If patient is non-depressed, consider preventive intervention for depression with escitalopram 10 mg (5 mg over 65) or problem-solving therapy.

Physical treatments

Antidepressants

Ten double-blind, randomized, placebo-controlled studies on treatment of PSD have been conducted. These trials are summarized in Table 12.3. Not all studies have found a significant difference in depression severity ratings between active and placebo treatment. The reason for most negative study outcomes was the high placebo response rate. Among three studies that reported negative findings, two found placebo response rates of 75% and 78%, respectively (20, 21). These high rates of placebo response would preclude any differentiation from active treatment.

Among the seven studies that reported that active treatment was superior to placebo, two documented that nortriptyline produced response rates of 100% and 77% compared with placebo response rates of 33% and 31% (22, 23). One study reported a significant treatment effect based on a 61% response rate to citalopram over 6 weeks compared with a 31% placebo response rate (24). The data on fluoxetine, however, have been mixed, with one study reporting a 62% response rate compared to 33% with placebo (25); three studies found that fluoxetine was not superior to placebo (20, 23, 26).

A recent meta-analysis included 1320 patients with PSD identified from 16 randomized controlled trials (27). Pooled response rates in the active groups (selective serotonin reuptake inhibitors [SSRIs], tricyclics, or other antidepressants) were significantly higher than in the placebo groups (i.e., 65.2% [234/359], and 44.4% [138/311], respectively) (rate difference, 0.23; 95% confidence interval [CI], 0.03 to 0.43). In addition, longer duration of treatment was positively correlated with the degree of improvement in depressive symptoms (Rho = -0.93, p = .001). Thus, there is empirical evidence supporting the efficacy and safety of antidepressants among patients with PSD. Among the SSRIs, the best evidence supports the use of citalopram 20 mg and 10 mg for those older than age 65. Among the tricyclics, the best data are available for nortriptyline 75 to 100 mg to treat PSD. In only one controlled study using stimulants, methylphenidate 30 mg was superior to placebo (28). The drug was well tolerated and might be used as an alternative treatment for those in whom treatment with other antidepressants fails, or for those who have severe psychomotor retardation or apathy.

Table 12.3 Treatment studies of post-stroke depression

Author (Ref.)	N	Medication (n) (max dose)	Duration	Evaluation method	Results	Response rate	Completion rate
Double-blind placebo-controlled studies							
Lipsey et al. (22)	34	Nortrip (14) (max 100 mg)	6 wk	HamD, ZDS	Nortrip > placebo int to treat and eff	Completers: 100% Nortrip 33% placebo	11 of 14 Nortrip 15 of 20 placebo
Reding et al. (41)	27	Traz (7) (max 200 mg) Placebo (9)	32+6 d	ZDS	Efficacy: Traz > placebo on Barthel ADL for pts abnl DST	NR	
Andersen et al. (42)	66	Cital (33) (20 mg, 10 mg > 65 yr) placebo (33)	6 wk	HamD, MES	Int to treat Cital > placebo	Completers: 61% Cital 29% placebo	26 of 33 Cital 31 of 33 placebo
Grade et al. (28)	21	Methylphen 30 mg (max 3 mg) placebo	3 wk	HamD	Int to treat Methyl > placebo	NR	9 of 10 Methyl 10 of 11 placebo
Wiart et al. (25)	31	Fluox (20 mg) placebo	6 wk	MADRS	Int to treat Fluox > placebo	62% Fluox 33% placebo	14 of 16 Fluox 15 of 15 placebo
Robinson et al. (23)	56	Fluox (23) (40 mg) Nortrip (16) (100 mg) placebo (17)	12 wk	HamD	Int to treat Nortrip > bo = Fluox = placebo	14% Fluox 77% Nortrip 31% placebc	14 of 23 Fluox 13 of 16 Nortrip 13 of 17 placebo
Fruehwald et al. (20)	54	Fluox (28) (20 mg) Placebo (26)	12 wk	Beck (BDF) HamD	HamD > 15 Fluox = placebo HamD scores	69% Fluox HamD≤13 75% placebo	26 of 28 Fluox 24 of 26 placebo
Rampello et al. (43)	31	Reboxetine (16) (4 mg) placebo (15)	16 wk	Beck HamD	Rebox > placebo for retarded dep pts	NR	NR
Murray et al. (21)	123	Sertraline (50–100 mg)	26 wk	MADRS	Sertral = placebo	76% sertraline 78% placebo	38 of 62 sertraline 31 of 61 placebo
Choi-Kwon et al. (26)	51	Fluox (20 mg)	12 wk	BDI	Fluox = placebo	NR	NR

Electroconvulsive therapy

Electroconvulsive therapy (ECT) was found useful in two retrospective chart reviews (29, 30). Currier et al. found that 19 of 20 elderly patients with PSD "markedly or moderately" improved (29). No patients developed exacerbations of stroke or new neurological deficits. Major complications, defined as requiring medical intervention, occurred in 25% of patients; prolonged postictal confusion and amnesia occurred in 15% of patients (30). Thus, ECT appears to be safe and possibly more effective than pharmacologic intervention for the treatment of post-stroke depression; however, rigorous clinical trials are needed to confirm these findings.

Effect of antidepressants on outcome

Recovery in activities of daily living

Most studies have failed to find a difference in recovery when comparing patients given antidepressants versus those given placebo. However, some studies have found a beneficial effect of treatment. For example, one study compared recovery in ADLs between patients whose depression remitted and those whose depression did not remit (31). Another study found that patients who were treated with antidepressants within the first month following stroke had significantly better recovery in ADLs by two years following stroke compared with patients who were treated after the first month post stroke (32).

Recovery in cognitive function

Similar to findings with recovery in ADLs, most treatment trials have failed to show a significant effect of active compared with placebo treatment on recovery in cognitive function. However, some studies have reported a beneficial effect.

For example, one study compared patients who responded to nortriptyline versus patients who failed to respond, and showed significantly higher Mini-Mental State Exam scores in responders at 75 and 100 mg of nortriptyline compared with non-responders (33). Another recent study found that treatment with escitalopram, 10 mg over 1 year, among non-depressed patients led to significantly greater recovery as measured by the Repeatable Battery for the Assessment of Neuropsychological Status (RBANS) compared with placebo (34).

Mortality

As indicated in the Background section, six studies have found that patients with post-stroke depression have increased mortality compared with non-depressed stroke patients. Two studies, however, reported that the use of antidepressants following stroke decreased the mortality rate as early as one year and as long as nine years following stroke (13, 35). Ried et al. (13) reported 8.0% mortality among 543 veterans with stroke and no antidepressant treatment compared with 4.8% mortality among 146 veterans with stroke who received antidepressants. An earlier study by Jorge et al. (35) reported that 67.9% of 53 patients given fluoxetine or nortriptyline in a double-blind study were alive at nine years follow-up compared with only 35.7% of the 28 patients given placebo. A logistic regression controlling for age, stroke severity, co-morbid diabetes, and recurrent depression showed that the use of antidepressants after stroke was an independent factor promoting survival.

Thus, available data support the conclusion that the administration of antidepressant medications following stroke not only is likely to improve depressive symptoms, but may benefit recovery in ADLs, cognitive function, and survival with relatively little risk to the patient with acute stroke.

Psychosocial interventions

Only two studies have used cognitive-behavioral therapy (CBT) to treat PSD (36). One included 23 patients given ten CBT sessions over three months and found no difference in depression rates between an attention-placebo group and a no-contact group (36).

Studies that have used a multi-disciplinary approach to treat PSD are limited. Recently, Williams and co-workers conducted a randomized trial of a care management intervention

(Activate-Initiate-Monitor intervention) versus usual care for treatment of PSD (37). It consisted of three main steps: (1) to "activate" stroke survivors and their families to understand and accept the diagnosis of depression and the need for treatment; (2) to initiate antidepressant medication; and (3) to monitor treatment effectiveness. The main finding was that care management resulted in greater remission of depression and reduction of depressive symptoms compared with usual care alone. Consistent with this study, a recent report presented an integrated care (IC) model consisting of a multi-faceted program that provided ongoing collaboration between a specialist stroke service and primary care physicians, using telephone tracking, a bi-directional information feedback loop, management of vascular risk factors, and regular screening for depressive symptoms. At 12 months, 30/91 (33%) of the treatment group had depressive symptoms, compared with 52/95 (55%) of the control group (p = .003) (38).

Another elegant study examined the impact of a physical exercise program on depressive symptoms in stroke survivors (39). Physical exercise during the sub-acute recovery phase of stroke had a beneficial effect on depressive symptoms. However, results of this study are limited by the lack of a formal psychiatric interview.

Preventive intervention

Because PSD has been associated with impaired recovery and increased mortality, consideration of a preventive intervention among non-depressed patients should be discussed with the patient, the family, and the treating physician. One study has recently demonstrated the utility of prevention for PSD (40).

Within three months of stroke, 59 patients were randomly assigned to escitalopram (10 mg age 65 years or younger, 5 mg age 66 years or older) for 12 months, 59 were assigned to problem-solving therapy (PST), and 58 were assigned to placebo. Depression developed in 22.4% of patients in the placebo group, 8.5% in the escitalopram group, and 11.9% in the PST group. Patients in the placebo group were 4.5 times (95% CI, 2.4 to 8.2; p < .001) and 2.2 times (95% CI, 1.4 to 3.5; p < .001) more likely to develop depression than those in the escitalopram and PST groups. Thus, when you are consulted on a patient who is ultimately found to not have depression, the potential benefits of a preventive intervention should be considered.

References

1. Robinson RG. The clinical neuropsychiatry of stroke. 2nd ed. Cambridge: Cambridge University Press; 2006.

2. Morris PLP, Robinson RG, Raphael B. Prevalence and course of depressive disorders in hospitalized stroke patients. Int J Psychiatr Med. 1990;20(4):349–64.

3. Astrom M, Adolfsson R, Asplund K. Major depression in stroke patients: a 3-year longitudinal study. Stroke. 1993;24(7):976–82.

4. Starkstein SE, Robinson RG, Price TR. Comparison of cortical and subcortical lesions in the production of poststroke mood disorders. Brain. 1987;110 (Pt 4): 1045–59.

5. Starkstein SE, Robinson RG, Price TR. Comparison of patients with and without poststroke major depression matched for size and location of lesion. Arch Gen Psychiatry. 1988;45(3):247–52.

6. Andersen G, Vestergaard K, Ingemann-Nielsen M, Lauritzen L. Risk factors for post-stroke depression. Acta Psychiatr Scand. 1995;92(3):193–8.

7. Angeleri F, Angeleri VA, Foschi N, et al. The influence of depression, social activity,

and family stress on functional outcome after stroke. Stroke. 1993;24(20):1478–83.

8. Paradiso S, Robinson RG. Gender differences in poststroke depression. J Neuropsychiatry Clin Neurosci. 1998; 10(1):41–7.

9. Tenev VT, Robinson RG, Jorge RE. Is family history of depression a risk factor for poststroke depression? Meta-analysis. Am J Geriatr Psychiatry. 2009;17(4):276–80.

10. Morris PL, Robinson RG, Raphael B, et al. The relationship between risk factors for affective disorder and poststroke depression in hospitalised stroke patients. Aust N Z J Psychiatry. 1992;26(2):208–17.

11. Morris PL, Raphael B, Robinson RG. Clinical depression is associated with impaired recovery from stroke. Med J Aust. 1992;157(4):239–42.

12. Bolla-Wilson K, Robinson RG, et al. Lateralization of dementia of depression in stroke patients. Am J Psychiatry. 1989;146: 627–34.

13. Ried LD, Tueth MJ, Jia H. A pilot study to describe antidepressant prescriptions dispensed to veterans after stroke. Res Social Adm Pharm. 2006;2(1):96–109.

14. Andersen G, Vestergaard K, Ingemann-Nielsen M, Lauritzen L. Risk factors for post-stroke depression. Acta Psychiatr Scand 1995;92(3):193–8.

15. Stenager EN, Madsen C, Stenager E, Boldsen J. Suicide in patients with stroke: epidemiological study [see comment]. BMJ. 1998;316(7139):1206.

16. U.S. Department of Health and Human Services Public Health Service. Agency for Health Care Policy and Research. Post-stroke rehabilitation: assessment, referral, and patient management. Clin Pract Guide Quick Ref Guide Clin. 1995; (16):i–iii, 1–32.

17. Paradiso S, Ohkubo T, Robinson RG. Vegetative and psychological symptoms associated with depressed mood over the first two years after stroke. Int J Psychiatry Med. 1997;27(2):137–57.

18. Whyte EM, Mulsant BH. Post stroke depression: epidemiology, pathophysio-logy, and biological treatment. Biol Psychiatry. 2002;52(3):253–64.

19. Eriksson M, Asplund K, Glader EL, et al. Self-reported depression and use of antidepressants after stroke: a national survey. Stroke. 2004;35(4):936–41.

20. Fruehwald S, Gatterbauer E, Rehak P, Baumhackl U. Early fluoxetine treatment of post-stroke depression – a three-month double-blind placebo-controlled study with an open-label long-term follow up. J Neurol. 2003;250(3):347–51.

21. Murray V, von Arbin M, Bartfai A, et al. Double-blind comparison of sertraline and placebo in stroke patients with minor depression and less severe major depression. J Clin Psychiatry. 2005;66(6): 708–16.

22. Lipsey JR, Robinson RG, Pearlson GD, et al. Nortriptyline treatment of post-stroke depression: a double-blind study. Lancet. 1984;i(8372):297–300.

23. Robinson RG, Schultz SK, Castillo C, et al. Nortriptyline versus fluoxetine in the treatment of depression and in short term recovery after stroke: a placebo controlled, double-blind study. Am J Psychiatry. 2000; 157(3):351–9.

24. Andersen G, Vestergaard K, Riis J. Citalopram for post-stroke pathological crying. Lancet. 1993;342(8875): 837–9.

25. Wiart L, Petit H, Joseph PA, et al. Fluoxetine in early poststroke depression: a double-blind placebo-controlled study. Stroke. 2000;31:1829–32.

26. Choi-Kwon S, Han SW, Kwon SU, et al. Fluoxetine treatment in poststroke depression, emotional incontinence, and anger proneness: a double-blind, placebo-controlled study. Stroke. 2006; 37(1):156–61.

27. Chen Y, Guo JJ, Zhan S, Patel NC. Treatment effects of antidepressants in patients with post-stroke depression: a meta-analysis. Ann Pharmacother. 2006; 40(12):2115–22.

28. Grade C, Redford B, Chrostowski J, et al. Methylphenidate in early poststroke

recovery: a double-blind, placebo-controlled study. Arch Phys Med Rehabil. 1998;79(9):1047–50.

29. Currier MB, Murray GB, Welch CC. Electroconvulsive therapy for post-stroke depressed geriatric patients. J Neuropsychiatry Clin Neurosci. 1992;4:140–4.

30. Murray GB, Shea V, Conn DK. Electroconvulsive therapy for poststroke depression. J Clin Psychiatry. 1986;47(5): 258–60.

31. Chemerinski E, Robinson RG, Arndt S, Kosier JT. The effect of remission of poststroke depression on activities of daily living in a double-blind randomized treatment study. J Nerv Ment Dis. 2001; 189(7):421–5.

32. Narushima K, Robinson RG. The effect of early versus late antidepressant treatment on physical impairment associated with poststroke depression: is there a time-related therapeutic window? J Nerv Ment Dis. 2003;191(10):645–52.

33. Kimura M, Robinson RG, Kosier T. Treatment of cognitive impairment after poststroke depression. Stroke. 2000;31(7): 1482–6.

34. Jorge RE, Robinson RG. Escitalopram enhances cognitive recovery following stroke. Arch Gen Psychiatry. 2010;67(2):187–96.

35. Jorge RE, Robinson RG, Arndt S, Starkstein S. Mortality and poststroke depression: a placebo-controlled trial of antidepressants. Am J Psychiatry. 2003;160(10):1823–9.

36. Lincoln NB, Flannaghan T. Cognitive behavioral psychotherapy for depression following stroke: a randomized controlled trial. Stroke. 2003;34(1):111–5.

37. Williams LS, Kroenke K, Bakas T, et al. Care management of poststroke depression: a randomized, controlled trial. Stroke. 2007;38(3):998–1003.

38. Joubert J, Joubert L, Reid C, et al. The positive effect of integrated care on depressive symptoms in stroke survivors. Cerebrovasc Dis. 2008;26(2):199–205.

39. Fitzgerald PB, Oxley TJ, Laird AR, et al. An analysis of functional neuroimaging studies of dorsolateral prefrontal cortical activity in depression. Psychiatry Res. 2006; 148(1):33–45.

40. Robinson RG, Jorge RE, Moser DJ, et al. Escitalopram and problem-solving therapy for prevention of poststroke depression: a randomized controlled trial. JAMA. 2008; 299(20):2391–400.

41. Reding MJ, Orto LA, Winter SW, et al. Antidepressant therapy after stroke: a double-blind trial. Arch Neurol. 1986;43: 763–5.

42. Andersen G, Vestergaard K, Riis JO, Lauritzen L. Incidence of post-stroke depression during the first year in a large unselected stroke population determined using a valid standardized rating scale. Acta Psychiatr Scand. 1994;90(8875):190–5.

43. Rampello L, Alvano A, Chiechio S, et al. An evaluation of efficacy and safety of reboxetine in elderly patients affected by "retarded" post-stroke depression: a random, placebo-controlled study. Arch Gerontol Geriatr. 2005;40(3): 275–85.

Chapter 13

Psychiatric aspects of Parkinson's disease

Joanne A. Byars and Laura Marsh

Typical consult question

"Our patient is a fifty-eight year old man with Parkinson's disease. Lately, he seems uninterested and doesn't seem motivated to do anything anymore. Even when something good happens, he doesn't crack a smile. Is he depressed?"

Background

Overview of Parkinson's disease

Parkinson's disease (PD) is a progressive neurodegenerative disease characterized by loss of dopaminergic neurons in the substantia nigra (1). Neurotransmission of serotonin, norepinephrine, and acetylcholine is also altered (2). The three principal motor symptoms of PD are rigidity, bradykinesia, and tremor (3). However, not all patients have all three motor symptoms. The classic tremor of PD is a rest tremor, but patients can have a postural or action tremor, or no tremor at all. Other early neurological signs include decreased facial expression (i.e., the masked face), or micrographia. Postural instability and autonomic dysfunction may occur later (4). About 1% of adults over age 60 have PD, with average age of onset in their sixties, although 5% to 10% of patients have young-onset PD, defined as onset before age 40 (5).

Although defined as a movement disorder, PD consists of overlapping motor, cognitive, and psychiatric features, which sometimes are difficult to distinguish. If a patient with PD has little emotional reactivity, is this the blunted affect of depression, an abulia characteristic of frontal-subcortical impairment, or the motor sign of facial masking? The frequency of psychiatric co-morbidities in PD and these phenomena of ambiguous origin often prompt psychiatric consultation.

Work-up

The term *Parkinson's disease* refers to the idiopathic form of the disease, but patients can have parkinsonism of other causes, such as medications or toxins (6). Other parkinsonian syndromes include progressive supranuclear palsy (PSP), dementia with Lewy Bodies (DLB), corticobasal ganglionic degeneration (CBGD), multiple system atrophy (MSA), fronto-temporal dementia with parkinsonism-17, vascular parkinsonism, Wilson's disease,

Psychosomatic Medicine: An Introduction to Consultation-Liaison Psychiatry, eds. James J. Amos and Robert G. Robinson. Published by Cambridge University Press. © Cambridge University Press 2010.

and Westphal variant of Huntington's disease (5, 6). Psychiatric symptoms are common in all parkinsonian disorders, but this chapter focuses on PD.

The first step in treating a patient with PD and psychiatric symptoms is ensuring that the patient actually has PD. Characteristic symptom patterns may distinguish PD from other forms of parkinsonism (4, 7). In PD, symptoms, or at least signs, begin unilaterally, progress asymmetrically, and improve with levodopa treatment. Early dementia (i.e., within the first year after motor symptom onset) or psychosis early in the illness course in the absence of dopaminergic treatment raises concern for DLB (6). Although antipsychotics are well-known causes of parkinsonism, non-psychiatric medications, such as antiemetics, also cause drug-induced parkinsonism that may be mistaken for new-onset PD, especially in older patients (5). Normal pressure hydrocephalus and degenerative spinal change are other causes of gait changes in the elderly that can be mistaken for PD.

Clinical decision-making and treatment

No disease-modifying treatments or neuroprotective drugs exist for PD (7). Symptomatic treatment for motor symptoms aims at restoring the dopamine no longer supplied by the substantia nigra. Treatments include levodopa; dopamine agonists such as pramipexole, ropinirole, and apomorphine; monoamine oxidase inhibitors such as seligiline and rasagaline; and glutamatergic antagonists such as amantadine. Anticholinergic agents may reduce tremor, but have prominent side effects (5). Deep brain stimulation (DBS) treats motor symptoms and the motor complications of dopaminergic therapy, namely, extreme motor fluctuations resulting from diminution, between doses, of the dopaminergic benefit on motor function (called "on-off" phenomena), dystonia, and hyperkinetic choreiform movements referred to as *dyskinesias* (3, 5). Physical exercise is an important component of disease management.

Psychiatric disturbances: background

Psychiatric symptoms are highly prevalent in PD, but are often unrecognized and under-treated, and are easily missed if not specifically investigated. Neuropsychiatric disturbances of PD fall into several main categories: mood and anxiety disorders, psychosis, behavioral changes including sexual disorders, impulse control disorders, abuse of dopaminergic medications, and sleep disorders.

Psychiatric disorders occur in PD from various causes. Some patients experience adjustment reactions to the stress of illness, but many psychiatric symptoms appear directly attributable to the neurobiology of PD or its treatment (3). PD disrupts frontal-subcortical circuits and alters neurotransmitters – dopamine, norepinephrine, and serotonin – involved in psychiatric symptoms (3). Dopaminergic treatment can induce psychiatric side effects, and anticholinergics can impair cognition. Complications of PD, such as a subdural hematoma and cognitive decline resulting from a PD-related fall, also trigger psychiatric problems. Depression and anxiety may represent risk factors for or prodromes of PD, as individuals who develop PD have elevated rates of pre-morbid depression and anxiety (6). The "on-off" phenomenon resulting from fluctuations in dopaminergic state can be associated with emotional lability in addition to motor fluctuations. Typically, such patients experience euphoria or euthymia in the "on" state and dysphoria or anxiety in the "off" state (3). Distress or affective worsening can precede motor worsening, suggesting that emotional changes are not due to the stress of motor fluctuations (2).

117

Most psychiatric disorders in PD are treatable, and lack of treatment has adverse consequences. Multiple studies show that psychiatric symptoms have a greater impact on quality of life than motor symptoms (8). Depression may have the largest effect on quality of life in PD and is linked to declines in cognitive functioning, activities of daily living, and motor functioning (8–10). Psychosis causes the most stress for caregivers and strongly predicts nursing home placement (11). The goal of treatment for psychiatric disorders in PD should be *remission* – it is essential to avoid undertreatment.

Work-up for the patient with Parkinson's disease and psychiatric illness

Clinicians should screen all patients with PD for psychiatric disorders, as patients may not mention psychiatric symptoms spontaneously. Collateral information from family or other associates can clarify symptoms, particularly when there is cognitive dysfunction or impulse control disorders and patients are less likely to provide an accurate history. As with all patients with psychiatric complaints, patients with PD should be assessed for potential dangerousness to self or others.

Medications used to treat PD, particularly dopaminergic and anticholinergic agents, can induce mental status changes. Medications should be reviewed and changes made as needed to reduce psychiatric side effects, with attention to the temporal context of when psychiatric symptoms developed relative to changes in PD medications.

Pain and fatigue occur commonly in PD and can be mistaken for somatization or symptoms of depression (2). Depression worsens pain and fatigue, but dyskinesias, dystonia, musculoskeletal problems, and the "off" state (2, 8) can directly cause hyperalgesia and fatigue in the absence of psychopathology.

Laboratory and imaging findings are usually unremarkable in PD, whether or not psychiatric symptoms are present. Abnormalities may indicate a supervening non-PD condition resulting in psychiatric complaints.

Neuropsychological testing can evaluate whether cognitive deficits are consistent with PD or point to another disorder, and can assess response to interventions intended to improve cognition. Neuropsychological testing and occupational therapy assessments help clarify level of cognitive functioning, and identify ways to compensate for deficiencies that capitalize on areas of preserved functioning.

Clinical decision-making and treatment

Few evidence-based guidelines have been put forth for treatment of psychiatric disorders in PD. Recommendations follow the general principles for treatment of idiopathic psychiatric disorders in geriatric or medically ill populations, with attention to avoiding negative side effects that could worsen PD symptoms. Medical treatment of PD should be optimized, as suboptimal treatment can worsen psychiatric symptoms. Psychotherapy is an evidence-based treatment for many idiopathic psychiatric disorders, and does not cause side effects or worsen motor symptoms. Educating patients, families, and clinicians about the psychiatric features of PD reduces misinterpretations of patients' behaviors, and may minimize avoidable interpersonal conflict (3).

Specific psychiatric disorders in Parkinson's disease

Mood disorders: background

Depression, apathy, and pseudobulbar affect

Depression occurs more commonly in PD than in other chronic illnesses; the severity of depressive symptoms in PD is not related to the duration of motor illness or the severity of motor symptoms (2). Even "sub-syndromal" forms of depression cause significant suffering and impairment (10). Depression exacerbates PD-related cognitive problems, and is often co-morbid with other psychiatric conditions (9, 10).

Work-up

Previous studies suggest that PD-related depression is characterized by more dysphoria and irritability, and less guilt and suicidality, than idiopathic depression, but individual cases show the range of depressive phenomena (2). Bradykinesia, or slowed motor movements, and reduced facial expression are prominent features of PD that resemble psychomotor slowing, which, along with PD symptoms like fatigue and sleep problems, overlap with *Diagnostic and Statistical Manual (DSM)-IV-TR* criteria for major depressive disorder (MDD) (9). Focusing on emotional rather than neurovegetative symptoms may aid in diagnosing depression in PD. One way to distinguish depressive syndromes from PD symptoms is to ask "How do you spend your time?" and see if patients brighten, engage in conversation, and describe recent activities that bring them pleasure (12).

Apathy is also common, possibly caused by dopamine depletion (13). Patients with apathy appear indifferent to their surroundings, show little interest in themselves or others, and engage in few activities, including spontaneous conversation (12). Apathy can be a feature of MDD or may represent a distinct disorder (14). Apathy should also be distinguished from facial masking or bradyphrenia. Low testosterone may exacerbate PD-related apathy (8).

Apathy worsens outcomes in PD, as patients are less likely to provide self-care, comply with treatment, and exercise (12). Apathy is often unrecognized. Apathetic patients do not complain, but their behavior often distresses families (9). Caregivers should be educated about apathy, to avoid misattributing the patient's behavior as deliberate. Patients with apathy benefit from an enriched, structured environment, as they rarely do much on their own initiative (15).

Pseudobulbar affect, also referred to as emotional incontinence or pathological laughing and crying, occurs in PD and other neurological diseases. Patients with pseudobulbar affect display excessive or spontaneous emotional reactions in the absence of a congruent mood state (9). As such, pseudobulbar affect represents a behavioral abnormality that potentially represents disrupted brain circuitry rather than a mood disturbance per se. Although the frequent tearfulness of pseudobulbar affect mimics depression, crying episodes in pseudobulbar affect are regarded by patients as excessive or "out of the blue," without accompanying feelings of sadness (16).

Clinical decision-making and treatment

To treat mood disturbances in PD, clinicians should optimize PD treatment, and treat any other potentially contributing medical conditions (15). Selective serotonin reuptake inhibitors (SSRIs) are generally considered first-line treatment for depression in PD, given their low risk of side effects. Tricyclic antidepressants (TCAs) and serotonin-norepinephrine reuptake inhibitors (SNRIs) may treat depression as well, and recent evidence suggests they may be more effective than SSRIs or placebo. However, TCAs cause an increased risk of delirium and falls (10). SSRIs and TCAs may improve pseudobulbar affect (16). Bupropion may help with depression, apathy, and possibly even motor symptoms (9). Selegiline, a monoamine oxidase (MAO)-B inhibitor, may treat both PD motor symptoms and depression; risk of serotonin syndrome occurs when combined with SSRIs/SNRIs, although in actual practice, this appears more theoretical (2). Stimulants may reduce apathy and amotivation (6). Non-stimulant dopamine agonists, such as pramipexole, may ameliorate depressive symptoms as well as motor symptoms (10). Electroconvulsive therapy (ECT) improves both mood and motor symptoms; however, patients with PD are at increased risk for ECT-induced delirium (1). Psychotherapy may represent a good first-line intervention for mild depression or as adjunctive treatment with medications and warrants further study in PD (9).

Mania

Mania and hypomania in PD typically occur as the result of dopaminergic or other PD treatment, not as the result of PD (15). However, some patients develop bipolar disorder long before onset of PD and subsequently develop PD later in life.

Mania due to medications or another medical condition requires treatment of the underlying cause. In mania due to dopaminergic medications, attempts should be made to adjust dopaminergic treatment. If no specific cause of mania can be identified, mood stabilizers may be considered, although they are not well studied in PD.

Anxiety disorders: background

Although patients with PD may have reactive worries from illness-related problems, most anxiety disturbances in PD are not related to motor severity. Rather, they appear related to the underlying neurobiological changes associated with the disease itself, which often present prodromally before PD is diagnosed (3). The most common anxiety disorders in PD are panic disorder, generalized anxiety disorder, and social phobia, but many anxiety disturbances in PD do not fall into classic *DSM* categories (9, 17).

Work-up

Obsessive-compulsive disorder (OCD) is not more prevalent in PD than in the general population. However, patients with PD, especially those with advanced disease, can exhibit repetitive, stereotyped behaviors known as "punding" that resemble OCD, but lack true obsessive or compulsive characteristics (18). Anxiety disorders in PD are often co-morbid with depression (9). The somatic symptoms of anxiety – tremor, poor sleep, impaired concentration, and diaphoresis – overlap with symptoms of PD, complicating diagnosis (19). Focusing on the emotional phenomena of anxiety disorders may improve their recognition.

Clinical decision-making and treatment

Anxiety treatments in PD have not been studied empirically; thus current approaches follow the general principles used with idiopathic anxiety in the elderly. Optimizing PD treatment and addressing co-morbid medical and psychiatric conditions are essential first steps. SSRIs are good first-line choices because of their favorable side effect profile. Starting with low doses and slowly titrating upwards may help reduce the risk of acute increases in anxiety that may occur with initiation of SSRI treatment. Benzodiazepines may reduce anxiety, but increase PD patients' already heightened risk for confusion and falls (15); they should be reserved for cases in which other interventions have failed. Psychotherapy, particularly cognitive-behavioral therapy, may be beneficial (9, 15).

Psychotic disorders: background

Except later in the illness course, psychotic symptoms in PD generally are associated with any of the antiparkinsonian medications. The diagnosis of DLB is a consideration when psychosis occurs before dopaminergic treatment is provided. Risk factors for psychotic symptoms in PD include poor vision; late-stage PD; and cognitive, mood, and sleep disorders (11). Psychotic symptoms may occur independently of other psychiatric manifestations, or as part of a mood disorder, dementia, or delirium (1).

Work-up

In PD, visual hallucinations are the most common psychotic symptom, in contrast to the idiopathic psychoses such as schizophrenia, in which most hallucinations are auditory. However, hallucinations in PD can occur in any sensory modality. Visual hallucinations can manifest as hallucinosis, occurring on a background of clear consciousness with retained insight. Visual hallucinations can be well formed and are often Lilliputian (2, 11). Delusions typically are paranoid, but may be of any type. Patients should be asked about the nature of their hallucinations and delusions; persecutory psychotic content may result in dangerous behaviors, especially if patients lack insight. Once psychotic symptoms develop, they tend to persist.

Clinical decision-making and treatment

The first step in treating PD-related psychosis is decreasing the dose of dopaminergic medications or changing to another dopaminergic agent. Dopamine agonists may be more likely than levodopa to cause psychosis. Co-morbid medical and psychiatric problems should also be treated.

If psychosis persists after changes are made in the dopaminergic regimen, or if these changes adversely impact motor symptoms, then antipsychotics can be used. In practice, the first-line antipsychotic for PD is quetiapine, as it is the second-least-likely antipsychotic to worsen motor symptoms. Clozapine is the least likely to cause extrapyramidal symptoms (EPS), but may cause agranulocytosis and requires weekly monitoring. Olanzapine, risperidone, and high-potency typical neuroleptics should be avoided, as they worsen motor symptoms. Other antipsychotics are not well studied in PD. Patients with PD show heightened sensitivity to antipsychotic side effects, including neuroleptic malignant syndrome (NMS); abrupt cessation of dopamine treatment can also cause an NMS-like syndrome (2, 20). Preliminary evidence suggests that cholinesterase inhibitors may reduce psychosis in PD (9). ECT is an option for psychosis in PD, particularly for psychotic depression or medication-refractory psychosis (11).

Cognitive disorders: background

The most common cognitive disorder in PD is the cognitive impairment subthreshold for dementia (15). PD-related cognitive problems often go unnoticed because patients remain relatively verbally intact, even as deteriorating executive functioning causes social and professional impairment (21). Even mild deficits cause substantial problems for patients. Cognitive disorders can occur from the neuropathology of PD itself, or as the result of medical and neurosurgical treatments for PD (6, 8, 21). PD-related dementia increases mortality and nursing home placement (1).

The pattern of cognitive impairment in PD differs from that seen in Alzheimer's dementia. Cognitive disorders in PD follow a frontal-subcortical pattern, with more executive dysfunction than memory loss. Symptoms include problems with planning and set-shifting, cognitive slowing, difficulties with memory retrieval in the context of relatively intact recognition memory, impairment of attention and working memory, and visuospatial dysfunction (6).

Work-up

The Mini-Mental State Exam (MMSE) lacks sensitivity to frontal-subcortical impairment, and often misses PD-related cognitive deficits. Focused questions about acquired executive dysfunction and other cognitive symptoms are often necessary. Formal neuropsychological testing may help in identifying PD-related cognitive decline, but performance on such tests can remain in the normal range despite dysfunction in everyday activities. This pattern is often seen earlier in the course, when executive dysfunction predominates, and in individuals with higher pre-morbid cognitive abilities.

Clinical decision-making and treatment

No specific treatment is known for PD-related cognitive changes (9, 15). Patients should be evaluated for treatable medical problems and psychiatric conditions, particularly depression, that can worsen cognition. Medications that impair cognition, like benzodiazepines and anticholinergics, should be eliminated. Preliminary data suggest that cholinesterase inhibitors and memantine may offer some benefit in PD-related cognitive disorders (2). Further general recommendations are found in the "Dementia" chapter of this handbook.

Other psychiatric symptoms in Parkinson's disease: background, work-up, and clinical decision-making and treatment

Delirium

The underlying brain changes of PD increase vulnerability to delirium. Dopaminergic and anticholinergic medications used to treat PD themselves can cause delirium (8, 22). In general, the same recommendations for delirium in other populations apply to delirium in PD. However, haloperidol should be avoided, as it can dangerously worsen motor symptoms. Additional management guidelines are found in the "Delirium" section of this handbook.

Sleep disorders

Sleep disorders occur frequently in PD. Insomnia and obstructive sleep apnea (OSA) are common and may cause daytime fatigue and excessive daytime sleepiness. Restless legs syndrome, periodic limb movements of sleep, and sleep fragmentation may disrupt sleep. Dopamine agonist therapy can provoke sleep attacks, in which patients suddenly fall asleep during daytime activities (23). Dopaminergic treatment may produce vivid dreams, potentially presaging the later development of daytime visual hallucinations (11).

REM behavior disorder (RBD) represents a dramatic parasomnia strongly correlated with parkinsonian syndromes. Patients with RBD physically act out their dreams instead of remaining paralyzed during REM sleep. RBD should *always* prompt work-up for a parkinsonian syndrome when diagnosed in patients not known to have one; in patients with PD who have RBD, RBD precedes the movement disorder up to 50% of the time (23).

In general, sleep disorders in PD are treated as in other geriatric or medically ill patients. Promoting good sleep hygiene is a first-line intervention (15). Optimizing PD treatment and treating co-morbid psychiatric conditions may improve sleep, as can addressing specific treatable sleep disorders like OSA. Avoiding medications that disrupt sleep or cause daytime somnolence may help significantly. Clonazepam may be specifically helpful for RBD (9). Many sedative/hypnotics have side effects that pose special concerns in patients with PD, as they may increase the likelihood of falls and delirium (19).

Clinicians should assess whether sleep-related problems endanger the patient or others. Patients should avoid driving if excessive daytime sleepiness or sleep attacks make this unsafe; the bed partners of patients with RBD may need to sleep in another room to maintain their safety (23).

Sexual disorders

Sexual problems in PD may result from autonomic dysfunction, motor difficulties, decreased dopamine levels, or psychological factors (24, 25). Common sexual disorders in PD include decreased libido, decreased arousal, erectile dysfunction, and impaired orgasm (1).

Optimizing treatment of PD may improve sexual disorders. Dopaminergic agents not only treat motor symptoms of PD, but may enhance libido. Minimizing medications that can inhibit sexual functioning, such as SSRIs, and treating comorbid medical and psychiatric problems can also help. If sexual disorders persist after these changes, the same interventions used in non-PD populations, like education, psychotherapy, or medications like sildenafil, can be used (24).

Behavioral changes and impulse control disorders

Behavioral changes and impulse control disorders (ICDs) generally occur as the result of PD treatments, not PD itself. Manifestations include pathological gambling, compulsive shopping, paraphilias, hypersexuality, and aggression. Although patients frequently lack insight into the problem, these behaviors can engender serious financial, legal, and social difficulties. Clinicians must ask specifically about these behaviors, because patients and families may not volunteer this sensitive information (18). Given patients' frequent lack of insight or denial, collateral information is essential.

The first step in treating behavioral changes and ICDs is ensuring that the patient and others are safe. This may involve providing a structured environment, increased supervision, or having the family assume control of the patient's affairs. Adjusting the dopaminergic regimen sometimes resolves behavioral problems, as some agents provoke these symptoms more frequently than others. No definitive pharmacologic treatments are available for behavioral disturbances and ICDs in PD. Treating any co-morbid psychiatric conditions such as mania and psychosis that could exacerbate these symptoms may help. Quetiapine and clozapine have been helpful in some patients.

Abuse of dopaminergic medications

Although dopaminergic medications are not typically viewed as drugs of abuse, some patients with PD develop a maladaptive pattern in which they compulsively take much more dopaminergic medication than is needed to control motor symptoms. Often, these patients show the craving and drug-seeking behaviors seen in more traditional addictions (15). Abuse of dopaminergic medications can lead to serious motor side effects and psychiatric problems (18).

Treatment of dopaminergic medication abuse involves limiting patients to the doses actually needed to control PD symptoms. Patients who abuse dopaminergic medications often resist attempts to limit drug use; they may require hospitalization to taper down their medications, and family members may need to administer outpatient medications (13, 18). Treating co-morbid psychiatric problems may reduce abuse of dopaminergic medications.

References

1. Lauterbach EC. The neuropsychiatry of Parkinson's disease. Minerva Med. 2005; 96(3):155–73.

2. Truong DD, Bhidayasiri R, Wolters E. Management of non-motor symptoms in advanced Parkinson disease. J Neurol Sci. 2008;266(1–2):216–28.

3. Marsh L. Neuropsychiatric aspects of Parkinson's disease. Psychosomatics. 2000;41(1):15–23.

4. Jankovic J. Parkinson's disease: clinical features and diagnosis. J Neurol Neurosurg Psychiatry. 2008;79(4):368–76.

5. Samii A, Nutt JG, Ransom BR. Parkinson's disease. Lancet. 2004;363(9423):1783–93.

6. Marsh L. In: Kaplan & Sadock's Comprehensive Textbook of Psychiatry. Sadock BJ, Sadock VA, Kaplan HI, editors. 8th ed. Philadelphia: Lippincott Williams & Wilkins; 2004. p. 403–23.

7. Davie CA. A review of Parkinson's disease. Br Med Bull. 2008;86:109–27.

8. Chaudhuri KR, Healy DG, Schapira AH. Non-motor symptoms of Parkinson's disease: diagnosis and management. Lancet Neurol. 2006;5(3):235–45.

9. Borek LL, Chou KL, Friedman JH. Management of the behavioral aspects of Parkinson's disease. Expert Rev Neurother. 2007;7(6):711–25.

10. Richard IH. Depression and apathy in Parkinson's disease. Curr Neurol Neurosci Rep. 2007;7(4):295–301.

11. Zahodne LB, Fernandez HH. Pathophysiology and treatment of psychosis in Parkinson's disease: a review. Drugs Aging. 2008;25(8):665–82.

12. Shulman LM. Apathy in patients with Parkinson's disease. Int Rev Psychiatry. 2000;12:298–306.

13. Ferrara JM, Stacy M. Impulse-control disorders in Parkinson's disease. CNS Spectr. 2008;13(8):690–8.

14. Marsh L, McDonald WM, Cummings J, et al. Provisional diagnostic criteria for depression in Parkinson's disease: report of an NINDS/NIMH Work Group. Mov Disord. 2006;21(2):148–58.

15. Ferreri F, Agbokou C, Gauthier S. Recognition and management of neuropsychiatric complications in Parkinson's disease. CMAJ. 2006;175(12):1545–52.

16. Rosen HJ, Cummings J. A real reason for patients with pseudobulbar affect to smile. Ann Neurol. 2007;61(2):92–6.

17. Pontone GM, Williams JR, Anderson KE, et al. Prevalence of anxiety disorders and anxiety subtypes in patients with Parkinson's disease. Mov Disord. 2009; 24(9):1333–8.

18. Lim SY, Evans AH, Miyasaki JM. Impulse control and related disorders in Parkinson's disease: review. Ann N Y Acad Sci. 2008; 1142:85–107.

19. Mercury MG, Tschan W, Kehoe R, et al. The presence of depression and anxiety in Parkinson's disease. Dis Mon. 2007;53(5): 296–301.

20. Ueda M, Hamamoto M, Nagayama H, et al. Susceptibility to neuroleptic malignant syndrome in Parkinson's disease. Neurology. 1999;52(4):777–81.

21. Levin BE, Katzen HL. Early cognitive changes and nondementing behavioral abnormalities in Parkinson's disease. Adv Neurol. 1995;65:85–95.

22. Leentjens AF, Van Der Mast RC. Delirium in elderly people: an update. Curr Opin Psychiatry. 2005;18(3):325–30.

23. De Cock VC, Vidailhet M, Arnulf I. Sleep disturbances in patients with parkinsonism. Nat Clin Pract Neurol. 2008;4(5):254–66.

24. Balami J, Robertson D. Parkinson's disease and sexuality. Br J Hosp Med (Lond). 2007; 68(12):644–7.

25. Meco G, Rubino A, Caravona N, et al. Sexual dysfunction in Parkinson's disease. Parkinsonism Relat Disord. 2008;14(6): 451–6.

Managing depression in traumatic brain injury

Oludamilola Salami and Vani Rao

Typical consult question

"Please consult on this young male with history of persistent mood and behavior problems, since head injury 1 year ago."

Background

Introduction

Traumatic brain injury (TBI) is damage to the brain stemming from trauma to the head from a source outside of the brain. Even though the terms *head injury* and *traumatic brain injury* are often used interchangeably, it is important to remember that trauma to the head injury does not always result in brain injury. The severity of traumatic brain injury may range from mild to severe. TBI is a significant cause of disability and functional impairment worldwide. In this chapter, we will discuss features of depression from mild to severe, in the context of post-TBI depression.

Epidemiology

In the United States, there is an estimated incidence of more than 1.5 million cases of head injury annually, resulting in over a quarter of a million hospitalizations and more than 50,000 fatalities (1). More than 80,000 patients will experience chronic disability (2). The risk of fatal head injury is four times greater in men than in women. The incidence of head injury has a bimodal pattern, peaking from ages 15 to 25, with a second peak in advanced age (3). It is estimated that the healthcare cost for a patient with minor TBI over a one-year period is greater than $8,100 and in excess of $105,350 for those with severe head or spinal cord injuries (4).

The prevalence of major depressive disorder within the first year of TBI ranges from 26% to 33% (5, 6). Other population-based studies have found rates of 18.3% (7). This variation in rates may be due to the use of different assessment instruments for diagnosis, selection biases, and the influence of co-morbid psychiatric and psychosocial disorders (8). In any case, the prevalence of depression following TBI is higher than rates of depression within the general population.

Psychosomatic Medicine: An Introduction to Consultation-Liaison Psychiatry, eds. James J. Amos and Robert G. Robinson. Published by Cambridge University Press. © Cambridge University Press 2010.

Table 14.1 Classification of head injury

Assessment method	Severity of head injury		
Glasgow Coma Scale (GCS)	Mild	Moderate	Severe
	13–15	9–12	Less than 8
Loss of consciousness (LOC)	Less than 30 minutes	1–24 hours	Greater than 24 hours
Posttraumatic amnesia (PTA)	Less than 1 hour	1–24 hours	Greater than 24 hours

Table 14.2 Mechanisms of TBI

Direct physiologic effect of trauma		Indirect consequence of trauma
Focal Injury	Diffuse Injury	
1. Contusion	1. Edema	1. Hypoxia
2. Hypoxic-ischemic injury	2. Hypoxic-ischemic injury	2. Anemia
3. Hemorrhage	3. Diffuse vascular injury	3. Metabolic dyscrasias
4. Hematoma	4. Diffuse axonal injury	4. Fat embolism
		5. Release of excitatory amino acids
		6. Release of oxidative free radicals
		7. Disruption of neurotransmitter circuits

Classification

The most common causes of TBI are motor vehicle accidents, falls, violence, and sports and recreational activities (9). Several systems are available for classifying both the head injury and the severity of the associated brain injury. Severity of head injury can be determined on the basis of any combination of the following: initial Glasgow Coma Scale (GCS), the duration of loss of consciousness (LOC), and the duration of posttraumatic amnesia (PTA) (10) (Table 14.1).

On the basis of the underlying pathophysiologic mechanism of damage, brain injury can be classified into primary injury from direct impact of trauma and secondary injury from factors indirectly associated with trauma (11) (Table 14.2).

Etiologic mechanisms

The underlying etio-pathogenesis of post-TBI depression is most likely multi-factorial and most likely involves biopsychosocial factors. The main underlying mechanism of depressive mood symptoms is neuronal cellular damage. This mechanism results in several secondary effects including an inflammatory response and subsequent molecular changes. These changes involve protease activation, calcium influx, free radical release, lipid peroxidation, and phospholipase activation, which may further harm neuronal cells. Studies suggest that dysfunction at specific locations in the brain, particularly the left dorsolateral frontal cortex and the left subcortical areas (especially the basal ganglia), most often was associated with acute presentations of depression (12). It has also been hypothesized that dysfunction may occur in the neurotransmitter systems including norepinephrine, serotonin, dopamine, and acetylcholine via disruption of the neurotransmitter circuits and pathways between the frontal cortex and the basal ganglia. Psychosocial factors including the presence or absence of family, community, or other social supports may play a role in perpetuating the symptoms.

Risk factors for post-TBI depression

Key elements that may increase the risk of developing major depression and other neuropsychiatric symptoms following TBI are previous history of psychiatric illness, particularly mood and anxiety disorders (6), pre-morbid history of poor social functioning, advanced age, history of alcoholism, and the presence of arteriosclerotic vascular disease.

Other less significant risk factors include higher severity of TBI, higher level of cognitive impairment, relationships and other interpersonal issues, level of education, and compensation claims (11).

Clinical features of post-TBI depression

Several psychiatric syndromes have been reported in individuals with TBI. These include disturbances of mood, cognition, personality, and behavior (13). A key point is the question of whether depressive symptoms occur as a direct physiologic consequence of the brain injury or arise as a result of a psychological "reaction" to the consequences of TBI, as increased awareness into physical and neuropsychological impairments develops (14). It is likely that depressive symptoms result from a combination of these factors. Acute onset of depressive symptoms post TBI may have a higher correlation with left anterior cerebral involvement and physical disability, although delayed-onset post-TBI depression may have a stronger association with psychological and psychosocial factors (12).

Post-TBI depression may present with a cluster of depressive symptoms similar to idiopathic dysthymia or as part of the clinical syndrome of major depression. Most patients who present with mood symptoms following TBI present with major depressive symptoms (6). Major depression is a clinical syndrome with features of sustained feelings of sadness or low mood and associated neurovegetative and cognitive disturbances. These disturbances include changes in sleep, appetite, energy, concentration, and interests; feelings of worthlessness, guilt, or hopelessness; or thoughts of suicide. Patients with depression also show impairment in attention, problem-solving ability, and cognitive flexibility. These symptoms clearly interfere with rehabilitation, productivity, and quality of life, and cause clinically significant distress or impairment in social, occupational, or other important areas of function. However, of greater concern is the increased risk of suicide after TBI (15). A recent review of the literature on suicide following TBI revealed an increased risk of suicide for people with severe TBI compared with mild TBI. Risk factors for suicide attempt included the presence of suicide ideation post TBI and psychiatric or emotional distress (16).

The onset of depressive symptoms may be acute (within 1 to 3 months of injury) or delayed (longer than 3 months after injury). Jorge et al. in a study of 66 patients with TBI found a relationship between onset of depression within the first 3 months of TBI and lesion location in the left dorsolateral frontal region and or left basal ganglia. However, this relationship was lost in those with onset of depression after 3 months post TBI (12). Depression following TBI may be transient, lasting for a few days to weeks, or persistent, with a chronic course of weeks to months (11). Gradual remission of symptoms may occur, and this process may be shortened with appropriate treatment. The presence of psychological disturbance exceeding the severity of injury and poor cooperation with rehabilitation may predispose patients to persistence of depressive symptoms (17). Recovery from the effects of brain injury may be prolonged and follow a complex course. The type of injury (focal or diffuse), as well as the location, size, site, and presence of hemorrhage, edema, and other pathophysiologic features, may impact the recovery process.

Post-TBI depression is co-morbid with anxiety in up to 60% of cases and may be associated with aggressive behaviors (18). Psychological symptoms, if present, such as changes in self-attitude, hopelessness, suicidal ideation, loss of interest, low self-worth, and lack of self-confidence, are important in differentiating depressed from non-depressed persons (19).

Work-up

A comprehensive assessment should be performed on any individual who presents with brain injury. This evaluation must include a diagnostic interview that comprises a detailed history obtained from the patient, collateral information from all pertinent available sources, and a thorough review of past medical records. A physical and neurological examination should be conducted. In addition, a mental status examination and screening of global cognitive function (using the Mini-Mental State Examination [MMSE] or the modified MMSE [3MS], for example) should be performed. Aspects of the initial evaluation should also attempt to elicit the risk factors for developing depression, the risk of harm to the patient or others as a consequence of depression, the level of pre-morbid function, the severity of functional deficits, and compensatory or adaptive strategies to cope with these deficits. It may be helpful, particularly when determining prognosis and planning treatment, to identify accessible psychosocial support systems available to the patient. A legal history related to the TBI should be elicited to guide formulation of the prognosis and treatment options.

Additional investigations may be warranted, based on findings from the diagnostic interview, or if the initial assessment is inconclusive. These investigations should include laboratory testing such as complete blood count, comprehensive metabolic panel, serum vitamin B12 and folic acid, serology to screen for syphilis, and thyroid function tests. Neuropsychological assessments should be performed to better characterize the presence of cognitive

Table 14.3 Aspects of diagnostic evaluation

A. History
   I. Demographic information
   II. Family history of psychiatric illness
   III. Personal history (birth, development and early childhood history, education, relationships, and pre-morbid function)
   IV. Drug and alcohol and other substance use history
   V. Pre- and post-injury legal history
   VI. Medical history and current medications
   VII. Past psychiatric history
   VIII. History of head injury (type, nature, and severity of brain injury, mechanism of injury, GCS at the time of injury, duration of loss of consciousness or posttraumatic amnesia, neuropsychiatric sequelae, treatment of surgical and/or medical complications, and stage of recovery).
B. Physical and neurological examination
C. Mental status examination and cognitive assessment
D. Laboratory tests
E. Neuroimaging studies
F. Neuropsychological tests
G. Occupational therapy assessment

Key:
GCS = Glasgow Coma Scale

deficits and may also assist in clarifying suspicion of malingering. Neurological imaging studies may be obtained to determine the location, severity, and extent of associated structural brain pathology. An occupational therapy evaluation may be performed to assess the patient's functional and motor skills as well as safety (Table 14.3).

Accurate diagnosis of post-TBI major depression is arduous because a number of symptoms of major depression, particularly the neuropsychiatric symptoms, are directly related to the brain injury itself. TBI depression should be differentiated from demoralization, pathological crying, and the primary syndrome of TBI-associated apathy. Depressed mood, feelings of hopelessness, feelings of helplessness, and poor self-worth are often prominent and sustained in post-TBI depression. These symptoms are transient and related to physical and psychosocial impairments and to demoralization, and often are absent in pathological crying and apathy. In addition, neurovegetative symptoms including changes in sleep, appetite, energy, and concentration usually are present in post-TBI depression and transient in demoralization, and often are absent in pathologic crying and apathy (17).

Clinical decision-making and treatment

Managing post-TBI depression is often challenging. The approach to management may follow a biopsychosocial model involving pharmacotherapy, psychotherapy, education, and support for caregivers or family members. Management should incorporate a collaborative interdisciplinary and multi-faceted effort. Based on the specific needs of the patient at any point in time, members of the team should represent psychiatry, neurology, rehabilitation medicine, occupational therapy, and physical therapy, among others.

Several key principles may be employed in formulating a treatment plan (10). First, it is important to devise a comprehensive plan that is feasible, realistic, and appropriate, and that is based on aspects of the work-up pertinent to the biopsychosocial needs of the patient. Consideration should be given to the severity of the head injury, the stage of recovery, the psychosocial situation, and psychiatric and medical complications. Second, one should educate the family members or caregivers and encourage their involvement in the treatment plan. Third, the clinician must identify and nurture the strengths of the patient, while anticipating and mitigating the problems, pitfalls, and challenges involved in achieving a favorable outcome. Finally, hope and motivation should be promoted and encouraged with the goal of improving function and limiting disability.

In post-TBI depression, unlike major depressive disorder, for which treatments target the underlying syndrome, interventions may be geared towards the specific symptoms causing distress or the underlying syndrome.

Pharmacologic treatments

An extensive and systematic review of the literature on the psychiatric aspects of TBI has concluded that the evidence base for treatment of post-TBI depression is poor (20, 21). For the most part, treatment of post-TBI depression is similar to treatment of idiopathic depression, except that treatment should be initiated at a low dosage and increases should be done gently and cautiously. Nevertheless, patients with TBI may end up on dosages similar to those of patients without brain damage. Patients with TBI often are more sensitive to medications than the general population; therefore it is important to exercise caution with pharmacologic agents. Indications, risks, and benefits of any medication should be discussed with the patient and family members before treatment is initiated. Consideration should be given to starting any agent at the lowest possible dose and increasing the dose slowly. In addition, side effects should be monitored closely and medications with known adverse CNS effects (e.g., sedation, strong anticholinergic activity) should be avoided or used cautiously if no alternatives are available.

Citalopram, fluoxetine, sertraline, and other selective serotonin reuptake inhibitors (SSRIs) may be considered as first-line agents, and several studies suggest their efficacy in treating depression (22–24). To achieve remission of symptoms, it may be necessary to optimize the dose or switch to another agent within the same class or across classes with venlafaxine, a serotonin-norepinephrine reuptake inhibitor, and mirtazapine, a pre-synaptic alpha-2-adrenergic/serotonin receptor antagonist, being reasonable options. Augmentation with buspirone and second-generation antipsychotics (other than clozapine) or psychostimulants, such as dextroamphetamine and methylphenidate, may be considered to achieve an adequate response if depressive symptoms persist despite adequate dosing and trial of a single agent. Second-generation antipsychotics may be used with antidepressants in cases of major depression with psychotic features. Monoamine oxidase inhibitors and tricyclic antidepressants, for the most part, should be avoided because of their anticholinergic side effects and their extensive interactions with food and other drugs. Bupropion and clozapine should also be avoided, given their potential for inducing seizures.

Somatic treatments

In treatment-resistant cases, electroconvulsive therapy (ECT) may be beneficial and has been shown to have a favorable efficacy and safety profile in patients with head injury (25). Data are insufficient regarding the efficacy or risks of other somatic therapies including vagus nerve stimulation and repetitive transcranial magnetic stimulation in the treatment of post-TBI depression.

Psychosocial treatments

Psychosocial interventions can be conceptualized on the basis of phase of post-TBI depression. In the acute phase (4 to 6 weeks following injury), early deficits associated with the location of injury should be taken into account. For example, domains of cognition such as abstraction, set-shifting, logical reasoning, sequencing and, introspection, which are crucial for successful treatment with traditional forms of cognitive therapy, may be impaired following injury to the left frontal cortex. Unfortunately, post-TBI depression is frequently associated with lesions affecting this area. As awareness of impairments sets in, fostering a therapeutic alliance with supportive counseling and education regarding the course and symptoms of depression is an important first step. In addition, improving accessibility and engaging family support may help facilitate physical and psychological rehabilitation and limit disability (14).

Several months post injury, as the residual cognitive capacity becomes clearer, other psychosocial interventions may be incorporated into the treatment plan as appropriate. These include occupational therapy, physical therapy, behavioral therapy, cognitive rehabilitation, speech therapy, social skills training, recreation therapy, vocational training, and substance abuse counseling. Adequate nutrition, regular exercise, and maintaining a regular routine and daily schedule should be recommended. If appropriate, patients should be encouraged to attend brain injury support groups, which create a support network and may be helpful in fostering adaptive and coping strategies to deal with functional limitations.

Conclusion

Depressive symptoms are common following traumatic brain. If left undiagnosed or untreated, post-TBI depression can lead to significant morbidity and mortality, and impairments in quality of life and daily function. The cause is likely multi-factorial and includes effects related to direct physiologic consequences of the brain injury and a reaction to the loss or physical disability resulting from the brain injury. Management of post-TBI depression should be multi-faceted and oftentimes multi-disciplinary. Unfortunately, there is a dearth of research focused on the pharmacologic treatment of post-TBI depression; this represents an avenue of tremendous potential for future research.

References

1. Rutland-Brown W, Langlois JA, Thomas KE, et al. Incidence of traumatic brain injury in the United States, 2003. J Head Trauma Rehabil. 2006;21(6):544–8.

2. Frankowski RF. Descriptive epidemiologic studies of head injury in the United States: 1974-1984. Adv Psychosom Med. 1986;16: 153–72.

3. Rao V, Lyketsos C. Neuropsychiatric sequelae of traumatic brain injury. Psychosomatics. 2000;41(2):95–103.

4. MacKenzie EJ, Shapiro S, Siegel JH. The economic impact of traumatic injuries: one-year treatment-related expenditures. JAMA. 1988;260(22):3290–6.

5. Fedoroff JP, Starkstein SE, Forrester AW, et al. Depression in patients with acute traumatic brain injury. Am J Psychiatry. 1992;149(7):918–23.

6. Jorge RE, Robinson RG, Moser D, et al. Major depression following traumatic brain injury. Arch Gen Psychiatry. 2004;61(1):42–50.

7. Deb S, Lyons I, Koutzoukis C, et al. Rate of psychiatric illness 1 year after traumatic brain injury. Am J Psychiatry. 1999;156(3): 374–8.

8. Bay E, Donders J. Risk factors for depressive symptoms after mild-to-moderate traumatic brain injury. Brain Inj. 2008;22(3):233–41.

9. McAllister TW. Neuropsychiatric sequelae of head injuries. Psychiatr Clin North Am. 1992;15(2):395–413.

10. Kraus MF: Neuropsychiatric sequelae: assessment and pharmacologic intervention. In: Marion DW, editor. Traumatic brain injury. Vol 14. New York: Thieme Medicine Publishers; 1999. p. 173–85.

11. Rao V, Lyketsos CG. Psychiatric aspects of traumatic brain injury. Psychiatr Clin North Am. 2002;25(1):43–69.

12. Jorge RE, Robinson RG, Arndt SV, et al. Comparison between acute- and delayed-onset depression following traumatic brain injury. J Neuropsychiatry Clin Neurosci. 1993;5(1):43–9.

13. Labbate LA, Warden DL. Common psychiatric syndromes and pharmacologic treatments of traumatic brain injury. Curr Psychiatry Rep. 2000;2(3):268–73.

14. Moldover JE, Goldberg KB, Prout MF. Depression after traumatic brain injury: a review of evidence for clinical heterogeneity. Neuropsychol Rev. 2004;14(3):143–54.

15. Wasserman L, Shaw T, Vu M, et al. An overview of traumatic brain injury and suicide. Brain Inj. 2008;22(11):811–9.

16. Simpson G, Tate R. Suicidality in people surviving a traumatic brain injury: prevalence, risk factors and implications for clinical management. Brain Inj. 2007;21(13–14):1335–51.

17. Jorge R, Robinson RG. Mood disorders following traumatic brain injury. Int Rev Psychiatry. 2003;15(4):317–27.

18. Rao V. Psychiatric aspects of neurologic diseases; practical approaches to patient care. In: Lyketsos CG, Rabins PV, Lipsey JR, Slavney PR, editors. New York (NY): Oxford University Press Inc; 2008. p. 84–8.

19. Jorge RE, Robinson RG, Arndt S. Are there symptoms that are specific for depressed mood in patients with traumatic brain injury? J Nerv Ment Dis. 1993;181(2): 91–9.

20. Kim E, Lauterbach EC, Reeve A, et al. Neuropsychiatric complications of traumatic brain injury: a critical review of the literature (a report by the ANPA Committee on Research). J Neuropsychiatry Clin Neurosci. 2007;19(2):106–27.

21. Neurobehavioral Guidelines Working Group, Warden DL, Gordon B, McAllister TW, Silver JM, Barth JT, et al. Guidelines for the pharmacologic treatment of neurobehavioral sequelae of traumatic brain injury. J Neurotrauma. 2006;23(10): 1468–501.

22. Rapoport MJ, Chan F, Lanctot K, et al. An open-label study of citalopram for major depression following traumatic brain injury. J Psychopharmacol. 2008;22(8): 860–4.

23. Lee H, Kim SW, Kim JM, et al. Comparing effects of methylphenidate, sertraline and placebo on neuropsychiatric sequelae in patients with traumatic brain injury. Hum Psychopharmacol. 2005;20(2):97–104.

24. Fann JR, Uomoto JM, Katon WJ. Sertraline in the treatment of major depression following mild traumatic brain injury. J Neuropsychiatry Clin Neurosci. 2000; 12(2):226–32.

25. Kant R, Coffey CE, Bogyi AM. Safety and efficacy of ECT in patients with head injury: a case series. J Neuropsychiatry Clin Neurosci. 1999;11(1):32–7.

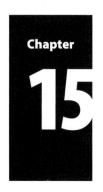

Chapter

15

Managing psychiatric aspects of seizure disorders

Alex Thompson

Typical consult question

"Would you please evaluate and treat the depression in our patient with refractory focal epilepsy on multiple antiepileptic drugs?"

What is "focal" epilepsy and how is it different from "localization-related" or "partial" epilepsy? What if the patient with refractory epilepsy seizes in my office? What happens when I add fluvoxamine to levetiracetam, valproic acid, and clobazam? These questions speak to the complications facing us when we help people with epilepsy (PWE) deal with co-morbid psychiatric disorders. It becomes much less complicated though when we work as a team alongside the patient and the neurologist. Being a good teammate requires having a basic understanding of epilepsy, its treatment, and the psychological and pharmacologic impact of our interventions. This chapter begins to address those skills.

Background

Definitions and classification

A seizure is a paroxysmal discharge of neurons; epilepsy is the condition of having recurrent, unprovoked seizures. A seizure may be **partial** or **general**, according to the point from which it starts. A partial seizure begins in one area (i.e., focus) of the brain with manifestations particular to the location affected. Symptoms may be motor, sensory, autonomic, or psychological. A partial seizure occurs with or without loss of consciousness (**complex** vs. **simple**) and may secondarily generalize into a tonic-clonic seizure. Complex partial seizures are the most common seizure type in adults. About two-thirds of complex partial seizures arise in the temporal lobes, with others arising from the frontal, occipital, and parietal lobes. A classic complex partial seizure consists of a simple partial onset (i.e., an aura such as epigastric fullness, foul odor, or strange taste), loss of consciousness, and automatisms. Partial epilepsy, focal epilepsy, and localization-related epilepsy are synonyms (1, 2).

A general seizure starts diffusely and involves both sides of the brain. Six types of generalized seizures have been identified: tonic-clonic, absence, myoclonic, tonic, clonic, and atonic. A tonic-clonic seizure starts with a 10- to 30-second tonic phase of flexion followed by extension. During the longer clonic phase, muscle relaxation intermittently disrupts tonic contraction, giving the rhythmic jerking appearance. An absence seizure involves the sudden onset of impaired consciousness and automatisms, and lasts about 10 seconds. Unlike complex partial seizures, absence seizures are not followed by confusion, can be precipitated

Psychosomatic Medicine: An Introduction to Consultation-Liaison Psychiatry, eds. James J. Amos and Robert G. Robinson. Published by Cambridge University Press. © Cambridge University Press 2010.

by hyperventilation, have a 3 Hz spike-and-wave EEG pattern, and usually go away by adulthood. Myoclonic seizures consist of sudden, brief muscle contractions that may be general, local, symmetric, or asymmetric. These are quick jerking movements that happen so fast they may be confused with tics or clumsiness. Juvenile myoclonic epilepsy (JME) is the most common cause of primarily generalized myoclonic and tonic-clonic seizures in adults. Carbamazepine, commonly used for partial epilepsies, may worsen the absence and myoclonic seizures of JME (1, 2).

Epidemiology

A seizure may be an acute symptomatic or unprovoked event. Acute symptomatic seizures have a cause such as brain trauma, infection, or drug withdrawal. The incidence of acute symptomatic seizures is 29 to 39 per 100,000 per year. The incidence of single unprovoked seizures is 23 to 61 per 100,000 per year. Like epilepsy, in general, both are more common in men, infants younger than one year, and adults older than 65 years of age (3). About 35% of those with a first unprovoked seizure have another one within the next five years (4). The cumulative incidence for all seizure disorders ranges from 10% to 20%, and the prevalence is about 0.5% to 1% (5). At least 50 million people live with epilepsy worldwide, most of them in developed countries. Despite cheap and effective treatments, much of the epilepsy in developing countries goes untreated (6).

Psychiatric disorders are very common in PWE and have a large negative impact on quality of life, suicide, and self-care. General risk factors for psychiatric and cognitive problems in PWE are poorly controlled seizures, multiple medications, high doses of medications, a past history of psychiatric problems, and comorbid medical conditions. The population-based Canadian Community Health Survey used a structured psychiatric interview to assess psychiatric morbidity in persons reporting diagnoses of epilepsy. The lifetime prevalence of mental disorders was 17.4% for major depression, 24.4% for any mood disorder, 22.8% for any anxiety disorder, and 25% for suicidal ideation (7). The incidence of psychiatric morbidity is even higher in PWE receiving care at tertiary epilepsy centers. One study examined 174 people with chronic epilepsy receiving care at university outpatient epilepsy centers. About half the patients had a current psychiatric diagnosis with the most common being major depression (17%). Current anxiety diagnoses, specifically, agoraphobia, generalized anxiety disorder, and social phobia, were also common. Most of the patients with depressive disorder also had anxiety disorders. Psychotic disorders were not common (8). Much of the psychiatric morbidity in those with epilepsy is not identified or treated.

Cognitive and psychiatric symptoms may be **preictal**, **ictal**, **postictal**, or **interictal**. Interictal symptoms are independent of seizures and make up the bulk of research and discussion in epilepsy psychiatry. Preictal mood and behavioral changes immediately precede the seizure or occur up to a few days before. Ictal psychiatric phenomena are simple partial seizures. The most common symptoms are fear, depression, and hallucinations. These are identified as ictal events by a careful history detailing their stereotyped presentation, brief duration relative to interictal psychiatric syndromes, and association with other seizure phenomena such as automatisms. Postictal (0 to 72 hours after the seizure) symptoms such as irritability, fatigue, worry, and suicidality are common, under-recognized, and strongly associated with interictal psychiatric disorders (9).

Depressive disorders are the most common psychiatric problem in persons with epilepsy. Factors associated with depression in epilepsy may include being male (10), having a low

IQ or learning disability (11), having a family history of major depression (12), being less physically active (13), and taking certain antiepileptic drugs (AEDs). Patients with epilepsy experience stigma in society and at work (14), which may be a risk factor for depression (15). A left-sided seizure focus (16) and frequent seizures (17) may also increase depression risk. **Bipolar disorders** and mania may be more common in those with epilepsy than in the general population. It is critical to determine the relationship of manic symptoms to seizures to make sure that what is seen is not resulting from ongoing seizures.

Anxiety disorders are the second most common psychiatric disorder in those with epilepsy and often occur along with a depressive disorder (18). Ictal fear may be misdiagnosed as a panic disorder. Epilepsy is an anxiety-provoking condition due to the loss of control inherent in having a brain disorder that often has no explanation and results in episodic loss of consciousness. **Postictal psychosis** occurs in adults with chronic epilepsy. A cluster of seizures, followed by a lucid interval of hours to days, leads to a psychosis that may last from hours to months. Mood symptoms are common, while "negative" symptoms of schizophrenia and "first-rank" symptoms are not. Chronic interictal psychosis looks like, and is managed as, chronic schizophrenia (19).

Cognitive disorders are very common in PWE and depend on the type of epilepsy, the severity and frequency of seizures, age of onset, the location of a lesion (if present), the epilepsy treatment (medicine and surgery), and chronic factors related to ongoing seizures and interictal brain changes. Memory loss is the most common deficit in epilepsy. Attention and concentration problems are also seen frequently (20). A large number of disordered **personality** traits ("viscosity," aggressiveness, religiosity, humorlessness) have been ascribed to PWE, especially those with temporal lobe epilepsy (21). Irritability may be a significant interictal feature in a PWE. That irritability, however, is probably part of an affective illness or anxiety disorder, or the effect of AEDs and psychotropics. A seizure rarely, if ever, explains a directed violent act.

Work-up

In addition to a thorough psychiatric evaluation, consider these questions:

1. Does the patient really have seizures?

Events described as seizures may be non-epileptic physiologic (e.g., syncope) or psychological events (e.g., panic attacks, psychogenic seizures). At least a third of patients undergoing video EEG monitoring have psychogenic non-epileptic events. Consider this diagnosis in a patient with refractory events, a past history of abuse, other unexplainable symptoms, symptom syndromes (e.g., irritable bowel syndrome, fibromyalgia), personality disorder, or financial factors supporting ongoing illness. Gather details about the seizure-like event from the patient and anyone else available. Find out who diagnosed the patient as having seizures or epilepsy and communicate with that person or review the record. Referral for a specialty neurological evaluation may be necessary if the diagnosis has never been clear.

2. If the patient has epilepsy, what is the type, is the cause known, what is the treatment, and is the epilepsy controlled?

Familiarize yourself with the patient's predominant seizure type including a description of the seizure from beginning to end. This seizure semiology includes details about the preictal,

ictal, and postictal states. With this understanding, it is much easier to clarify the relationship of mood, anxiety, and psychotic symptoms to the patient's seizures. If the patient has had a detailed neurological evaluation, seizure descriptions may be detailed clearly for you. Treatment compliance is important to discuss.

3. What psychiatric symptoms are present, do they represent a psychiatric syndrome, and what is their relationship to seizures (i.e., are the symptoms preictal, postictal, or interictal) and epilepsy treatment?

Psychiatric disorders in epilepsy may present differently than in the general population. Depressive disorders are a good example. An intermittent and pleomorphic dysphoric disorder was described by Kraepelin. This "interictal dysphoric disorder" consists of depression in addition to irritability, anxiety, phobic fear, anergia, pain, and occasional euphoric mood (22). Find out whether psychiatric symptoms started after antiepileptic drug changes.

4. How is the patient handling epilepsy?

The list of risk factors for depression in epilepsy alludes to the multiple biopsychosocial stresses borne by these patients. Discussions about the individual, interpersonal, professional, and social impacts of having epilepsy will help you tailor treatment and may be therapeutic for the patient. Ask how the patient and his loved ones understand epilepsy and its treatment. Determine whether there are communication problems between the patient and other care providers around diagnoses and treatment goals. Consider the role that cultural differences may play and how this could impact care in a Western medical institution.

5. Are AEDs playing a role in cognitive and psychiatric symptoms?

Psychiatric and cognitive functioning usually improve when an AED decreases or stops seizures. But AEDs also contribute to psychiatric problems through direct (e.g., GABA potentiation) and indirect (e.g., forced normalization) mechanisms (23). Patients with a previous psychiatric or cognitive problem and those taking high doses of AEDs or more than one AED are going to be at higher risk for AED-related problems. Phenobarbital and primidone increase the risk for depression and other psychiatric disturbances (24, 25). Levetiracetam, vigabatrin, and topiramate often precipitate depression, anxiety, and psychosis (26). Tiagabine does not frequently cause psychosis but may increase the risk for depression (25). One author's review of this literature led to the following conclusions: avoid phenobarbital, primidone, vigabatrin, and tiagabine in depression; avoid lamotrigine, felbamate, and levetiracetam in anxiety; and avoid vigabatrin, topiramate, and ethosuximide in psychosis (23). The AEDs most likely to cause cognitive problems are phenobarbital, primidone, and topiramate. Among other older AEDs (phenytoin, valproic acid, and carbamazepine), conflicting data describe absolute and relative cognitive side effects. Some of the newer AEDs, especially lamotrigine and levetiracetam, cause few cognitive problems (27).

6. Is the patient suicidal?

Suicide is a major cause of death in people with epilepsy. The major risk factor is psychiatric illness. Another risk factor may be AED use. The U.S. Food and Drug Administration (FDA) issued a warning that patients taking AEDs had twice the risk of suicidal behavior or ideation as those not taking AEDs. The FDA analysis was based on 199 placebo-controlled

Table 15.1 Antiepileptic drug recommendations by seizure type and patient group

		Healthy Adolescent or Adult	Elderly or Medically Ill	Co-morbid Depression
Idiopathic Generalized Epilepsy	**Generalized Tonic-clonic Seizures**	Valproate Lamotrigine Topiramate	Lamotrigine Levetiracetam	Lamotrigine Valproate
	Absence Seizures	Valproate Ethosuximide Lamotrigine		
	Myoclonic Seizures	Valproate		
Partial Epilepsy		Carbamazepine Oxcarbazepine Lamotrigine Levetiracetam		Lamotrigine Carbamazepine Oxcarbazepine

trials of patients taking AEDs for epilepsy and for other reasons like migraine and psychiatric conditions. Four suicides were reported (28). Overall, the increased risk appears quite small, the mechanisms by which AEDs might increase suicidality are not clear, and the risk may be peculiar to those with epilepsy rather than all users of AEDs (29). Given the high co-morbidity of psychiatric disorders in persons with epilepsy, the need for AED use, and the frequent use of antidepressants, it is important to ask about suicidal thoughts and behaviors both at initial evaluation and at follow-up.

7. Was neuropsychological testing completed?

Patients with epilepsy who are referred to you (especially in tertiary care settings) often have refractory epilepsy that has required multiple medications and evaluations. Neuropsychological testing may have been done and is a fountain of well-described relevant information including past history, treatment course, cognitive and psychiatric functioning, and psychosocial treatment recommendations.

Clinical decision-making and treatment

Psychiatric disorders in PWE are best managed by avoiding the ictus altogether. Although AED decision-making should be guided by a neurologist, it is important to understand basic treatment strategies along with the potential for rash and fetal malformations.

Epilepsy treatment

Experts agree that monotherapy is the treatment of first choice for partial and generalized epilepsies. If the first antiepileptic drug fails, neurologists prescribe monotherapy with a second AED. The following table is a useful summary of expert opinions for first-line epilepsy treatment for different seizure types and patient groups (30) (Table 15.1).

- **AED use in pregnancy and the risk for a major malformation:** Valproic acid use increases the risk of major malformations and should be avoided during the first trimester. Carbamazepine use is probably not associated with major malformations, and there is not yet enough evidence to describe the risk for LTG, although it appears to be the same as for CBZ (31).

- **Rash:** All AEDs present some risk for rash (usually a diffuse, red, itchy maculopapular eruption) that may advance to the life-threatening Stevens-Johnson syndrome or toxic epidermal necrolysis. Risk of rash appears to be highest in those taking phenytoin, carbamazepine, and lamotrigine and may be lower with levetiracetam, gabapentin, and valproic acid. Any prior AED-induced rash increases the risk of another rash (32), and the risk of rash is elevated in certain groups like the Han Chinese because of the presence of the HLA-B*1502 allele (33).

Psychiatric disorder treatment

The indications for psychotropic use in someone with epilepsy are the same as in the general population. Make treatment decisions as a team including the patient, patient's family (if appropriate), neurologist, primary care doctor, and on-line medication database. Your most frequent decision will involve starting an antidepressant for a depressive or anxiety disorder in the presence of one or more AED(s). My recommendations for psychiatric treatment in patients with epilepsy include the following:

1. Start with low medication doses and provide close follow-up to assess for treatment effect and any change in seizure activity.
2. Patients and families often have dealt with numerous drug trials and are leery of adding yet another medication. I meet this by going over the exact reason I am recommending a medication and by reviewing (using an on-line tool that provides patient handouts, like Micromedex) side effects and drug interactions.
3. Although no robust evidence supports psychological treatment in epilepsy (34), I do refer higher functioning patients with depression and anxiety for cognitive-behavioral therapy. I encourage safe exercise. Exercise may counter drug-induced weight gain, and there is some evidence that it improves seizure control (35).
4. For depressive and anxiety disorders, start with selective serotonin reuptake inhibitors (SSRIs) that have limited pharmacologic interactions, like citalopram or escitalopram. If one does not work, I will try another SSRI. After that, I move to venlafaxine, duloxetine, or mirtazapine, depending on the clinical situation.
5. Manage bipolar disorders with lamotrigine, valproic acid, or carbamazepine in a manner that complements seizure treatment. Lithium is effective but may not be acceptable because of cognitive and physical side effects and the need for blood level monitoring.
6. When psychotic disorders are treated, there is little evidence to support the use of one antipsychotic over another (36). Risperidone is a good choice with little impact on AED clearance, although carbamazepine may lower risperidone levels.

In addition to those opinions, consider the following based on two reviews of psychotropic medication use in epilepsy (37, 38):

- Psychotropics may worsen seizures directly.
  - Bupropion, clomipramine, amoxapine, and maprotiline should be avoided. Clozapine, chlorpromazine, and loxapine have the highest seizure risk among antipsychotics, although all the typical agents may lower seizure threshold. In general, antidepressants, stimulants, and atypical antipsychotic agents are safe to use in PWE. Lithium and the benzodiazepines do not appear to increase seizure risk.

- Psychotropics and AEDs may interact pharmacokinetically.

  ○ Phenytoin, phenobarbital, primidone, and carbamazepine are CYP isoenzyme inducers and may lead to decreased levels of many drugs including antidepressants, antipsychotics, and anxiolytics.

  ○ Oxcarbazepine and topiramate may induce CYP isoenzymes at higher doses.

  ○ Valproic acid is a CYP isoenzyme inhibitor.

  ○ Fluoxetine and fluvoxamine inhibit CYP isoenzymes and may increase levels of phenytoin.

  ○ Levetiracetam, lamotrigine, gabapentin, pregabalin, tiagabine, and zonisamide do not induce or inhibit CYP isoenzymes.

- Psychotropic drugs may compound adverse effects of AEDs.

  ○ Lithium does not interact pharmacokinetically with AEDs. But its combination with AEDs may exacerbate cognitive problems, tremor, and weight gain. Benzodiazepines may also worsen cognitive slowing, energy, mood, and behavior when combined with AEDs. Antipsychotic agents may precipitate or worsen metabolic disorders. The risk for neuroleptic malignant syndrome and tardive movement disorders may be greater when it is used in someone with CNS lesions.

Conclusion

Epilepsy is not a psychiatric disorder or a sacred disease brought on by demons or miasma. Epilepsy is a symptom of many different brain disorders and is often psychologically taxing for patients and providers. Psychiatrists help patients and their neurologists when we team up with them to create behavioral, pharmacologic, and psychological treatments. Thank you to Beatrice Tannous, MD, for her thoughtful review and suggestions.

References

1. Elger CE, Schmidt D. Modern management of epilepsy: a practical approach. Epilepsy Behav. 2008;12(4):501–39.

2. Brown TR, Holmes GL. Handbook of epilepsy. 4th ed. Philadelphia: Lippincott Williams & Wilkins; 2008.

3. Hauser WA, Beghi E. First seizure definitions and worldwide incidence and mortality. Epilepsia. 2008;49(Suppl 1): 8–12.

4. Hauser WA, Rich SS, Lee JR, et al. Risk of recurrent seizures after two unprovoked seizures. N Engl J Med. 1998;338(7):429–34.

5. Hesdorffer DC, Hauser WA. Epidemiological considerations. In: Ettinger AB, Kanner AM, editors. Psychiatric issues in epilepsy. 2nd ed.

Philadelphia (PA): Lippincott Williams & Wilkins; 2007. p. 1–16.

6. de Boer HM, Mula M, Sander JW. The global burden and stigma of epilepsy. Epilepsy Behav. 2008;12(4): 540–6.

7. Tellez-Zenteno JF, Patten SB, Jette N, et al. Psychiatric comorbidity in epilepsy: a population-based analysis. Epilepsia. 2007;48(12):2336–44.

8. Jones JE, Hermann BP, Barry JJ, et al. Clinical assessment of Axis I psychiatric morbidity in chronic epilepsy: a multi-center investigation. J Neuropsychiatry Clin Neurosci. 2005;17(2):172–9.

9. Kanner AM. Peri-ictal psychiatric phenomena: clinical characteristics and implications of past and future psychiatric

disorders. In: Ettinger AB, Kanner AM, editors. Psychiatric issues in epilepsy. 2nd ed. Philadelphia (PA): Lippincott Williams & Wilkins; 2007. p. 321–45.

10. Septien L, Gras P, Giroud M, et al. Depression and temporal epilepsy: the possible role of laterality of the epileptic foci and of gender. Neurophysiol Clin. 1993;23(4):327–36.

11. Lund J. Epilepsy and psychiatric disorder in the mentally retarded adult. Acta Psychiatr Scand. 1985;72(6):557–62.

12. Hermann BP, Whitman S. Psychosocial predictors of interictal depression. J Epilepsy. 1989;2(4):231–7.

13. Roth DL, Goode KT, Williams VL, Faught E. Physical exercise, stressful life experience, and depression in adults with epilepsy. Epilepsia. 1994;35(6):1248–55.

14. Jacoby A, Austin JK. Social stigma for adults and children with epilepsy. Epilepsia. 2007;48(Suppl 9):6–9.

15. Hermann BP, Whitman S, Wyler AR, et al. Psychosocial predictors of psychopathology in epilepsy. Br J Psychiatry. 1990;156:98–105.

16. Altshuler LL, Devinsky O, Post RM, Theodore W. Depression, anxiety, and temporal lobe epilepsy: laterality of focus and symptoms. Arch Neurol. 1990;47(3):284–8.

17. Trostle JA, Hauser WA, Sharbrough FW. Psychologic and social adjustment to epilepsy in Rochester, Minnesota. Neurology. 1989;39(5):633–7.

18. Kanner AM. Psychiatric issues in epilepsy: the complex relation of mood, anxiety disorders, and epilepsy. Epilepsy Behav. 2009;15(1):83–7.

19. Nadkarni S, Arnedo V, Devinsky O. Psychosis in epilepsy patients. Epilepsia. 2007;48(Suppl 9):17–9.

20. Carreno M, Donaire A, Sanchez-Carpintero R. Cognitive disorders associated with epilepsy: diagnosis and treatment. Neurologist. 2008;14(6 Suppl 1):S26–S34.

21. Bear DM, Fedio P. Quantitative analysis of interictal behavior in temporal lobe epilepsy. Arch Neurol. 1977;34(8):454–67.

22. Blumer D, Montouris G, Davies K. The interictal dysphoric disorder: recognition, pathogenesis, and treatment of the major psychiatric disorder of epilepsy. Epilepsy Behav. 2004;5(6):826–40.

23. Mula M, Monaco F. Antiepileptic drugs and psychopathology of epilepsy: an update. Epileptic Disord. 2009;11(1):1–9.

24. Barry JJ, Lembke A, Gisbert PA, Gilliam F. Affective disorders in epilepsy. In: Ettinger AB, Kanner AM, editors. Psychiatric issues in epilepsy. 2nd ed. Philadelphia (PA): Lippincott Williams & Wilkins; 2007. p. 219.

25. Mula M, Sander JW. Negative effects of antiepileptic drugs on mood in patients with epilepsy. Drug Saf. 2007;30(7):555–67.

26. Sussman N, Ettinger AB. Psychotropic properties of antiepileptic drugs. In: Ettinger AB, Kanner AM, editors. Psychiatric issues in epilepsy. 2nd ed. Philadelphia (PA): Lippincott Williams & Wilkins; 2007. p. 67–82.

27. Mula M, Trimble MR. Antiepileptic drug-induced cognitive adverse effects: potential mechanisms and contributing factors. CNS Drugs. 2009;23(2):121–37.

28. U.S. Food and Drug Administration. Information for healthcare professionals: suicidality and antiepileptic drugs. January 1, 2008; cited 2009 May 1. Available from: http://www.fda.gov/Cder/Drug/InfoSheets/HCP/antiepilepticsHCP.htm.

29. Bell GS, Mula M, Sander JW. Suicidality in people taking antiepileptic drugs: what is the evidence? CNS Drugs. 2009;23(4):281–92.

30. Karceski S, Morrell MJ, Carpenter D. Treatment of epilepsy in adults: expert opinion, 2005. Epilepsy Behav. 2005;7(Suppl 1):S1–S64.

31. Harden CL, Meador KJ, Pennell PB, et al. Practice parameter update: management issues for women with epilepsy – focus on pregnancy (an evidence-based review): teratogenesis and perinatal outcomes. Report of the Quality Standards Subcommittee and Therapeutics and

Technology Subcommittee of the American Academy of Neurology and American Epilepsy Society. Neurology. 2009;73(2):126–32.

32. Arif H, Buchsbaum R, Weintraub D, et al. Comparison and predictors of rash associated with 15 antiepileptic drugs. Neurology. 2007;68(20):1701–9.

33. Miller JW. Of race, ethnicity, and rash: the genetics of antiepileptic drug-induced skin reactions. Epilepsy Curr. 2008;8(5):120–1.

34. Ramaratnam S, Baker GA, Goldstein LH. Psychological treatments for epilepsy. Cochrane Database Syst Rev. 2008;(3): CD002029.

35. Nakken KO. Physical exercise in outpatients with epilepsy. Epilepsia. 1999;40(5):643–51.

36. Farooq S, Sherin A. Interventions for psychotic symptoms concomitant with epilepsy. Cochrane Database Syst Rev. 2008;(4):CD006118.

37. Kanner AM, Gidal BE. Pharmacodynamic and pharmacokinetic interactions of psychotropic drugs with antiepileptic drugs. Int Rev Neurobiol. 2008;83: 397–416.

38. Kanner AM. The use of psychotropic drugs in epilepsy: what every neurologist should know. Semin Neurol. 2008;28(3):379–88.

Chapter 16

Distress and depression in cancer care

Janeta Tansey and Donna Greenberg

Typical consultation questions

1) *"The patient is very distressed during her oncology appointments. Please evaluate for depression."*
2) *"The patient is enrolled in an effective treatment protocol for his cancer, but has started questioning whether he wants to continue. Please evaluate for depression."*

Background

Both of these questions reflect the impetus that often lies behind the referral of a cancer patient for psychiatric evaluation – namely, that the patient's mental state is negatively affecting participation in treatment. And although this is certainly sufficient cause for a referral, it reflects only a small portion of those who would benefit from psychiatric evaluation and care. Psychiatric disorders are common in the setting of oncology. One of the earliest studies in the subspecialty of psychooncology found that in a random sample of hospitalized and ambulatory cancer patients, 47% had diagnosable psychiatric disorders. Within that group, 68% had adjustment disorders with mood or anxiety symptoms, 13% had major depression, 8% had an organic mental disorder, 7% had personality disorders, and 4% had a pre-existing anxiety disorder (1). More recent reviews looking at depression and major depression in patients with cancer report that prevalence varies widely from 0% to 58% for depressive syndromes, and from 0% to 38% for major depression (2), with identified prevalence probably at least partially impacted by the diagnostic criteria used (3), as well as by cancer types, prognosis, advanced stage of disease, and a number of psychosocial variables. Generalizing the risk of depression is difficult because of the diversity of the cancer population; many studies on the incidence of depression in patients with cancer have focused on certain types of cancer, such as breast or lung. Nevertheless, the rule of thumb is that approximately 25% of patients will suffer from clinically significant depression at some point in their cancer journey.

It is also worth noting special barriers to the identification of depression in the patient with cancer, including the tendency to normalize what would otherwise be considered pathological mood symptoms to the extraordinary circumstances of a cancer diagnosis, as in "Well, it's normal to be depressed when you have cancer," patient denial that persistent low mood is present because of an implicit and overvalued prescription to remain upbeat, as in "Try to stay positive, or you'll never be able to beat this cancer" (4), and misattribution of symptoms of depression to the physical impact of cancer or cancer therapies. Exactly because of

Psychosomatic Medicine: An Introduction to Consultation-Liaison Psychiatry, eds. James J. Amos and Robert G. Robinson. Published by Cambridge University Press. © Cambridge University Press 2010.

the high risk of depression and such barriers to identification, screening and education of patients, families, and clinicians about the risk of depression are needed, followed by appropriate psychosocial interventions.

Screening for distress and the Mental Health Evaluation

In 1998, when the National Comprehensive Cancer Network (NCCN) turned its attention to improving and systematizing psychosocial cares for patients with cancer (5), the multidisciplinary panel suggested that asking about patient "distress" was less stigmatizing and more sensitive than asking about "psychiatric, psychosocial or emotional" problems.

Distress is a multi-factorial, unpleasant emotional experience of a psychological (cognitive, behavioral, emotional), social, and/or spiritual nature that may interfere with the ability to cope effectively with cancer, its physical symptoms, and its treatment. Distress extends along a continuum, ranging from common normal feelings of vulnerability, sadness, and fears to problems that can become disabling, such as depression, anxiety, panic, social isolation, and existential and spiritual crisis (5).

The term *distress* has been successfully used in screening and triage of patients with psychosocial concerns in a wide variety of care settings in the past decade and is increasingly become the screening term of choice in many cancer centers and clinics.

Influenced by the success of the 1–10 pain scale as the "fifth vital sign" (6), the NCCN recommended the use of a similarly scaled distress thermometer (DT) (7) as a "sixth vital sign" (Figure 16.1). In the time since its recommendation by the NCCN, the DT has been validated against other brief screening tools, such as the Beck Depression Inventory, the Patient Health Questionnaire-9, and the Hospital Anxiety and Depression Scale. Findings suggest that the DT, similar to other brief screening instruments, can be completed in minutes and has high sensitivity but relatively lower specificity (8). As with the pain scale, the efficient and accessible format of the DT makes it an effective first-line tool for frequent screening throughout a patient's cancer journey, although insufficient for making a psychiatric diagnosis.

A score of 4 or higher on the DT scale has been validated against other psychological instruments as indicating moderate to severe distress. Patients screening at 4 or more should be evaluated further by the primary oncology team, often with referrals to mental health, social work, and/or pastoral service, depending on the patient's identified concerns.

Those patients referred for mental health care should be particularly evaluated for mood, anxiety, cognitive, substance abuse, and personality disorders. Medication lists should be reviewed carefully, as multiple cancer agents or drug interactions can impair mental status. Pre-cancer psychiatric disease and risk factors will have implications for prognosis and psychiatric treatment. Patient safety must be assessed as cancer is a risk factor for suicide and deliberate self-harm, particularly in the first few months of diagnosis or with the perception of poor prognosis (9). In a recent study of two large databases completed over a 30-year period, patients with cancer had nearly twice the rate of suicide as non-cancer patients, with highest rates reported in older white men; suicide rates varied by cancer site, with higher rates seen among lung, stomach, oropharyngeal, and laryngeal carcinomas (10). Finally, psychiatric evaluation is an appropriate way to assess decision-making capacity and to explore patient values with respect to treatment options and life goals.

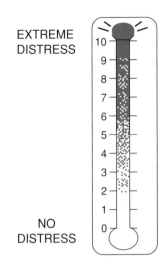

EXTREME
DISTRESS

10
9
8
7
6
5
4
3
2
1
0

PLEASE CIRCLE THE NUMBER (0–10) THAT BEST DESCRIBES HOW MUCH DISTRESS YOU HAVE BEEN EXPERIENCING IN THE PAST WEEK, INCLUDING TODAY.

NO
DISTRESS

PLEASE TICK WHICH OF THE FOLLOWING IS A CAUSE OF DISTRESS

PRACTICAL PROBLEMS
CHILDCARE ☐
HOUSING ☐
MONEY ☐
TRANSPORT ☐
WORK/SCHOOL ☐

FAMILY PROBLEMS
DEALING WITH PARTNER ☐
DEALING WITH CHILDREN ☐

EMOTIONAL PROBLEMS
DEPRESSION ☐
FEARS ☐
NERVOUSNESS ☐
SADNESS ☐
WORRY ☐
ANGER ☐

SPIRITUAL/RELIGIOUS CONCERNS
LOSS OF FAITH ☐
RELATING TO GOD ☐
LOSS OF MEANING OR ☐
PURPOSE IN LIFE

PHYSICAL PROBLEMS
PAIN ☐
NAUSEA ☐
FATIQUE ☐
SLEEP ☐
GETTING AROUND ☐
BATHING/DRESSING ☐
BREATHING ☐
MOUTH SORES ☐
EATING ☐
INDIGESTION ☐
CONSTIPATION ☐
DIARRHEA ☐
CHANGES IN URINATION ☐
FEVERS ☐
SKIN DRY/ITCHY ☐
NOSE DRY/CONGESTED ☐
TINGLING IN HANDS/FEET ☐
METALLIC TASTE IN MOUTH ☐
FEELING SWOLLEN ☐
SEXUAL ☐
HOT FLUSHES ☐
IS THERE ANYTHING IMPORTANT
YOU WOULD LIKE TO ADD TO THE
LIST?

Figure 16.1 Distress thermometer. Reproduced with permission from Hodder & Stoughton.

Physical symptom burden and distress

Although a distress scale represents a one-dimensional assessment of the patient, the causes of distress in cancer are multi-dimensional, with a significant burden of co-existing physical symptoms. It has been well established that patients with cancer report distress from unremitting or severe physical symptoms such as pain, fatigue, nausea, shortness of breath, sleep disturbances, and diminished mobility (11–13). It can sometimes be unclear, particularly in the face of suspected or reported mood changes, whether these physical symptoms are caused or exacerbated by a depressive disorder. Ongoing assessment is often indicated to clarify the diagnosis, particularly if depressed mood could be related to the effects of cancer drugs or cytokine therapies, or to the neurological, hormonal, hematological, or metabolic disturbances of the cancer itself.

Because patients with cancer often have malaise of physical illness with or without depressive disorder, researchers have explored clusters of symptoms in hopes of clarifying the presentation of malaise and the diagnostic validity of depressive disorder. A *symptom cluster* has been defined as two or more concurrent symptoms that co-occur in a stable fashion, but that may not have a common cause (14, 15). It has been anticipated that symptom clusters might describe the subjective complaints associated with the animal model of cytokine-mediated "sickness behavior" (16). Inquiry into symptom complexes has yielded important information about the co-variance of depression with other physical complaints such as fatigue and insomnia. Donovan and Jacobsen (17) provided a review of 16 studies with correlations between these symptoms, and found that, on average, measures of depression and fatigue administered concurrently to patients with cancer shared 30% of their variance, and measures of depression and insomnia shared 20% (17). Clinicians should be aware of the high co-variance of these conditions and should aim to provide symptom relief with customized therapies.

This is not at all to say that the process of improving diagnostic validity is unimportant. Clarifying whether a patient has a primary mood disorder has significant implications for treatment options, outcomes, and prognosis. General rules have been developed for discriminating major depressive disorder in the patient with cancer from generalized distress related to the physical symptom burden. It is believed that the diagnosis of a major depressive disorder in medically ill patients has higher validity in the presence of helpless or hopeless beliefs, anhedonia, guilt and worthlessness, and suicidal ideation (18). That is, cognitive symptoms of depression have stronger face value than physical symptoms of depression in the physically ill population. Another study of sleep disturbances in patients with cancer found that late insomnia or early awakening, coupled with agitation, anxiety, and diurnal mood variation, were more likely in the depressed cancer patient, whereas middle awakening and a relative lack of agitation were more common in the non-depressed cancer patient (19).

Pharmacologic treatments for depression in cancer – A cautionary tale

Antidepressant medication therapy is considered appropriate treatment for depressive disorders co-occurrent with cancer, although only a small number of trials are sufficiently rigorous, given high dropout rates and limited information about adverse drug reactions. The studies that are available too often measure a decrease in depressive symptoms rather than recovery from major depression (20). Antidepressants are often chosen for their side effect profile to help moderate symptoms such as insomnia, anergia, and anorexia. For depression with co-variant fatigue and/or insomnia, judicious augmentation with psychostimulants, sleep agents, and benzodiazepines has been employed. Particular care must be taken to address possible interactions of psychiatric medications with cancer treatment agents.

For example, tamoxifen, a selective estrogen receptor modulator often used in patients with breast cancer, is metabolized by cytochrome P450 into its active form via CYP2D6-mediated hydroxylation. The active metabolite of tamoxifen is antiestrogenic in the breast, but estrogenic in the bone, liver, and uterus; hot flashes are a common side effect, and depression and anxiety have also been reported. Clinical trials with selective serotonin reuptake inhibitors (SSRIs) and serotonin-norepinephrine reuptake inhibitors (SNRIs) have been found effective in decreasing hot flashes by as much as 60%, as compared with 24% to 35% with placebo (21). But in a study looking at concurrent administration of paroxetine, an inhibitor of CYP2D6, the levels of tamoxifen's active metabolite were diminished, and even more so in tissue samples showing inactivating genotypic polymorphisms of CYP2D6, which can range from decreased to absent CYP2D6 activity (22, 23). Concomitant use of drugs that strongly inhibit CYP2D6, including fluoxetine and paroxetine, should be avoided for patients on tamoxifen (21). Although genotypic testing for CYP2D6 variations is available, it is not currently the standard of care for customizing tamoxifen therapies, despite research suggesting that breast cancer patients with CYP2D6-inhibiting polymorphisms have increased risk of recurrence and diminished likelihood of disease-free survival (24). Perhaps even weak inhibitors of CYP2D6 are problematic for the subset of patients who have an unidentified genotypic variation of inhibited or absent CYP2D6 activity. Specific pharmacologic studies to this point suggest that venlafaxine, citalopram, and mirtazapine are the better antidepressants for use with hot flashes, depression, or anxiety during tamoxifen therapy because of their minimal effect on CYP2D6.

The take-home point of this specific illustration is that as individualized assessments of genotypes, tumor markers, and environmental risks are performed more often, and as new cancer therapies are developed, the pharmacologic treatments for depression must be reassessed and studied for both efficacy and harm unique to the cancer patient and the treatment protocol. Determination of whether specific antidepressants are particularly helpful for patients with depression and certain kinds of cancer or cancer therapies, or for patients with related co-variant symptom complexes, requires additional study.

Non-pharmacologic therapies for depression in cancer

Psychotherapy

Psychotherapy is helpful for cancer patients with depression and distress, although what type of psychotherapy is most effective at various points in the cancer journey or per cancer type is not well established. A meta-analysis of psychological treatments in patients with breast cancer suggested that short-term therapy focusing on coping was more effective for depression in early cancer care, while longer-term therapy focusing on support has improved efficacy for advanced cancer care (25). Findings for cognitive-behavioral therapy are largely positive, but mixed, with some small studies indicating benefit and others suggesting less benefit or lack of sustained effectiveness (20). It is not clear whether psychotherapeutic modalities have a direct impact on cancer survival. In a study reviewing cognitive-behavioral, supportive-expressive, and psychoeducational therapies, survival times for breast cancer and melanoma were not extended; instead, decreased survival was associated with greater social disparity and untreated depression. (21).

Existential and spiritual care

These therapeutic modalities have received greater attention in the palliative and pastoral care literature, but the topics often arise for consulting psychiatrists during bedside encounters (26). A resource for support and assessment of existential issues is the article by Skalla and McCoy, in which clinicians are coached in using their MorVAST model to explore patients' beliefs about **Mor**al Authority and **V**ocational, **A**esthetic, **S**ocial, and **T**ranscendent meanings, towards gaining better understanding and support, and enhancing incorporation of patient values into the healing process (27). The NCCN Practice Guidelines encourage pastoral care as a key resource for cancer patients, suggesting that topics particularly appropriate for assessment include concerns about death and the afterlife, conflicted or challenged belief systems, conflicts between religious beliefs and recommended treatments, hopelessness, guilt, isolation from religious community, loss of faith, concerns about relationship with deity, concerns about meaning and purpose of life, and grief. The NCCN suggests referrals to pastoral care services, where interventions might include spiritual counseling, bibliotherapy, prayer, reconciliation rituals, and referral to the patient's faith community.

Exercise and movement

Indications suggest that exercise can be significantly helpful for the symptom complex of sleep disturbances (28) and fatigue (29, 30). It is less clear whether exercise is efficacious for the treatment of depression, although as interest in the use of yoga and physical therapies in cancer centers around the country has increased, reports have described diminished distress and improved quality of life.

Nutrition and supplements

Although significant attention is given to nutrition and nutritional supplements in the alternative medicine literature, findings in the scientific literature are very limited and often cause concern. It has been established that in the general population, vitamin and supplement use can have unforeseen negative consequences. In the cancer population, several recent studies showed no benefit for nutrient supplementation (31–34). And in a study of folic acid supplementation versus placebo over a 10-year period, the estimated probability of being diagnosed with prostate cancer was 9.7% in the folic acid group compared with 3.3% in the placebo group (35). Another study showed no correlation between serum levels of omega-3 fatty acid and the incidence of depression in patients with lung cancer (36). What role nutrition and supplements might have in managing depression is even less robust in the literature. However, attention to sound nutritional practices, nourishing food, and digestive health are common-sense cares for a cancer patient's overall health and quality of life.

Care for the caregivers

Depression may be present in up to 50% of the spouses and family members who are caregivers of patients with cancer. This is not simply due to anticipatory grief or stress from caregiving responsibilities. Caregivers may have depressive disorders with high morbidity and mortality (37). In a study of the caregivers of 64 patients with prostate cancer, 40.7% reported high anxiety, 36.7% had sleep disturbances, and 12.1% reported depression. Patients with distressed caregivers had lower levels of functioning and reported lower quality of life (38). In another study looking at depression in caregivers of terminal cancer patients, caregivers' depression was not dependent on the degree of care demanded, but was associated with caregiver age and the time between diagnosis and death of the patient. Those caregivers aged 45 to 54 reported more depressive symptoms, while caregivers aged 35 to 44 reported more difficulty with feelings of abandonment. Patients who died very quickly after diagnosis had caregivers who reported the highest level of depressive symptoms and burden in the cohort (39). Screening caregivers for depression and distress can be a very important psychosocial intervention, both for the caregiver and for the cancer patient. A variety of screening mechanisms have been used successfully for caregivers, including the distress thermometer.

Although distress of family members of cancer patients has been evaluated, what has not been so well acknowledged or measured in terms of clinical impact is the distress of healthcare providers. It is clear that medical caregivers experience significant distress in their own right. In 1991, a survey of 1000 members of the American Society of Clinical Oncology found that 56% of them fulfilled the criteria for burnout syndrome (40). In 2008, a meta-analysis of 10 studies (N = 2375) looked at symptoms of burnout in cancer professionals and found on self-report that 36% had emotional exhaustion, 35% experienced depersonalization of others as objects, and 25% had low personal satisfaction (41). While teaching cancer patients a comprehensive model of cancer care, ironically, medical caregivers may have difficulty in taking care of themselves. What impact the distress and burnout of cancer professionals have had on the distress or outcomes of patient care has not been evaluated in the medical literature. However, in the evaluation of patients with cancer, consulting psychiatrists may have an opportunity to provide education, empathy, and care for medical caregivers as well as the family caregivers.

Cancer survivorship

Depression and other psychiatric illnesses are not incidental or trivial, but are causally related to features of the cancer survivor's life journey, from pre-diagnosis, to diagnosis and treatment, and beyond into ongoing survivorship. Psychosocial studies have largely focused on care for patients in the initial diagnosis and treatment stages, but as survival continues to improve and the long-term consequences of cancer are better investigated, it has been suggested that 20% to 30% of cancer survivors who are 5 or more years from diagnosis continue to have psychosocial consequences of their cancer (42). The experience of cancer has lasting existential impact, as many patients moving out of acute treatment struggle to make meaning of the experience and its impact on their lives and relationships. Lasting signs of the cancer journey may provoke depressive symptoms in cancer survivors. For example, correlation has been observed between the prevalence of depression and negative perceptions of body image and sexuality following mastectomy for breast cancer (43). Chronic fatigue can be an impairment in cancer survivors, especially in those with co-morbid depression (44, 45). Risks of suicide remain elevated compared to the general population (10). In patients with a history of cancer, the consultation psychiatrist must be mindful of personal trauma and medical consequences associated with that experience.

References

1. Derogatis LR, Morrow GR, Fetting J, et al. The prevalence of psychiatric disorders among cancer patients. JAMA. 1983; 24:751–7.

2. Massie MJ. Prevalence of depression in patients with cancer. J Natl Cancer Inst Monogr. 2004;32:57–71.

3. Kathol R, Muigi A, Williams J, et al. Diagnosis of major depression according to four sets of criteria. Am J Psychiatry. 1990; 147:1021–4.

4. Endicott J. Measurement of depression in patients with cancer. Cancer. 1984;53 (10suppl):2243–9.

5. National Comprehensive Cancer Network, Inc. Clinical practice guidelines in oncology: distress management. Vol 1. 2008. Available from: www.nccn.org/ professionals/physician_gls/f_guidelines.asp [on-line].

6. Berry PH, Chapman CR, Covington EC, et al., editors. Pain: current understanding of assessment, management and treatments. National Pharmaceutical Council and the Joint Commission for the Accreditation of Healthcare Organizations; 2001.

7. Roth AJ, Kornblith AB, Batel-Copel L, et al. Rapid screening for psychologic distress in men with prostate carcinoma: a pilot study. Cancer. 1998;82:1904–8.

8. Mitchell A. Pooled results of from 38 analyses of the accuracy of distress thermometer and other ultra-short methods of detecting cancer-related mood disorders. J Clin Oncol. 2007;25(29): 4670–81.

9. Camidge DR, Stockton DL, Frame S, et al. Hospital admissions and deaths relating to deliberate self-harm and accidents within 5 years of a cancer diagnosis: a national study in Scotland, UK. Br J Cancer. 2007; 96(5):752–7.

10. Misono S, Weiss NS, Fann JR, et al. Incidence of suicide in persons with cancer. J Clin Oncol. 2008;26(29):4731–8.

11. Kaasa S, Malt U, Hagen S, et al. Psychological distress in cancer patients with advanced disease. Radiother Oncol. 1993;27:193–7.

12. Stone P, Hardy J, Broadley K, et al. Fatigue in advanced cancer: a prospective controlled cross-sectional study. Br J Cancer. 1999;79:1479–86.

13. Sateia MJ, Lang BJ. Sleep and cancer: recent developments. Curr Oncol Rep. 2008;10(4):309–18.

14. Dodd MJ, Miaskowski C, Paul SM. Symptom clusters and their effect on the functional status of patients with cancer. Oncol Nurs Forum. 2001;28: 465–70.

15. Kim HJ, McGuire DB, Tulman L, et al. Symptom clusters: concept analysis and clinical implications for cancer nursing. Cancer Nurs. 2005;28:270–84.

16. Cleeland CS, Bennett GJ, Dantzer R, et al. Are the symptoms of cancer and cancer treatment due to a shared biologic mechanism? A cytokine-immunologic model of cancer symptoms. Cancer. 2003;97:2919–25.

17. Donovan KA, Jacobsen PB. Fatigue, depression, and insomnia: evidence for a symptom cluster in cancer. Semin Oncol Nurs. 2007;23:127–35.

18. Miller K, Massie MJ. Depression and anxiety. Cancer J. 2006;12(5):388–97.

19. Guo Y, Musselman DL, Manatunga AK, et al. The diagnosis of major depression in patients with cancer: a comparative approach. Psychosomatics. 2006;47: 376–84.

20. Williams S, Dale J. The effectiveness of treatment for depression/depressive symptoms in adults with cancer: a systematic review. Br J Cancer. 2006; 94:372–90.

21. Henry NL, Stearns V, Flockhart DA, et al. Drug interactions and pharmacogenomics in the treatment of breast cancer and depression. Am J Psychiatry. 2008;165(10): 1251–5.

22. Stearns V, Johnson MD, Rae JM, et al. Active tamoxifen metabolite plasma concentrations after coadministration of tamoxifen and the selective serotonin

reuptake inhibitor paroxetine. J Natl Cancer Inst. 2003;95(23):1758–64.

23. Goetz MP, Kama Al, Ames MM. Tamoxifen pharmacogenomics: the role of CYP2D6 as a predictor of drug response. Clin Pharmacol Ther. 2008;83(1):160–6.

24. Goetz MP, Rae JM, Suman VJ, et al. Pharmacogenetics of tamoxifen biotransformation is associated with clinical outcomes of efficacy and hot flashes. J Clin Oncol. 2007;25:5187–93.

25. Naaman S, Radwan K, Fergusson D, et al. Status of psychological trials in breast cancer patients: a report of three meta-analyses. Psychiatry. 2009;72(1): 50–69.

26. Kissane D. Beyond the psychotherapy and survival debate: the challenge of social disparity, depression and treatment adherence in psychosocial cancer care. Psychooncology. 2009;18(1):1–5.

27. Skalla K, McCoy JP. Spiritual assessment of patients with cancer: the moral authority, vocational, aesthetic, social, and transcendent model. Oncol Nurs Forum. 2006; 33(4):745–51.

28. Payne JK, Held J, Thorpe J, et al. Effect of exercise on biomarkers, fatigue, sleep disturbances, and depressive symptoms in older women with breast cancer receiving hormonal therapy. Oncol Nurs Forum. 2008;35(4):635–42.

29. Mitchell S, Beck S, Hood L, et al. Evidence-based interventions for fatigue during and following cancer and its treatment. Clin J Oncol Nurs. 2007;11(1): 99–113.

30. Kirshbaum MN. A review of the benefits of whole body exercise during and after treatment for breast cancer. J Clin Nurs. 2007;16(1):104–21.

31. Gaziano JM, Glynn RJ, Christen WG, et al. Vitamins E and C in the prevention of prostate and total cancer in men. The Physicians' Health Study II Randomized Controlled Trial. JAMA. 2009;301(1): 52–62.

32. Lippman SM, Klein EA, Goodman PJ, et al. Effect of selenium and vitamin E on risk of prostate cancer and other cancers. The Selenium and Vitamin E Cancer Prevention Trial (SELECT). JAMA. 2009;301(1):39–51.

33. Zhang SM, Cook NR, Albert CM, et al. Effect of combined folic acid, vitamin B6, and vitamin B12 on cancer risk in women: a randomized trial. JAMA. 2008;300(17): 2012–21.

34. Lin J, Cook NR, Albert CM, et al. Vitamins C and E and beta carotene supplementation and cancer risk: a randomized controlled trial. J Natl Cancer Inst. 2009;101(1): 14–23.

35. Figueiredo JC, Grau MV, Haile RW, et al. Folic acid and risk of prostate cancer: results from a randomized clinical trial. J Natl Cancer Inst. 2009;101:432–5.

36. Kobayakawa M, Yamawakii S, Hamazaki K, et al. Levels of omega-3 fatty acid in serum phospholipids and depression in patients with lung cancer. Br J Cancer. 2005;93: 1329–33.

37. Rivera HR. Depression symptoms in cancer caregivers. Clin J Oncol Nurs. 2009;13(2):195–202.

38. Fletcher BS, Paul SM, Dodd MJ, et al. Prevalence, severity, and impact of symptoms on female family caregivers of patients at the initiation of radiation therapy for prostate cancer. J Clin Oncol. 2008;26(4):599–605.

39. Given B, Wyatt G, Given C, et al. Burden and depression among caregivers of patients with cancer at end of life. Oncol Nurs Forum. 2004;31(6):1105–15.

40. Whippen DA, Canellos GP. Burnout syndrome in the practice of oncology: results of a random survey of 1000 oncologists. J Clin Oncol. 1991;9: 1916–20.

41. Trufelli DC, Bensi CG, Garcia JB, et al. Burnout in cancer professionals: a systematic review and meta-analysis. Eur J Cancer Care. 2008;17(6):524–31.

42. Foster C. Psychosocial implications of living 5 years or more after cancer diagnosis: a systematic review of the research evidence. Eur J Cancer Care. 2009;18(3):223–47.

43. Reich M, Lesur A, Pedrizet-Chevallier C. Depression, quality of life and breast cancer: a review of the literature. Breast Cancer Res Treat. 2008;110(1):9–17.

44. Minton O, Richardson A, Sharpe M, et al. A systematic review and meta-analysis of the pharmacological treatment of cancer-related fatigue. J Natl Cancer Inst. 2008;100(16):1155–66.

45. Butler LD, Koopman C, Cordova MJ, et al. Psychological distress and pain significantly increase before death in metastatic breast cancer patients. Psychosom Med. 2003;65(3):416–26.

Depression in the patient with hepatitis C

Joseph A. Locala

Typical consult question

"My patient has a history of depression and chronic hepatitis C. Is it safe to start interferon? If so, how do I manage him/her, from a psychiatric standpoint, during the treatment course?"

Introduction

Current recommended therapy for hepatitis C viral infection (HCV) consists of pegylated interferon-alpha and ribavirin, a combination associated with significant risk for development of depressive disorders, other mood disorders, and anxiety. In the early days of interferon (IFN) therapy, patients were screened for psychiatric co-morbidity with the intent to exclude them from treatment. High rates of psychiatric illness and substance use disorders in the HCV population effectively denied many patients care. Current guidelines allow for treatment of patients with psychiatric history or recent mood symptoms; however, screening for pre-existing mood disorders and careful monitoring for emergence of psychiatric problems during therapy remain critical for safe and efficacious treatment of chronic HCV. This chapter will

- Review pre-treatment considerations and risk factors for development of psychiatric side effects
- Discuss prophylactic antidepressant therapy during interferon therapy
- Suggest a treatment algorithm for IFN-induced depression
- Propose causes of IFN-induced psychiatric symptoms

Background

Hepatitis C infection is a serious global health issue that affects 170 million people worldwide and approximately 4 million individuals in the United States (1). Patients with chronic HCV are prone to develop significant morbidity and mortality, often at an early age. Up to 20% of persons with untreated chronic HCV will develop cirrhosis within 20 to 25 years and are at increased risk for end-stage liver disease and hepatocellular carcinoma (2, 3). However, treatment with pegylated interferon and ribavirin in combination results in 50% of patients with undetectable levels of HCV in the blood 6 months after therapy ends (3). With such an efficacious response, management of adverse effects and optimal enrollment of eligible patients into therapy become paramount. Interferon-induced depression is a major obstacle to successful treatment and must be addressed.

Psychosomatic Medicine: An Introduction to Consultation-Liaison Psychiatry, eds. James J. Amos and Robert G. Robinson. Published by Cambridge University Press. © Cambridge University Press 2010.

Table 17.1 Reasons for psychiatric consultation prior to IFN therapy

Current depression or anxiety symptoms

Current suicide or homicide ideation

History of IFN-induced psychiatric symptoms

History of depressive disorder, bipolar disorder, or anxiety disorder, or other major psychiatric disorder

History of prior suicidal thoughts or attempts

Strong family history of mood disorders

Personal history of substance use disorders

Patients with HCV have higher rates of baseline psychiatric disorders. In a recent study of HCV patients treated at a university hospital in Brazil, 49% had at least one psychiatric diagnosis as assessed by the Mini-International Neuropsychiatric Interview. Of that subgroup, 59% had current psychiatric symptoms and 85% had gone undiagnosed. Thirty-six percent had two or more psychiatric diagnoses, 29% had co-morbid substance abuse/dependence, and 19% had current mood disorder (4). In another sample, higher prevalence rates for depression (26%) and anxiety disorders (24%) were demonstrated in untreated HCV populations (5). Depression in this study was associated with methadone maintenance, poor work and social adjustment, lower acceptance of illness, higher illness stigma, reports of poor cognition and concentration, and more subjective physical symptoms. Significant prevalence rates for HCV have been reported in psychiatric patients. Screening for HCV must be considered for patients in psychiatric practice, particularly when risk factors exist, and in older, less educated males with substance use histories (5). Dinwiddie et al. screened 1556 admissions to a public sector psychiatric hospital and found HCV seroprevalence rates of 8.5% (6). Not only is this important for recognition and treatment of undiagnosed liver disease, but prevalence of HCV and potential cirrhosis will impact psychopharmacology practice in this population.

In general terms, one can estimate the rate of depression caused by interferon-alpha/ribavirin therapy to average one in three patients. This estimate is based upon recent, prospective studies that utilized screening instruments and structured interviews to identify the prevalence of depression at 23% to 45% (7). Rates of depression appear related to dose and duration of therapy, and IV interferon appears to cause higher depression ratings than subcutaneous IFN (8). The addition of ribavirin to the regimen appears to independently increase risk for depression (9).

Close collaboration with a psychiatrist is recommended for patients with co-morbid psychiatric history. In a recent study from France, a retrospective survey showed that 19% of patients with a psychiatric diagnosis had not received optimal treatment for HCV and less than half of managing clinicians were working in collaboration with a psychiatrist or psychologist (10). Table 17.1 outlines circumstances in which referral to psychiatry is critical during interferon therapy. Past history significant for major mental disorders, suicidality, interferon-induced neuropsychiatric disorders, or substance use disorders, as well as current psychiatric symptoms, necessitates ongoing psychiatric monitoring. The optimal setting for treatment of HCV should include use of standardized assessments to identify at-risk patients, adequate staffing to permit ongoing close psychosocial monitoring and symptom evaluation, clinical expertise to initiate pharmacologic intervention in a timely fashion, and a close working relationship with mental health providers experienced with interferon-induced psychiatric disorders (11).

Although depression is the most widely reported neuropsychiatric side effect of IFN therapy, clinicians should be aware that other symptoms, such as simple fatigue, anxiety, insomnia, irritability, cognitive impairment, and mania, may occur. Suicide is a real threat for patients in treatment for HCV. Suicidal thoughts are a common complication of interferon therapy and stem from a combination of depressive symptoms along with anxiety, agitation, and irritability. Dieperink et al. reported rates of suicidal ideation as high as 27% in HCV patients who were not on interferon, and 43% of patients on interferon endorsed suicide ideation at some point during therapy (12). Screening for suicide ideation must occur at regular, closely spaced intervals.

Screening and assessment

Diagnosis of a significant depressive disorder in patients on IFN is confounded by other adverse effects of this medication, including fatigue, sleep disturbance, irritability, and anxiety symptoms. Although the depressive disorder in this instance is most accurately labeled a substance-induced mood disorder, depressed or mixed, the criteria for major depressive disorder are used clinically to determine need for treatment. Patients respond best when treatment for depression is initiated early, so the threshold for starting an antidepressant should be low. Onset of depression typically occurs within the first three months of therapy (highest in the first eight weeks) and prevalence increases for the initial six months of therapy (13, 14).

All candidates cleared for IFN medically should receive psychosocial screening, which at a minimum must include past psychiatric history and current assessment for mood or anxiety symptoms, substance use, and suicidality. It is useful to employ depression screening tools such as the Beck Depression Inventory (BDI), the Zung Self-Rating Depression Scale, or the Center for Epidemiologic Studies Depression Scale (CES-D). In a study of patients receiving interferon-alpha 2b for chronic HCV, use of the seven items in the Zung vegetative-depressive subscale at four weeks of therapy successfully predicted 95% of emerging depressions (15). At the time of initial evaluation, patients (and families if present) must be educated about the risk of IFN-induced neuropsychiatric disorders and how to recognize symptoms. Explain that treatment options are available if these problems emerge, and encourage patients to self-report. Significant pressure exists to complete a full round of therapy. Patients have been known to minimize symptoms for fear that interferon will be terminated.

Clinical decision-making and treatment

Proposed mechanisms for interferon-induced depression

Understanding the mode in which substances iatrogenically cause depressive disorders may lead to greater appreciation of mechanisms for depression occurring in the natural state. Loftis et al. demonstrated an association between severity of depressive symptoms and expression of pro-inflammatory cytokines (tumor necrosis factor [TNF]-alpha and interleukin [IL]-1 beta) in HCV patients *in the absence of* IFN therapy (16). Multiple theories for biological mechanisms of IFN-induced mood disorders have been presented, each of which warrants separate recognition. For a concise summary, see Table 17.2.

Table 17.2 Proposed mechanisms for interferon-induced depression

Serotonin (5-HT) abnormalities: serotonin depletion due to shunt from tryptophan pathway
Genetic differences in the serotonin reuptake transporter promoter (5-HTTLPR): interaction with inflammatory cytokines may contribute to depression
Polymorphism of 5-HT receptor gene: IFN alters encoding for the 5-HT_{2c} receptor
HPA axis dysfunction: IFN stimulates CRH and increases ACTH
Increase in inflammatory cytokines (e.g., IL-6) linked to depression
ICAM-1: increased levels; increased blood-brain barrier permeability
Increased nitric oxide production associated with depression
Over-stimulation of hippocampal NMDA receptors: results in apoptosis and neuronal atrophy
Diminished dopaminergic function
Thyroid dysfunction: hypothyroidism secondary to IFN

Key:
ACTH = adrenocorticotropic hormone
CRH = corticotropin releasing hormone
HPA = hypothalamic-pituitary axis
ICAM = intercellular adhesion molecule
IFN = interferon
IL = interleukin
NMDA = N-methyl-D-aspartate

Immune system activation causes tryptophan to shunt from the serotonin pathway to the kynrenine pathway, with a resultant decrease in overall serotonin (17). Decreases in plasma tryptophan have been demonstrated to correlate with increased depression during interferon-alpha therapy (18). Interferon-alpha has been demonstrated in human glioblastoma cells to alter encoding for the 5-HT_{2c} receptor, with the suggestion that this is relevant to the development of depression (19). Genetic differences in the serotonin reuptake transporter promoter (5-HTTLPR) have been associated with major depressive disorder during interferon-alpha treatment, highlighting a possible interaction between inflammatory cytokines and 5-HTTLPR variability (20). The efficacy of serotinergic antidepressants for IFN-induced depression may be explained by diminished serotonergic function in IFN-induced depression. Interferon-alpha therapy has been found to alter other monoamines, such as dopamine (21) and norepinephrine; these changes may play a causal role in depression.

Interferon-alpha activates other pro-inflammatory cytokines. Cytokines are frequently regulated in cascades, where earlier cytokines serve to increase production of later cytokines. Pro-inflammatory cytokines, such as IL-1, IL-6, and TNF augment the immune response to speed elimination of pathogens and resolve inflammatory challenge, whereas anti-inflammatory cytokines, such as IL-4, IL-10, and IL-13 serve to dampen the immune response (22). It is interesting to note that some studies have linked hyperactivity of the hypothalamic-pituitary axis and parallel increases in pro-inflammatory cytokines to the presence of major depression (23). Sickness behaviors often associated with infection, such as increased sleep, decreased appetite, and decreased sex drive, may also be attributed to effects of the cytokines (22). During treatment with IFN, a rise in IL-6 was correlated with development of depression and anxiety symptoms. Interferon-alpha activates the hypothalamic-pituitary-adrenal axis through direct stimulation of corticotropin-releasing hormone, which subsequently increases adrenocorticotropic hormone (ACTH) production (24). Both of these hormones have been found to be elevated in major depressive disorder.

One theory is that IFN causes increased permeability of the blood-brain barrier as a result of increased levels of the intercellular adhesion molecule (ICAM)-1, which also is found in higher amounts in post-mortem analysis of depressed patients (25). A recent study demonstrated higher serum ICAM-1 levels and depression scores after three months of interferon therapy (25).

Interferon may be associated with overstimulation of N-methyl-D-aspartate (NMDA) receptors in the hippocampus, which results in apoptosis and neuronal atrophy (26, 27). One small study found efficacy in treating patients with HCV on interferon therapy with amantadine, an NMDA receptor antagonist and dopaminergic agent, with resultant diminished depression scores on the Hospital Anxiety and Depression Scale (28). Additional double-blind placebo-controlled studies will be necessary before clear conclusions can be drawn.

Other causes have been proposed in a theoretical sense with less research to back them. These include the link to interferon-induced hypothyroidism, depressive symptoms exacerbated by IFN-induced anemia (more common with the combination of IFN and ribavirin) (29), and the relation between increased nitric oxide and depression onset (30). These all warrant closer investigation.

Pretreatment and the debate over prophylactic medications

Many clinicians advocate prophylactic antidepressants for patients with a history of severe depression or previous depression with IFN therapy, this author included. Evidence to support general use of antidepressants to minimize psychiatric side effects is lacking at this time.

For those who receive higher dose IFN, such as in the treatment of melanoma, preventative medication seems to have greater utility. Indeed, a double-blind, placebo-controlled trial of patients receiving high-dose IFN-alpha for malignant melanoma found that pretreatment with paroxetine reduced the incidence of depression from 45% to 11% (13). However, research is still unclear as to the merit of prophylactic antidepressants for all patients with HCV, including those without psychiatric history. Two double-blind studies using prophylactic paroxetine for prevention of IFN-induced depression came to different conclusions. One study found no decrease in the likelihood of depression with prophylactic antidepressants (36% paroxetine group and 32% placebo group) (31). However, investigators did note that open-label treatment with paroxetine in the rescue arm of the study helped to reduce symptoms of depression in 10 of 11 patients. Another study demonstrated that pre-treatment with paroxetine decreased the likelihood of development of moderate to severe depressive symptoms during a six-month trial of pegylated interferon-alpha 2b and ribavirin (32).

Treatment of depression symptoms during IFN therapy

The primary treatment for IFN-induced depression is traditional antidepressant therapy; however, a number of adjuvant medications have been utilized to assist with symptomatic relief. An overview of medications is provided in Table 17.3. This is meant to be a short list of options and is by no means inclusive of all possible therapies. Guidelines for screening and ongoing monitoring and specific treatment recommendations for IFN-induced depression are reviewed in Table 17.4.

Selective serotonin reuptake inhibitors (SSRIs) clearly appear to be the optimal first-line therapy for IFN-induced depressive disorders. Case reports and limited studies can be found

Table 17.3 Common medications used for treatment of neuropsychiatric complications of interferon (IFN)

Medication Class	Specific Medications to Consider	Target Disorder or Symptom	Comments
Selective serotonin reuptake inhibitors (SSRIs)	citalopram, paroxetine, escitalopram, sertraline	Depression Anxiety Irritability	SSRIs are a good first-line treatment.
Serotonin-norepinephrine reuptake inhibitors (SNRIs), dopaminergic or other antidepressants	bupropion venlafaxine duloxetine mirtazapine	Depression Irritability (SNRIs)	Bupropion has potential for seizure in combo with IFN. Duloxetine may be problematic in patients with chronic liver disease. Mirtazapine may assist with insomnia and poor appetite.
Stimulants	modafinil methylphenidate	Adjuvant for Depression Fatigue	May cause heightened anxiety or insomnia in some patients. Traditional stimulants such as methylphenidate may exacerbate psychotic symptoms.
Anxiolytics	lorazepam		Use short half-life meds (glucuronidated) because of liver disease: use caution with addictive medications in this population.
Dopamine agonists	amantadine	Depression	Still experimental and with limited evidence
Hypnotics	zolpidem trazodone mirtazapine	Insomnia	Zolpidem has potential for abuse, albeit lower than benzodiazepines.
Mood stabilizers	quetiapine olanzapine	Hypomania Mania	First-line treatment would be atypical antipsychotics, pending further psychiatric evaluation.

for many of the SSRIs, including sertraline, citalopram, and paroxetine. This author has experienced excellent results with sertraline, potentially because of the serotinergic and dopaminergic effects of this medication. Sertraline can be somewhat activating for some patients and may induce additional anxiety, which is less common with citalopram or escitalopram. Kraus et al. reported a randomized, double-blind, placebo-controlled study of citalopram for patients who became depressed during IFN therapy (peg-IFN alpha-2b plus ribavirin), which led to reduced scores on the Hospital Anxiety and Depression Scale for all those receiving medication (33). The blind was broken for the placebo group because of severe depression, and all citalopram patients were able to complete the planned course of interferon therapy.

Other options include the serotonin-norepinephrine reuptake inhibitors (SNRIs) (venlafaxine, desvenlafaxine, and duloxetine), bupropion, and mirtazapine. SNRIs have utility in the treatment of pain, which is a common side effect of antiviral therapy. Bupropion has an activating effect and is strongly dopaminergic, both of which are advantages in treating IFN-induced depression. IFN has been associated with potential seizure, and bupropion theoretically will have an additive risk for lowering seizure threshold when used concomitantly. Mirtazapine has utility for patients with significantly diminished appetite and insomnia. Antidepressants with serotonergic activity and benzodiazepines also have value in the treatment of irritability associated with IFN therapy (34).

Table 17.4 Suggested guidelines for treatment of interferon (IFN)-induced depressive disorders

1. All candidates cleared for IFN medically should receive psychiatric screening:
   a. Past psychiatric history
   b. Current screening for mood or anxiety symptoms – useful to employ screening tools such as Beck Depression Inventory (BDI), Zung Self-Rating Depression Scale, or Center for Epidemiologic Studies Depression Scale (CES-D)
   c. Inquire about substance use.
   d. Educate patients about the risk of IFN-induced neuropsychiatric disorders and how to recognize symptoms.
   e. Explain that treatment options are available if these problems emerge.
2. Patients require psychiatric management in the following circumstances:
   a. Complex psychiatric history (severe depression, suicide ideation, bipolar disorder, schizophrenia, anxiety disorders, etc)
   b. History of alcohol or substance use disorder
   c. Patient in ongoing psychiatric treatment
   d. History of significant psychiatric hospitalizations
3. In patients with current depression or anxiety of moderate or severe intensity **or** patients with history of severe depression or IFN-induced depression who are currently asymptomatic:
   a. Offer pre-treatment with antidepressant at least 4 weeks before interferon.
   b. Delay interferon therapy for patients whose symptoms remain significant after 4 weeks.
   c. Monitor at a minimum every two weeks during first three months of treatment (frequency may decrease after that time to every two to four weeks).
4. For patients who do not require pre-treatment:
   a. Initiate interferon.
   b. Monitor at a minimum every 2 weeks during the first three months, then every 2 to 4 weeks thereafter – perform psychiatric screens and ask about suicidal thoughts at every visit.
   c. If depressive symptoms occur, initiate antidepressant therapy immediately.
   d. Be aware that some patients may minimize symptoms because of concern regarding discontinuation of treatment.
   e. During IFN therapy, physical symptoms may be secondary to IFN and not frank depression. Focus especially on more psychological symptoms such as depressed mood, anhedonia, ruminatory thoughts, helpless and hopeless feelings, crying spells, irritability, social withdrawal, and guilt.
5. If depression or anxiety symptoms worsen during treatment, increase antidepressant dosage and consider augmentation with second antidepressant from a different class. Refer immediately for emergent psychiatric assessment/hospitalization and discontinue IFN for the following circumstances:
   a. Suicide or homicide ideation
   b. Hypomania, mania
   c. Severe depression, anxiety, or other psychiatric symptoms
   d. Psychosis
6. Throughout treatment, closely monitor patients with concurrent or previous substance use disorders for relapse.

Patients should continue antidepressants through the entire IFN course, and only after symptoms have fully resolved should the medications be tapered off. Antidepressants should be continued for a minimum of 1 to 3 months after IFN therapy ends.

Antidepressants offer little relief from IFN-induced fatigue, and often patients successfully treated for depression have residual physical symptoms that can be equally debilitating. Often fatigue is due to anemia, and growth factors to promote increased hemoglobin levels demonstrate effectiveness (35). Psychostimulants (such as methylphenidate) have been used extensively in patients with other medical co-morbidities to treat fatigue, and may be used as an adjuvant therapy for depressed patients and solo for treatment of isolated fatigue. Modafinil, a non-stimulant promoter of wakefulness, also has potential value in treating fatigue in this population. As with all addictive medications, caution should be exercised in the HCV population to avoid relapse into substance use.

Insomnia is another significant adverse effect of IFN therapy, and traditional benzodiazepines and hypnotics again present concern for addiction. Non-benzodiazepine hypnotics such as zolpidem and zopiclone are less addictive and efficacious. Sedating antidepressants such as mirtazapine and trazodone (in low dosage, 25 to 50 mg) are also helpful. If benzodiazepines must be given, use of those metabolized by glucuronidation such as lorazepam, temazepam, and oxazepam is best in patients with liver disease.

Mania may emerge with IFN therapy, during discontinuation of IFN, and with the addition of antidepressants during the treatment course. Mania should trigger an immediate psychiatric evaluation, and clinicians should have a low threshold for psychiatric admission in this setting. First-line treatment may be initiated with atypical antipsychotics upon recognition of mania. Other mood stabilizers may be considered for the longer term after the immediate crisis has abated.

Future directions

A conclusion of recent studies has been the association of interferon-induced depression and improved treatment response with regard to HCV. One group of researchers has proposed that depression may be a marker for optimal IFN dosing and a positive predictor of antiviral response (7). This may serve as a small consolation for those patients afflicted with severe substance-induced depression.

Once the causes of interferon-induced depression and neuropsychiatric symptoms are better elucidated, we may be in a position to develop a "cocktail" of adjuvant medications to minimize side effects. The jury is still out as to whether medications given prophylactically will lessen the severity of depressive symptoms and other neuropsychiatric effects. Different types of IFN may have lesser rates of adverse events. It is thought that pegylated IFN-alpha causes less depression than IFN-alpha, and IFN-beta has been used very little in this country, but may offer the same efficacy with fewer side effects; this remains to be determined. Clearly, much additional research is necessary for a better understanding of IFN-induced disorders and their management, and perhaps a glimpse into the fundamental cause of depression itself might be obtained in the process.

References

1. Alter MJ, Kruszon-Moran D, Nainan OV, et al. The prevalence of hepatitis C virus infection in the United States, 1988 through 1994. N Engl J Med. 1999;341(8):556–62.

2. Management of hepatitis C: 2002. NIH Consens State Sci Statements. 2002;19:1–46.

3. Strader DB, Wright T, Thomas DL, et al. Diagnosis, management, and treatment of hepatitis C. Hepatology. 2004;39(4):1147–71.

4. Batista-Neves SC, Quarantini LC, de Almeida AG, et al. High frequency of unrecognized mental disorders in HCV-infected patients. Gen Hosp Psychiatry. 2008;30(1):80–2.

5. Golden J, O'Dwyer AM, Conroy RM. Depression and anxiety in patients with hepatitis C: prevalence, detection rates and risk factors. Gen Hosp Psychiatry. 2005;27(6):431–8.

6. Dinwiddie SH, Shicker L Newman T. Prevalence of hepatitis C among psychiatric patients in the public sector. Am J Psychiatry. 2003;160(1):172–4.

7. Asnis GM, De La Garza R. Interferon-induced depression in chronic hepatitis C: a review of its prevalence, risk factors, biology and treatment approaches. J Clin Gasroenterol. 2006;40(4):322–35.

8. Capuron L, Ravaud A, Dantzer R. Timing and specificity of the cognitive changes induced by interleukin-2 and interferon-alpha treatments in cancer patients. Psychosom Med. 2001;63(3):376–86.

9. Asnis GM, De LaGarza R Miller AH, et al. Ribavirin may be an important factor in IFN-induced neuropsychiatric effects. J Clin Psychiatry. 2004;65(4):581–2.

10. Lang JP, Michel L, Melin P,, et al. Management of psychiatric disorders and addictive behaviors in patients with viral hepatitis C in France. Gastroenterol Clin Biol. 2009;33(1 pt 1):1–7.

11. Raison CL, Afdal NH. Neuropsychiatric side effects associated with interferon-alfa plus ribavirin therapy: treatment and prevention. UpToDate 2009. Available from: www.uptodate.com. Accessed 5/29/2009.

12. Dieperink E, Ho SB, Tetrick L, et al. Suicidal ideation during interferon – alpha 2b and ribavirin treatment of patients with chronic hepatitis C. Gen Hosp Psychiatry. 2004;26(3):237–40.

13. Musselman DL, Lawson DH, Gumnick JF, et al. Paroxetine for the prevention of depression induced by high dose interferon alpha. N Engl J Med. 2001;344(13):961–6.

14. Horikawa N, Yamazaki T, Izumi N, et al. Incidence and clinical course of major depression in patients with hepatitis type c undergoing interferon alpha therapy: a prospective study. Gen Hosp Psychiatry. 2003;25(1):34–8.

15. Robaeys G, De Bie J, Wichers MC, et al. Early prediction of major depression in chronic hepatitis c patients during peg-interferon alpha 2b treatment by assessment of vegetative depressive symptoms after four weeks. World J Gastroenterol. 2007;13(43):5736–40.

16. Loftis JM, Huckans M, Rulmy S, et al. Depressive symptoms in patients with chronic hepatitis C are correlated with elevated plasma levels of interleukin 1 beta and tumor necrosis factor alpha. Neurosci Lett. 2008;430(3):264–8.

17. Bonaccorso S, Marino V, Puzella A, et al. Increased depressive ratings in patients with hepatitis C receiving interferon-alpha-based immunotherapy are related to interferon-alpha-induced changes in the serotonergic system. J Clin Psychopharmacol. 2002;22(1):86–90.

18. Capuron L, Neurauter G Musselman Dl, et al. Interferon-induced changes in tryptophan metabolism: relationship to depression and paroxetine treatment. Biol Psychiatry. 2003;54(9):906–14.

19. Yang W, Wang Q, Kanes SJ, et al. Altered RNA editing of serotonin 5-HT2c receptor induced by interferon: implications for depression associated with cytokine therapy. Mol Brain Res. 2004;124(1):70–8.

20. Lotrich FE, Ferrell RE, Rabinovitz M,, et al. Risk for depression during interferon alpha treatment is affected by the serotonin transporter polymorphism. Biol Psychiatry. 2009;65(4):344–8.

21. Shuto H, Kataoka Y, Horikawa T, et al. Repeated interferon-alpha administration inhibits dopaminergic neural activity in the mouse brain. Brain Res. 1997;747(2):348–51.

22. Kronfol Z, Remick D: Cytokines and the brain: implications for clinical psychiatry. Am J Psychiatry. 2000;157(5):683–94.

23. Maes M, Meltzer H, Bosmans E, et al. Increased plasma concentrations of interleukin-6, soluble interleukin-6 receptor soluble interleukin-2 receptor and transferrin receptor in major depression. J Affect Disord. 1995;34(4):301–9.

24. Gisslinger H, Svoboda T, Clodi M, et al. Interferon alpha stimulates the hypothalamic-pituitary adrenal axis in vivo and in vitro. Neuroendocrinology. 1993;57(3):489–95.

25. Schaefer M, Horn M, Schmidt F, et al. Correlation between sICAM-1 and depressive symptoms during adjuvant treatment of melanoma with interferon-alpha. Brain Behav Immun. 2004; 18(6):555–62.

26. Behan WM, McDonald M, Darlington LG, et al. Oxidative stress as a mechanism for quinolinic acid-induced hippocampal damage: protection by melatonin and deprenyl. Br J Pharmacol. 1999;128(8):1754–60.

27. Wu HQ, Guidetti P, Goodman JH, et al. Kynurenergic manipulations influence excitatory synaptic function and excitotoxic vulnerability in the rat

hippocampous in vivo. Neuroscience. 2000;97(2):243–51.

28. Quarantini LC, Miranda-Scippa A, Schinoni MI, et al. Effect of amantadine on depressive symptoms in chronic hepatitis C patients treated with pegylated interferon: a randomized, contolled pilot study. Clin Neuropharmacol. 2006;29(3):138–43.

29. Sulkowski MS. Anemia in the treatment of hepatitis C viral infection. Clin Infect Dis. 2003;37(Suppl 4):S315–S322.

30. Suzuki E, Yoshida Y, Shibuya A, et al. Nitric oxide involvement in depression during interferon-alpha therapy. Int J Neuropsychopharmacol. 2003;6(4):415–9.

31. Morasco BJ, Rifai MA, Loftis JM, et al. A randomized trial of paroxetine to prevent interferon alpha induced depression in patients with hepatitis C. J Affect Disord. 2007;103(1-3):83–90.

32. Raison CL, Woolwine BJ, Demetrashvili MF, et al. Paroxetine for prevention of depressive symptoms induced by interferon-alpha and ribavirin for hepatitis C. Aliment Pharmacol Ther. 2007;25(10): 1163–74.

33. Kraus MR, Schaffer A, Schottker K, et al. Therapy of interferon-induced depression in chronic hepatitis C with citalopram: a randomized, double-blind, placebo-controlled study. Gut. 2008;57(4): 531–6.

34. Maddock C, Baita A, Orru MG, et al. Psyhcopharmacological treatment of depression, anxiety, irritability and insomnia in patients receiving interferon-alpha: a prospective case series and a discussion of the biological mechanisms. J Psychopharmacol. 2004;18(1):41–6.

35. Afdhal NH, Dieterich DT, Pockros PJ, et al. Epoetin alfa maintains ribavirin dosage in HCV-infected patients: a prospective, double-blind, randomized controlled study. Gastroenterology. 2004;126(5): 1302–11.

Chapter 18

Psychiatric aspects of AIDS

Mary Ann Cohen

Typical consult questions

- *"Mr. A. is a forty-one year old man with AIDS who reports that he is seeing frightening faces – evaluate for visual hallucinations."*
- *"Mr. B. is a thirty-seven year old man who does not believe he has AIDS and is refusing to stay in the nursing home – he is an elopement risk."*
- *"Mr. C. is a fifty-eight year old man with HIV and hepatitis C (HCV) who is depressed and suicidal."*
- *"Ms. D. is a thirty-eight year old woman with HIV in her eighth month of pregnancy who is actively using cocaine."*
- *"Mr. E. is a sixty-eight year old man with AIDS, diabetes mellitus, hypertension, and coronary artery disease who was admitted with chest pain – please evaluate for depression."*

Mr. A. is a forty-one year old construction worker who was not diagnosed with HIV until his first hospital admission for odynophagia, weakness, wasting, and weight loss. He was found to have esophageal *Candida*, an opportunistic infection (OI) and AIDS-defining illness, and late-stage AIDS (CD4 count of 2 and an elevated viral load); he was treated for esophageal *Candida*, and was transferred to a long-term care facility for nutritional resuscitation and reconditioning, as well as combination antiretroviral medication (CART). One month later, Mr. A. was transferred back to the hospital with a fever and abnormal chest X-ray and was diagnosed with *Mycobacterium avium-intracellulare* (MAC).

When he reported that he was seeing frightening faces, his HIV clinician requested a psychiatric consultation. My psychiatric assessment revealed no psychiatric symptoms or signs to suggest delirium or an underlying thought or mood, substance dependence, or anxiety disorder that could account for his visual hallucinations. Because Mr. A. also complained of decreased visual acuity, I recommended ophthalmologic consultation. This revealed a diagnosis of the third OI, cytomegalovirus (CMV) retinitis. Mr. A.'s visual hallucinations were resolved on ganciclovir, although his visual acuity was not fully restored.

A comprehensive biopsychosocial approach (1–4) to assessment of psychiatric symptoms is needed in persons with HIV and AIDS.

Mr. B. is a thirty-seven year old disabled investment banker with AIDS (CD4 112 and elevated viral load) who was admitted to a nursing home when he was no longer able to care for himself in the community or perform activities of daily living (ADLs). On initial psychiatric consultation, Mr. B. denied being ill or needing care and wanted to return home. He had impaired memory, abstract thinking, and executive function, as well as anosognosia,

Psychosomatic Medicine: An Introduction to Consultation-Liaison Psychiatry, eds. James J. Amos and Robert G. Robinson. Published by Cambridge University Press. © Cambridge University Press 2010.

and constructional apraxia on clock and Bender drawings, psychomotor retardation, and profoundly diminished intellectual functioning relative to his educational and occupational levels. He was incontinent of urine and feces. His diagnosis was HIV-associated dementia.

After two years of direct observation CART in the nursing home setting, dementia could not be detected on psychiatric examination. Mr. B. was able to resume independent living and went from disabled young man with dementia to dapper investment banker.

Dementia can occur at any age in persons with HIV infection. Early recognition of HIV-associated dementia and treatment with CART can lead to reversal of cognitive impairment and restoration of function in some persons with AIDS.

Mr. C. is a fifty-eight year old married grandfather and disabled chef who is a long-term non-progressor with HIV, CD4 of 1382, and undetectable viral load (never treated with antiretroviral medications). He has been depressed and suicidal since his HIV diagnosis. He has multimorbid medical illnesses, as well as a prior history of depression.

Mr. C. is followed in an ambulatory AIDS center and has oxygen-dependent chronic obstructive pulmonary disease with mild cyanosis and severe emphysema, pulmonary hypertension, rheumatic heart disease, untreated hepatitis C, Paget's disease, and benign prostatic hypertrophy. He is addicted to cigarette smoking, although dependent on oxygen. He has a longstanding history of major depressive disorder and recurrent suicide ideation. Mr. C.'s suicidal thoughts rarely leave him and are related to the HIV stigma.

Mr. C. was diagnosed with major depressive disorder recurrent, severe, with chronic suicide ideation and active nicotine cigarette dependence. He engaged easily in weekly psychotherapy and agreed to attempt smoking cessation. He responded well to dynamic psychotherapy, family therapy, and medication with venlafaxine XR, 150 mg hs, and quetiapine, 25 mg at bedtime for augmentation. Bupropion XL, 150 mg, was added for smoking cessation, as well as augmentation. He responded to a recommendation to use jigsaw puzzles to keep occupied and prevent cigarette cravings but refused nicotine substitution. After two years of smoking cessation, he has been acyanotic and has convinced other family members to give up smoking as well.

Mr. C. was able, in individual and family therapy, to accept that he was not a burden to his family but a beloved, productive, valued member, and a reliable caregiver to his grandchildren. Although he remains intermittently suicidal, he is gradually working on the development of a sense of meaning and purpose; he is less depressed and is adherent to medical and psychiatric care.

Suicide is a tragic, prevalent, and risky complication of depression and of HIV and its stigma, AIDSism (5). Every person with HIV should be evaluated for depression and suicide ideation. Suicide is preventable if depression is diagnosed and adequately treated.

Ms. D. is a thirty-eight year old divorced unemployed woman with HIV who is pregnant and actively using cocaine. She was found to have posttraumatic stress disorder due to early childhood trauma and intimate partner violence and responded well to twice-weekly psychodynamic psychotherapy and placement in a structured residential drug treatment facility for pregnant and addicted women and their children. She was escorted to her psychotherapy, discontinued cocaine use, received antiretrovirals in direct observation therapy, and delivered a healthy HIV-negative baby. She continued in psychotherapy for a total of three years and began to attain her goals before relapsing to cocaine after discharge to the community and becoming non-adherent to medical and psychiatric care.

PTSD is often overlooked in persons with HIV and AIDS because it may be overshadowed by other psychiatric diagnoses. A biopsychosocial approach and integrated psychiatric and medical care are essential in AIDS psychiatry (1–3) and are necessary in the prevention of perinatal transmission of HIV infection.

Mr. E. is a sixty-eight year old married disabled attorney admitted with chest pain who has diabetes mellitus, hypertension, coronary artery disease, HIV (CD4 1100, viral load undetectable), and hepatitis C and was referred for depression. Psychiatric consultation revealed psychomotor slowing, confusion, disorientation to time and place, fluctuating levels of consciousness, emotional incontinence, and no evidence of depression. The diagnosis was hypoactive delirium. A comprehensive medical evaluation, including urine and blood cultures, was recommended and revealed a urinary tract infection with *Escherichia coli* sepsis.

Hypoactive delirium is prevalent in persons with HIV and AIDS, can masquerade as depression, and is easily resolved when the underlying cause is identified and treated.

Background

Since the development of CART in 1995, persons with access to medical care and CART are no longer dying of AIDS but are dying of other multimorbid and severe medical illnesses, as are comparable populations with HIV infection. However, when psychiatric disorders interfere with adherence to care, persons with HIV and AIDS are dying, as they did early in the pandemic before the development of antiretrovirals (6). This can happen to children with AIDS as they transition from adolescence to adulthood and rebel against following a carefully prescribed regimen; to persons with substance dependence who prioritize cocaine, crystal methamphetamine, or heroin over medical care; or to persons with depression, mania, post-traumatic stress disorder (PTSD), psychosis, or cognitive disorders. AIDS is a paradigm for psychosomatic medicine.

- AIDS is a multimorbid, severe, complex medical and psychiatric illness.
- Figure 18.1 provides a graphic representation of the complexity and severity of AIDS psychiatry.

AIDS is a paradigm of a psychosomatic illness. AIDS psychiatry has become a subspecialty of psychosomatic medicine, similar to psychonephrology, psychooncology, and transplant psychiatry. A body of AIDS psychiatry literature includes two textbooks, one edited by Cohen and Gorman (6) and the other by Fernandez and Ruiz (7), as well as thousands of articles and chapters. The Organization of AIDS Psychiatry (OAP) has a growing membership of national and international members. Founded as a Special Interest Group of the Academy of Psychosomatic Medicine in 2004, the OAP meets annually and is dedicated to providing a network and forum for AIDS psychiatrists and other mental health clinicians. It can be accessed on the Web (8).

- Although AIDS is similar to other severe and complex medical illnesses, AIDS presents special challenges, such as its public health implications, that make it a very different illness.
- AIDS is a highly stigmatized illness.
- These differences are summarized in Table 18.1.

AIDS stigma and discrimination against persons with HIV and AIDS were described in 1989 (5) as "AIDSism." AIDSism results from a multiplicity of prejudicial and discriminatory factors and is built on a foundation of racism, homophobia, ageism, addictophobia, misogyny, and discomfort with mental and medical illness, poverty, and sexuality, as well as fears of contagion and death in many communities throughout the world and in the United States.

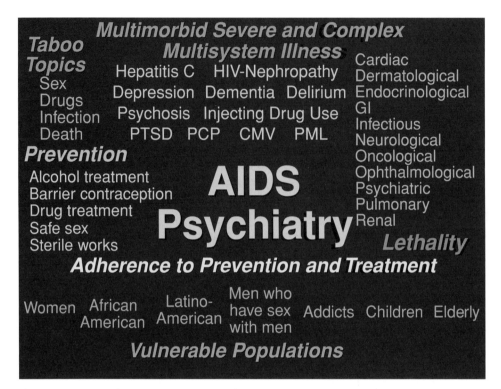

Figure 18.1 AIDS psychiatry as psychosomatic medicine paradigm.

Although the medical profession has made great strides against discrimination and stigma, AIDSism still exists. In February of 2009, a fifty-two year old New York teacher with HIV was refused excision of a facial lipoma by a dermatologist who told the patient that he was concerned about HIV infection. On May 12, 2009, Lambda Legal filed suit in U.S. federal court on behalf of a seventy-five year old university provost who fulfilled all criteria for admission to an Arkansas assisted living facility but was forced to leave the facility on the day after arrival when a detailed review of his medical records indicated HIV seropositivity (11).

Work-up

The five consultations that I have chosen represent the gamut of painful and complex medical, psychiatric, and psychosocial issues that result in severe distress and non-adherence to medical care and CART, as well as to reduction in the risk behaviors that lead to HIV transmission. These illustrative examples provide clinicians with some of the most frequent, salient, and potentially risky presenting problems in AIDS psychiatry in different medical settings:

Mr. A. – new-onset visual hallucinations in late-stage AIDS due to CMV retinitis

- Mr. A. was not diagnosed with HIV or treated with CART until he had late-stage AIDS. His hallucinations were due to CMV retinitis, an opportunistic infection with CMV that could have been prevented.
- New-onset visual hallucinations in a person with HIV or AIDS are rarely caused by underlying psychiatric disorders and most often are caused by medical conditions or delirium.

Table 18.1 How AIDS differs from most other severe and complex medical illnesses

Pathophysiology
- Infectious origin
- Modes of transmission: unsafe sex, sharing of needles in injection drug use, perinatal

Public Health Implications
- AIDS is preventable and contagious
- Disinhibition induced by HIV-associated dementia, substance use, or other psychiatric disorders can lead to HIV, HBV, HCV, and STD transmission
- Recognition and treatment of psychiatric disorders can prevent HIV transmission as well as AIDS progression and can ameliorate suffering throughout the course of illness

Unique Issues
- AIDS stigma and discrimination, or AIDSism (5)
- Age of onset from birth to old age
- Treatment, stabilization, or prevention with antiretrovirals is possible
- Exacerbation by treatment with antiretrovirals can occur – IRIS (9)
- Multiple infections and complex medical multi-morbidities
- Complex psychiatric multi-morbidities
- High prevalence of psychiatric disorders including substance use and its consequences
- High prevalence of delirium due to infectious, respiratory, cardiac, and metabolic illnesses
- High prevalence of delirium due to end-stage renal and liver disease
- High prevalence of HIV-associated dementia
- HIV is the most frequent cause of treatable dementia is persons younger than 50 [10]
- Unique neurological deficits, paresis, paralysis, pain
- Unique behavioral manifestations

Key:
HBV = hepatitis B virus
HCV = hepatitis C virus
IRIS = immune reconstitution inflammatory syndrome
STD = sexually transmitted disease

It is possible that Mr. A. was made more vulnerable to both MAC and CMV retinitis when he was started on CART in late-stage AIDS shortly after his first opportunistic infection with esophageal *Candida*. New Centers for Disease Control and Prevention (CDC) recommendations suggest that beginning CART in a treatment-naïve individual within weeks following a first opportunistic infection may unmask another subclinical opportunistic infection (such as CMV, toxoplasmosis, MAC, or cryptococcosis) by causing an immune reconstitution inflammatory syndrome (IRIS) (9).

- The differential diagnosis of visual hallucinations in late-stage AIDS is summarized in Table 18.2.
- This vignette illustrates the need for early recognition of risk behaviors, early and accurate diagnosis of new-onset psychiatric symptoms, and early diagnosis and treatment of HIV infection to prevent tragic complications such as blindness. It also validates the need for integrating mental health care into the care of persons with HIV and AIDS for both prevention of HIV infection and alleviation of suffering.

Mr. B – a young man with HAD that was reversed with CART in a nursing home setting

- HAD is prevalent long-term care settings.
- This vignette illustrates that although CART has had a major impact on both morbidity and mortality in persons with AIDS, HAD is still prevalent and is the most common treatable cause of dementia in persons younger than 50 years of age (10).

Table 18.2 Differential diagnosis of visual hallucinations in late-stage AIDS

Medical causes
- Infectious
- Cytomegalovirus (CMV) retinopathy
- Sepsis
- Fungemia
- Immune reconstitution inflammatory syndrome (IRIS)

Neurological causes
- Space-occupying lesions of brain: CNS lymphomas, toxoplasmosis, progressive multi-focal leukoencephalopathy (PML)
- Seizures: ictal, interictal, and postictal states

Psychiatric causes
- Substance use disorders
- Alcohol withdrawal
- Benzodiazepine withdrawal
- Hallucinogens
- Amphetamine and other stimulants
- Delirium – see Table 18.3 for specific causes of delirium in persons with HIV

Metabolic encephalopathy

Medications that cause delirium such as anticholinergics – see Table 18.3
- Psychotic disorders
- Schizophrenia
- Schizoaffective disorder
- Mood disorders
- Major depressive disorder with psychotic features
- Mania
- Anxiety disorders
- Posttraumatic stress disorder with psychotic features

- It is important to diagnose HIV infection early and to begin CART, because evidence suggests that HIV begins to damage the brain within months of infection.
- Every person with HIV infection needs a comprehensive evaluation for cognitive impairment at baseline and at least twice yearly to ensure early diagnosis of HIV and of HAD. Comprehensive psychiatric assessment for HAD and other psychiatric disorders in persons with HIV and AIDS is described in Chapter 6 of the *Comprehensive Textbook of AIDS Psychiatry* (4).
- HAD is a prevalent diagnosis in young persons as well as in elderly persons with AIDS.
- CART reduces the severity and slows the progression of HAD. CART that reduces the cerebrospinal fluid (CSF) viral load can induce full recovery in some persons with HAD (12).
- HAD leads to non-adherence if patients are not supervised and cannot remember to take medication or to keep appointments. Direct observation therapy in the nursing home setting led to a full reversal of Mr. B.'s dementia.
- This vignette illustrates the reversibility of HAD as well as the role of AIDS psychiatrists in its prevention and treatment.

Mr. C. – depression, suicide, and HIV infection

- Mr. C. had depression and suicide ideation and was seen in the outpatient setting of an AIDS clinic.
- Depression and suicide are prevalent in persons with HIV and AIDS (6, 7).

Table 18.3 Differential diagnosis of delirium in persons with HIV and AIDS

Toxic or drug-induced delirium
- Intoxication: sedative/hypnotics, alcoholic hallucinosis, opiates
- Drugs: antibiotics, anticholinergics, anticonvulsants, antineoplastic drugs, antiretrovirals, ketamine, lithium, narcotic analgesics
- Withdrawal: alcohol, sedative/hypnotics

Metabolic encephalopathy
- Hypoxia
- Hepatic, renal, pulmonary, pancreatic insufficiency
- Hypoglycemia

Disorders of fluid, electrolyte, and acid-base balance
- Dehydration
- Lactic acidosis (secondary to antiretroviral treatment)
- Hypernatremia, hypokalemia, hypocalcemia, hypercalcemia, alkalosis, acidosis
- Endocrine disorders
- Hypothyroidism
- Pancreatitis and diabetes mellitus

Infections
- Systemic: bacteremia, septicemia, infective endocarditis, bacterial pneumonia
- *Pneumocystis jerovici* pneumonia, cryptococcal pneumonia
- Herpes zoster
- Disseminated *Mycobacterium avium-intracellulare* complex
- Disseminated candidiasis
- Intracranial: cryptococcal meningitis, HIV encephalitis, tuberculous meningitis, toxoplasmosis

Malnutrition and vitamin deficiency
- Protein-energy undernutrition
- Vitamin B12 deficiency
- Thiamine deficiency and Wernicke's encephalopathy
- Wasting and failure to thrive

Neoplastic
- Space-occupying lesions: CNS lymphoma, CNS metastases, cryptococcoma, toxoplasmosis
- Paraneoplastic syndromes associated with lung and other neoplasms

Neurological
- Seizures: ictal, interictal, postictal states
- Head trauma
- Space-occupying lesions of brain: CNS lymphomas, toxoplasmosis, cytomegalovirus infection, abscesses, cryptococcoma

Hypoxia
- *Pneumocystis jerovici* pneumonia
- Pulmonary hypertension
- Cardiomyopathy
- Coronary artery disease
- End-stage pulmonary disease
- Anemia

- It is extremely important to take a suicide history in every person with HIV and AIDS. For details on suicide history taking in persons with HIV, see Chapter 6 in Cohen and Chao (4).
- It is also important to incorporate smoking cessation as well as nutrition, relaxation, and exercise as part of an effort to maximize life potential in persons with HIV and AIDS.
- Psychotherapy, crisis intervention, family therapy, and medication can alleviate depression and prevent the tragic complication of suicide in persons with HIV and AIDS.

Ms. D. – pregnant woman with HIV who has PTSD and active cocaine dependence

- PTSD is often overlooked in persons with HIV and AIDS because it may be overshadowed by other psychiatric diagnoses such as substance dependence and depression, which often are multimorbid with PTSD. Furthermore, early trauma may lead to substance dependence to numb the anguish of traumatic memories and to escape from intrusive thoughts. In AIDS, the diagnosis of PTSD has been associated with risky behavior and non-adherence to risk reduction and medical care (1).
- Early childhood trauma–induced PTSD is prevalent in persons with HIV and responds well to psychodynamic psychotherapy and medication (1).
- Ms. E. responded well to a structured rehabilitation residential treatment program.
- Psychiatric care and an integrated multi-disciplinary team approach to prenatal and other care of persons with HIV and AIDS can make a difference in the prevention of perinatal, sexual, and injection drug–related HIV transmission, as well as illness progression and the morbidity and mortality of AIDS.

Mr. E. – delirium due to urosepsis in a person with AIDS

- Mr. E. had multimorbid medical illness and was found to have hypoactive delirium due to urosepsis.
- Delirium is rarely recognized by HIV clinicians and is rarely mentioned in reasons for consultation, although it is the most common reason for consultation in the inpatient medical setting (see Chapter 4 of this textbook).
- It is often possible to identify a specific cause in persons with HIV and AIDS.
- Delirium may be overlooked in persons with HIV and AIDS because it can be prevalent in any age group; in other illnesses, it is more prevalent in older individuals.
- Delirium is a prevalent diagnosis in the inpatient medical setting in persons with AIDS and may be overlooked because it often mimics other psychiatric disorders. Hypoactive delirium often masquerades as depression; hyperactive or agitated delirium often masquerades as mania or psychosis.
- Delirium may be superimposed on HIV-associated dementia. (See Chapter 4 of this handbook for a full discussion of delirium.)
- A differential diagnosis of delirium in AIDS is presented in Table 18.3.

Clinical decision-making and treatment

Clinical decision-making in persons living with HIV and AIDS takes into account not only the multimorbid medical and psychiatric illnesses but also the need for prevention of HIV transmission and alleviation of the distress and suffering of persons infected and affected by the illness. Psychiatric illness is prevalent in persons with HIV infection, and HIV infection is prevalent in persons with severe mental illness. The most important factors in clinical decision-making include the following:

- Psychosomatic medicine and prevention of HIV transmission
    - Prevention of early childhood trauma through prenatal and parenting education
    - Designing educational programs for children and adolescents to prevent unsafe sex and substance abuse and other risky behaviors
    - Recognition of, education about, and treatment of risky behaviors and their causes

- Education of clinicians
  - Encouraging availability of condoms in inpatient and outpatient settings
  - Education of staff about offering testing for HIV
  - Education about reduction of risk behavior, harm reduction
  - Training about sexual and drug history taking
- Recognition and treatment of psychiatric disorders – diagnostic mnemonic A, B, C, D
  - Anxiety and PTSD
  - Bereavement
  - Bipolar disorder and mania secondary to HIV
  - Cognitive disorders – delirium and HIV-associated dementia
  - Drug and alcohol dependence
  - Depression
  - Demoralization
- Comprehensive psychiatric evaluation (4)

Each person with AIDS who is referred for psychiatric consult should be carefully evaluated at baseline and evaluated periodically for the following:

- Risk behaviors and histories– relational patterns, sexual behaviors, and drug use
- Depression
- Suicide ideation and history
- Cognitive impairment

Treatment issues

- Psychotherapeutic modalities – full range of modalities tailored to needs
  - Individual, couple, family, and group psychotherapy
  - Crisis intervention
  - Palliative psychiatry
  - Bereavement therapy
  - Spiritual support
  - Relaxation response
  - Wellness interventions including exercise, yoga, keeping a journal or writing a life narrative, reading, artwork, movement therapy, and listening to music or books on tape

Psychopharmacology and AIDS psychiatry (12–14)

- General principles
  - Accurate diagnosis and awareness of drug-drug and drug-illness interactions are of primary importance in AIDS psychiatry; it is important to become familiar with resources in the literature (12–14) as well as those on-line that are updated regularly (15, 16).
  - The principle of geriatric psychopharmacology is even more significant in AIDS psychiatry: START VERY LOW and GO VERY SLOW.
  - Persons with AIDS are exquisitely vulnerable to extrapyramidal and anticholinergic side effects of psychotropic medications.

Psychopharmacology and addictive disorders (12–15)

- Become familiar with medications that are cytochrome p 450 3A4 inducers because these medications can lower levels of methadone in persons on agonist treatment and will lead to opioid withdrawal symptoms, discontinuation of antiretrovirals, or relapse to heroin
- Cytochrome P450 3A4 inducers include the following:
  - Carbamazepine
  - Efavirenz
  - Nevirapine
  - Ritonavir
  - St. John's wort

- When a person with AIDS and pain is maintained on a standing dose of methadone or is treated with methadone for heroin withdrawal, pain should be treated as a separate problem with additional opioids including methadone.
- The patient's methadone maintenance dose cannot be thought of as analgesia, but rather as agonist therapy for relapse and withdrawal prevention. Methadone for relapse prevention will target opioid tolerance needs and prevent withdrawal but will not provide analgesia for pain.

Psychopharmacology and other psychiatric disorders (12–15) – includes results of OAP Consensus Survey (12) – with examples of medicines and doses

- Citalopram, 10 to 40 mg, or escitalopram, 10 to 20 mg
- Quetiapine, 25 to 100 mg, or olanzapine, 2.5 to 10 mg
- Bupropion, 150 to 300 mg
- Clonazepam, 1 to 2 mg bid

Conclusion

Psychosomatic medicine psychiatrists, AIDS psychiatrists, geriatric psychiatrists, child psychiatrists, other psychiatrists, and mental health clinicians can play a vital role in the prevention of HIV transmission, the care of persons with HIV and AIDS, the leadership of multidisciplinary teams, and prevention of the stigma of AIDS or AIDSism.

References

1. Cohen MA, Alfonso CA. AIDS psychiatry: psychiatric and palliative care, and pain management. In: Wormser GP, editor. AIDS and other manifestations of HIV infection. 4th ed. San Diego: Elsevier Academic Press; 2004. p. 537–76.

2. Cohen MA, Weisman H. A biopsychosocial approach to AIDS. Psychosomatics. 1986;27:245–9.

3. Cohen MA. History of AIDS psychiatry – a biopsychosocial approach – paradigm and

paradox. In: Cohen MA, Gorman JM, editors. Comprehensive textbook of AIDS psychiatry. New York (NY): Oxford University Press; 2008. p. 3–14.

4. Cohen MA, Chao D. Comprehensive psychosocial and psychiatric diagnostic consultation in persons with HIV and AIDS. In: Cohen MA, Gorman JM, editors. Comprehensive textbook of AIDS psychiatry. New York (NY): Oxford University Press; 2008. p. 61–73.

5. Cohen MA. AIDSism, a new form of discrimination. Am Med News. 1989;32:43.

6. Cohen MA, Gorman JM. Comprehensive textbook of AIDS psychiatry. New York (NY): Oxford University Press; 2008.

7. Fernandez F, Ruiz P. Psychiatric aspects of HIV/AIDS. Philadelphia: Lippincott Williams & Wilkins; 2006. p. 39–47.

8. Organization of AIDS Psychiatry. Available from: http://www.apm.org/sigs/oap/.

9. CDC. Guidelines for prevention and treatment of opportunistic infections in HIV- infected adults and adolescents. Recommendations from CDC, the NIH and the HIV Medicine Association of the Infectious Diseases Society of America. MMWR. 2009;58:1–5.

10. Ances BM, Ellis RJ. Dementia and neurocognitive disorders due to HIV-1 infection. Semin Neurol. 2007;27:86–92.

11. Available from: http://www.lambdalegal.org/publications/articles/protecting-our-seniors.html.

12. OAP Consensus Survey. Available from: http://www.apm.org/sigs/oap/.

13. Ferrando SJ. Psychopharmacologic treatment of patients with HIV/AIDS. Curr Psychiatry Rep. 2009;11:235–42.

14. Cozza KL, Williams SG, Wynn GH. Psychopharmacologic treatment issues in AIDS psychiatry. In: Cohen MA, Gorman JM, editors. Comprehensive textbook of AIDS psychiatry. New York (NY): Oxford University Press; 2008. p. 455–85.

15. Drug interactions. Available from: http://hivinsite.ucsf.edu.

16. Drug interactions. Available from: http://www.hiv-druginteractions.org.

Chapter 10

Managing depression and renal failure

Thomas W. Heinrich

Typical consult question

"We have a sixty-two year old gentleman with renal failure on our service who is requesting that we stop dialysis. We are concerned that the patient is depressed and is trying to commit suicide. Please help!"

Background

Individuals with renal impairment suffer from significant rates of psychological co-morbidity. Of the myriad of potential mental health issues experienced by these complex patients, it has been commonly acknowledged that depressive disorders are the most common. Depression may complicate the course of an already significant medical condition by adversely affecting morbidity and mortality rates. It is therefore, imperative that psychiatrists caring for patients with renal disease be aware of the significance of depression in this at-risk population. Clinicians must also be familiar with possible treatment options for depression and the potential complications that renal insufficiency or failure imparts onto the pharmacologic management of depression in these patients.

Types and epidemiology of renal disease

Renal disease represents a major health issue. It has been estimated that almost 20 million Americans suffer from renal insufficiency of various degrees of severity (1). This number includes the approximately 470,000 individuals in the United States with renal failure (2). It is important to note that end-stage renal disease (ESRD) appears to disproportionately affect the African American community with a prevalence rate 4.4 times higher than that of Caucasian Americans (3). This increased prevalence appears to be due to higher rates of hypertension and diabetes in the African American population.

Impaired renal function has many potential causes. Patients may manifest renal dysfunction as a consequence of a multi-system disease (hypertension or diabetes) or a disease process localized to the kidneys (membranous glomerulonephritis). Depending on the underlying condition and treatment, kidney function may recover completely after the initial insult or may suffer continued progressive deterioration leading to ESRD and the need for renal replacement therapies. Once patients develop ESRD, they are at high risk of co-morbid medical problems and increased mortality rates.

Psychosomatic Medicine: An Introduction to Consultation-Liaison Psychiatry, eds. James J. Amos and Robert G. Robinson. Published by Cambridge University Press. © Cambridge University Press 2010.

Renal replacement therapies

Once an individual's renal function declines significantly and the kidneys are no longer able to function effectively, patients and clinicians are often faced with the dilemma of initiating dialysis or seeking renal transplantation. The choice of renal replacement therapy is very patient dependent and must take into account many factors including psychosocial support systems, community resources, co-morbid medical conditions, and the patient's psychological state.

In dialysis, the body's toxins are removed via osmosis across a semi-permeable membrane. In hemodialysis (HD), removal of toxins occurs outside the patient's body in the dialysis machine, where a semi-permeable membrane separates the dialysate fluid from the patient's blood, allowing for removal of toxins. In peritoneal dialysis (PD), the patient's peritoneal lining serves as the semi-permeable membrane that permits osmosis once the dialysate is introduced into the peritoneal cavity.

Regardless of the type of renal replacement therapy utilized, the patient experiences significant lifestyle modifications. Patients may find living on dialysis a constant challenge with many dietary restrictions and a demanding therapy schedule. Patients with renal disease who require renal replacement therapy need to be educated about each potential treatment option. They, in consultation with their nephrologist, should then be allowed to choose the treatment that is best suited for their medical illness, social situation, and personality style.

Epidemiology of renal disease and depression

It is well recognized that depression represents a significant co-morbidity for patients already confronted with chronic medical conditions. Individuals with kidney disease are not an exception to this observation. It is, however, difficult to obtain an accurate rate of depression in this population because of issues involving study methods. Research issues most often implicated as contributing to this problem include the population studied, the assessment tool administered, and the criteria for depression utilized in the study. Regardless of these methodologic issues, major depressive disorder and sub-syndromal symptoms of depression appear to be frequent occurrences in the ESRD population. The prevalence of major depressive disorder appears to range around 20%, and the prevalence of sub-syndromal depression has been estimated to be between 9% and 45% (4). It has been suggested that individuals receiving PD may experience less depression than those on HD (5). The potential severity of the psychological distress in this patient population is evident in a study by Kimmel et al., in which 9% of a population of 175,000 Medicare patients with ESRD were hospitalized psychiatrically over a one-year period (6).

Despite the high prevalence, depression in this patient population appears to be poorly recognized and under-treated in the clinical setting. Comparisons between depression screening tools and clinical records indicate that depressive symptoms frequently may go unrecognized and under-treated by the clinician (7).

Work-up

Cause of depression in renal failure

Many potential psychological, social, and biological contributions to the high rate of depression in patients with ESRD have been identified. The mechanism underlying this complex relationship between depression and renal disease is unclear but likely is multi-factorial and bi-directional.

Patients with ESRD experience psychological stressors that may have a profound impact on the development of depressive symptoms. Depression in patients with ESRD may occur secondary to the experience of loss, whether actually present or merely anticipated. Patients with ESRD on dialysis often suffer the loss of work status and time, health, and independence. Patients are also confronted with a sense of uncertainty regarding their future and often have an acute sense of their own mortality as medical complications develop. The individual's emotional response to the need for long-term renal replacement therapy is varied and often is linked to the maturity of the patient's coping mechanisms. Depression, however, does not appear to be merely related to the psychological impact associated with initiation of dialysis, but rather is a chronic problem in this patient population that may occur throughout the disease process.

Various physiologic factors have also been linked to the occurrence of depression in patients experiencing renal failure. Although studies are inconsistent, activation of the inflammatory response system may be related to the onset of depressive symptoms in patients with ESRD (8). The presence of uremia itself may pre-dispose patients to the development of depression. This may be due to the adverse impact of uremia on various neurotransmitters within the CNS (9). When attempting to determine the potential etiologies of depressive symptoms one must also consider the contribution of co-morbid medical conditions. Patients with ESRD are often prescribed many medications the may account for adverse effects on mood.

Consequences of depression and renal failure

It is essential that patients with ESRD suffering from a depressive disorder are identified and treated, as depression appears to be associated with significant morbidity and the potential for increased mortality. Ideally, one of the therapeutic goals in the identification and treatment of depression in this medically ill population is to prevent these additive and potentially avoidable adverse outcomes.

The presence of depression in patients with ESRD has been shown to adversely affect measures of quality of life. Depressive symptoms may, in fact, be the best predictor of an impaired quality of life in a population of patients with ESRD (10). The impairment in quality of life may have numerous dire psychological effects in depressed ESRD patients and may lead to reduced motivation to engage in medical care or even to maintain simple self-care.

Studies have linked depression with markers of poor treatment adherence in dialysis patients (11). Non-adherence with medical therapy has been shown to be three times more common in depressed patients than in patients without concurrent depression (12). The presence of depression in patients with ESRD has also been associated with significant medical co-morbidity. In a study of Veterans Administration patients on HD, depression was associated with a greater number of hospitalizations and increased duration of hospitalization even when demographic and medical factors were controlled (13). Increased rates of peritonitis, a dangerous complication of PD, have been found in depressed patients (14). Depression has also been associated with poor nutritional status and has been shown to precede the decline in serum albumin levels often seen in patients with ESRD (15).

Depressive disorders represent a risk factor for suicide, and this remains true of depression in patients with renal disease. Studies have shown suicide in patients with ESRD to occur at a rate 84% higher than in the general U.S. population (16). This study found that alcohol or drug dependence and a history of psychiatric hospitalization were strongly associated with an increased risk of suicide in the ESRD population. This study also revealed that the risk of suicide was highest in the first three months following initiation of dialysis and lessened considerably thereafter. It should be remembered that patients undergoing dialysis have potential means to harm themselves readily available. They may commit suicide by non-compliance with dialysis and/or medical and dietary prescriptions.

It is important for the physician to distinguish between suicidal intent and elective dialysis withdrawal. Approximately one in four patients with ESRD choose to voluntarily discontinue dialysis treatment (17). This decision is based on multiple individual patient factors such as co-morbid medical conditions and perceived quality of life. Because of the consequences of this decision, it is not uncommon for a concerned nephrologist to request psychiatrist consultation to help determine the patient's motives. One of the psychiatrist's duties in this situation is to screen for the presence of a depressive disorder. A recent study revealed that depression represented a significant risk factor for withdrawal for HD, even after age and other clinical variables were controlled (18). The psychiatrist must also determine whether dementia or delirium is interfering with the patient's capacity to make such a life-and-death decision.

Although not all studies agree, depression does appear to negatively impact the prognosis of renal disease itself, as an association between depression and increased mortality rates in ESRD patients has been demonstrated (19, 20). It remains unclear whether depression represents an independent risk factor for increased mortality, or whether depression influences other biopsychosocial variables that may adversely impact survival.

Clinical decision-making and treatment

It appears that a wide variety of effective treatments are available for patients with ESRD and co-morbid depression. The current standard of care involves the use of antidepressant medications and/or a range of psychotherapy techniques. Despite the variety of treatment modalities available to the clinician, treatment of depression is often dictated by the patient's acceptance of medication and/or psychiatric referral. It must also be remembered that although treatment of a depressive disorder can result in improvement in depressive symptoms, it remains unclear whether such therapy will translate into improvement in medical outcomes.

The effective treatment of depression in patients with renal disease represents a challenge because of several factors (21). First, the diagnosis of depression is often difficult because of the fact that the symptoms of renal failure and uremia may produce somatic signs and symptoms that overlap with those of major depression. Second, patients with ESRD may refuse psychiatric assessment because of an underlying stigma regarding the diagnosis of depression. Third, patients' compliance with prescribed therapies is often suboptimal because of institutional barriers, financial concerns, co-morbid medical conditions, medication side effects, or other psychiatric disorders such as substance abuse and dependence or personality disorders.

Pharmacologic therapy in renal failure

Most antidepressants appear to be safe and effective in the treatment of depression concurrent with renal disease. To provide safe and effective pharmacotherapy to the ESRD patient who is experiencing depression, the physician must take into account the potential for altered pharmacokinetic and pharmacodynamic parameters in patients with impaired renal function.

Pharmacokinetic and pharmacodynamic issues in renal failure

Patients with acute and chronic renal insufficiency experience alterations in the pharmacokinetic and pharmacodynamic properties of many commonly used drugs. Even with drugs that are metabolized primarily through the liver, patients with renal failure are at risk for adverse drug reactions or toxicity, as the pharmacologically active metabolites may require the kidney for excretion. The potential for toxic drug accumulation and adverse drug effects can develop if drug dosages are not adjusted according to impaired renal function. Knowledge of the potential for pharmacokinetic and pharmacodynamic interactions when the medication regimen is altered will help reduce significant morbidity. These medication issues are significant in that medication-related problems were identified in 130 of 133 (98%) HD patients who were suffering from a mean of six co-morbid illnesses and were taking a mean of 11 different drugs (22).

Pharmacodynamic

Pharmacodynamic drug properties refers to the pharmacologic effects of drugs. Patients with renal disease often have other chronic medical conditions for which they take medications. This potential for polypharmacy necessitates careful consideration of pharmacodynamic drug interactions when one is prescribing antidepressants. Orthostatic hypotension can occur during and after HD and may be exacerbated by concurrent administration of antidepressants that are alpha-adrenergic antagonists. Many patients on dialysis experience constipation, so exposure to drugs with anticholinergic properties should be minimized. The prescribing clinician should also be aware of the high co-morbidity of cardiac disease in patients with ESRD, so antidepressants with the potential to induce cardiac side effects should be prescribed with caution. ESRD may contribute to a lower seizure threshold; therefore, care should be exercised in using drugs that may further contribute to the risk of seizures.

Pharmacokinetic

Pharmacokinetic properties of a drug refers to the absorption, distribution, metabolism, and excretion of the parent drug and its metabolites. The presence of renal insufficiency or failure may alter several of the factors that constitute the pharmacokinetic properties of antidepressant medications.

Drug absorption refers to how much of the medication actually enters the body. Absorption is not commonly impacted by renal disease, but may be delayed in cases of gastroparesis or edema of the gastrointestinal tract.

Renal insufficiency and failure may adversely impact the distribution of the drug throughout the body following absorption. Increased volume status in patients with ESRD may increase the volume of distribution of medications. Most psychotropic medications are highly protein bound, with the most common binding protein being albumin. Patients with renal failure often have decreased amounts of albumin to bind the medications, thereby leaving more of the drug unbound and pharmacologically available for therapeutic efficacy or toxicity.

The metabolism of most psychotropic medications is not seriously affected by renal failure, as most psychiatric medications are metabolized by the liver. A general slowing of chemical reduction and of hydrolysis has been reported, but rates of glucuronidation, microsomal oxidation, and conjugation appear to be unaffected (23). The issue of drug-drug interactions, however, must remain a concern in this population because most patients with renal disease often have co-morbid conditions requiring pharmacotherapy.

The excretion of psychotropic medications through the urine may be affected to varying degrees depending on the significance of the renal dysfunction. The elimination of drugs can also be affected by the type of renal replacement therapy utilized in the case of patients with ESRD. Drugs with a large molecular weight and highly protein bound medications are not amenable to removal by HD. Minimal drug removal occurs in PD because of slow flow rates. Therefore, the parent medication or metabolites that remain pharmacologically active may be retained in patients with renal insufficiency or undergoing dialysis. The resulting impaired drug clearance can then result in pharmacologic adverse effects or toxicity. It is fortunate that a majority of psychiatric medications are eliminated in the bile after hepatic metabolism and eventually are excreted from the body in the feces.

Antidepressant medications in renal failure

Despite the small number of studies examining the treatment of depression in patients with ESRD, some evidence suggests that antidepressant medications are efficacious in this population (24). However, studies of antidepressant pharmacotherapy in patients with ESRD are limited by study design and small size.

Many different classes of antidepressants have been used in this complex patient population (Table 19.1). The medications most often utilized include the selective serotonin reuptake inhibitors (SSRIs) and the serotonin-norepinephrine reuptake inhibitors (SNRIs). The older tricyclic antidepressants (TCAs) and monoamine oxidase inhibitors (MAOIs), along with herbal supplements, such as St. John's wort, are sub-optimal in these patients because of increased risk of drug interactions and adverse effects (25).

The SSRIs represent the class of antidepressants with the most data available for use in patients with ESRD (26, 27). SSRIs appear to be effective in the alleviation of depressive symptoms and are well tolerated in this population. It is important to note that the SSRIs, with the exception of paroxetine, appear to require little dose adjustment, as pharmacokinetics appears minimally impacted by renal impairment. Paroxetine concentrations are increased in individuals with severe renal impairment, so dose reduction is appropriate (28). An additional potential beneficial effect of SSRIs in patients with ESRD is that they may limit HD-related hypotension (29).

The SNRI venlafaxine exhibits altered pharmacokinetics in patients with moderate to severe renal impairment. Clearance of both venlafaxine and its metabolite, O-desmethyl-venlafaxine, were decreased by 55% in the ESRD cohort, while clearance values for the mild renal impairment cohort were similar to those of normal subjects (30). Consequently, it is recommended that the daily dose of venlafaxine be decreased by 25% to 50% in patients with renal impairment and in those undergoing dialysis (31). Venlafaxine may also increase blood pressure, so careful monitoring of blood pressure is important, as

Table 19.1 Common antidepressant doses in renal insufficiency and failure

Antidepressant	Starting Adult Dose in Renal Failure	Adult Dose Range Mild to Moderate Renal Failure	Adult Dose Range Severe Renal Failure – ESRD
Fluoxetine	10 mg	10–40 mg	20 mg
Paroxetine IR	10 mg	10–30 mg	10–20 mg
Sertraline	25 mg	50–200 mg	50–150 mg
Citalopram	10 mg	20–60 mg	10–40 mg
Escitalopram	10 mg	10–20 mg	10–20 mg
Venlafaxine ER	37.5 mg	75–225 mg	37.5–112.5 mg
Desvenlafaxine	50 mg	50 mg qd	50 mg qod
Duloxetine	20 mg	20–40 mg	Do not use
Mirtazapine	7.5 mg	15–30 mg	7.5–22.5 mg
Bupropion	100 mg	150–300 mg	150 mg

Although many of these medications do not require final dose adjustment for renal insufficiency or failure, a cautious approach with dosing and titration is encouraged.

From Cohen LM, Tessier EG, Germain MJ, Levy NB. Update on psychotropic medication use in renal disease. Psychosomatics. 2004;45(1):34–48.

hypertension is a very common co-morbidity is in this patient population. Desvenlafaxine also requires dose adjustment for moderate to severe renal insufficiency, with a maximum recommended daily dose of 50 mg in this population, and in the case of ESRD, no more than 50 mg every other day (32). The manufacturer of duloxetine does not recommend its use in patients with creatinine clearance less than 30 ml/min or in those receiving dialysis (33).

The kidney is responsible for a majority of the excretion of bupropion and its metabolites. Pharmacokinetic considerations, therefore, dictate a reduced dose in patients with ESRD and in those receiving dialysis (23). Bupropion has also been associated with a decreased seizure threshold. In patients with renal disease, the risk of seizures may be further exacerbated by the electrolyte abnormalities that often complicate the management of renal insufficiency and failure. The pharmacokinetics of mirtazapine are also altered by changes in renal function, thereby requiring a decrease in dosage. Clearance of mirtazapine is reduced by 30% in patients with a creatinine clearance less than 40 ml/min, and by 50% in patients receiving dialysis (34).

The administration of TCAs in patients with renal disease is rife with potential complications. Through their actions on multiple neurotransmitters, the TCAs are associated with multiple pharmacodynamic adverse effects such as orthostatic hypotension, sedation, and anticholinergic toxicity. The TCAs also have the potential to induce cardiac arrhythmias in susceptible individuals. In addition, concentrations of the metabolites of various TCAs were found to be elevated in subjects at various stages of renal failure (35). These pharmacodynamic and pharmacokinetic issues make the administration of TCAs a challenge in the medically ill and in those with ESRD. This class of antidepressants should be used very cautiously, with significant dose reduction and slow dose titration in the ESRD population.

The MAOIs are rarely administered to patients with renal disease. Information on the pharmacokinetic properties of MAOIs in patients with renal disease is lacking. MAOIs can exacerbate the orthostatic hypotension commonly experienced following HD.

Psychostimulants are commonly used to address the neurovegetative symptoms of depressive disorders in the medically ill. They offer the benefits of a rapid onset of action and minimal abuse potential when used in patients with co-morbid medical illnesses (36). Methylphenidate, a common stimulant used in this population, does not appear to require dose adjustment in the presence of renal dysfunction (37).

In summary, it has been suggested that when using antidepressants in ESRD or significant renal insufficiency, the prescriber should initiate therapy at about half the usual starting dose (38). Once pharmacotherapy is started, it is imperative to monitor for side effects, therapeutic efficacy, and the potential for drug interactions as new medications are added to treat co-morbid illnesses. If dose escalation is necessary, a cautious approach is advised with gradual titration over time. If clinically appropriate, drug levels may be obtained to determine appropriate dosing.

Nonpharmacologic therapy for depression in renal failure

In light of the potential problems surrounding pharmacotherapy in patients with renal impairment, non-pharmacologic approaches should always be considered for patients with renal disease and depressive disorders. Electroconvulsive therapy has been used in patients with ESRD, and although data are limited, it appears well tolerated and effective in this patient population. Evidence exploring the effectiveness of psychosocial interventions in patients with ESRD is also sparse, but suggests that various types of psychotherapeutic interventions may play an important role in the treatment of depressive disorders.

Available evidence suggests that cognitive-behavioral therapy (CBT) and supportive therapy are effective in relieving depression in patients undergoing dialysis (39). Group therapy, focusing on social support, may also be beneficial in HD patients (40). Exercise rehabilitation programs have been shown to significantly decrease depressive symptoms in patients with ESRD on HD (41). Programs that focus on education may also be of benefit to patients and their caregivers. Many patients with ESRD rely on family and friends to help manage the disease process, potential complications, and required therapy. The needs of these caregivers are often neglected, but they also experience emotional distress and anxiety (42). Interventions that help support these important caregivers may improve their quality of life, which therefore may indirectly improve medical and psychosocial outcomes of the patient with ESRD.

Conclusion

Renal disease has a significant impact on the lives of patients. Individuals with renal disease, their families, and the professionals caring for them need to be aware of the problem of co-morbid depression. They need to be aware of the high incidence of concurrent depression and the increased morbidity and mortality likely associated with depression in patients with this medical condition, who are already burdened by significant adverse outcomes. They need to be informed of the importance of monitoring their mental health. It is only through clinical diligence that the identification, treatment, and support of patients experiencing these dangerous co-morbid conditions will result in improved outcomes and a reduced burden of illness.

References

1. Coresh J, Astor BC, Greene T, et al. Prevalence of chronic kidney disease and decreased kidney function in the adult US population: Third National Health and Nutrition Examination Survey. Am J Kidney Dis. 2003;41:1–12.

2. U.S. Renal Data Systems. USRDS 2006 annual data report: atlas of end-stage renal disease in the United States. Bethesda (MD): National Institutes of Health, National Institute of Diabetes and Digestive and Kidney Diseases; 2007.

3. U.S. Renal Data Systems. USRDS 2004 annual data report: atlas of end-stage renal disease in the United States. Bethesda (MD): National Institutes of Health, National Institute of Diabetes and Digestive and Kidney Diseases; 2004.

4. Kimmel PL, Cukor D, Cohen SD, et al. Depression in end-stage renal disease patients: a critical review. Adv Chr Kidney Dis. 2007;14:328–34.

5. Kalender B, Ozdemir AC, Dervisoglu E, et al. Quality of life in chronic kidney disease: effects of treatment modality, depression, malnutrition and inflammation. Int J Clin Pract. 2007;61:569–76.

6. Kimmel PL, Thamer M, Richard CM, et al. Psychiatric illness in patients with end-stage renal disease. Am J Med. 1998;105:214–21.

7. Lopes AA, Albert JM, Young EW, et al. Screening for depression in hemodialysis patients: associations with diagnosis, treatment, and outcomes in the DOPPS. Kidney Int. 2004;66:2047–53.

8. Finkelstein FO, Wuerth D, Troidle LK, et al. Depression and end-stage renal disease: a therapeutic challenge. Kidney Int. 2008;74:843–5.

9. Smogorzewski M, Ni Z, Massry SG. Function and metabolism of brain synaptosomes in chronic renal failure. Artif Organs. 1995;18:795–800.

10. Steele TE, Baltimore D, Finkelstein SH, et al. Quality of life in peritoneal dialysis patients. J Nerv Ment Dis. 1996;184:368–74.

11. Cukor D, Rosenthal DS, Jindal RM, et al. Depression is an important contributor to low medication adherence in hemodialyzed patients and transplant recipients. Kidney Int 2009;75(11):1223–9.

12. DiMatteo MR, Lepper HS, Croghan TW. Depression is a risk factor for noncompliance with medical treatment. Arch Intern Med. 2000;160:2101–7.

13. Hedayati SS, Grambow SC, Szczech LA, et al. Physician-diagnosed depression as a correlate of hospitalizations in patients receiving long-term hemodialysis. Am J Kidney Dis. 2005;46:642–9.

14. Troidle L, Watnick S, Wuerth DB, et al. Depression and its association with peritonitis in long-term peritoneal dialysis patients. Am J Kidney Dis. 2003;42:350–4.

15. Friend R, Hatchett L, Wadhwa NK, et al. Serum albumin and depression in end-stage renal disease. Adv Perit Dial. 1997;13:155–7.

16. Kurella M, Kimmel PL, Young BS, et al. Suicide in the United States end-stage renal disease program. J Am Soc Nephrol. 2005;16:774–81.

17. Cohen LM, Germain MJ, Poppel DM. Practical considerations in dialysis withdrawal: "to have that option is a blessing." JAMA. 2003;289:2113–9.

18. McDade-Montez EA, Christensen AJ, Cvengros JA, et al. The role of depression symptoms in dialysis withdrawal. Health Psychol. 2006;25:198–204.

19. Einwohner R, Bernardini J, Piraino B. The effect of depression on survival in peritoneal dialysis patients. Perit Dial Int. 2004;24:256–63.

20. Hedayati SS, Bosworth HB, Briley LP, et al. Death or hospitalization of patients on chronic hemodialysis is associated with physician-based diagnosis of depression. Kidney Int. 2008;74:930–6.

21. Wuerth D, Finkelstein SH, Finkelstein FO. The identification and treatment of depression in patients maintained on hemodialysis. Semin Dial. 2005;18:142–6.

22. Manley HJ, McClaren ML, Overbay DK, et al. Factors associated with medication-

related problems in ambulatory hemodialysis patients. Am J Kidney Dis. 2003;41:386–93.

23. Cohen LM, Tessier EG, Germain MJ, et al. Update on psychotropic medication use in renal disease. Psychosomatics. 2004;45:34–48.

24. Wuerth D, Finkelstein SH, Ciarcia J, et al. Identification and treatment of a cohort of patients maintained on chronic peritoneal dialysis. Am J Kidney Dis. 2001;37:1011–7.

25. Cohen SD, Morris L, Acquaviva K, et al. Screening, diagnosis, and treatment of depression in patients with end-stage renal disease. Clin J Am Soc Nephrol. 2007;2: 1332–42.

26. Blumenfield M, Levy NB, Spinowitz B, et al. Fluoxetine in depressed patients on dialysis. J Psychiatry Med. 1997;27:71–80.

27. Kalender B, Ozdemir AC, Yalug I, et al. Antidepressant treatment increases quality of life in patients with chronic renal failure. Ren Fail. 2007;29:817–22.

28. Doyle GD, Laher M, Kelly JG, et al. The pharmacokinetics of paroxetine in renal impairment. Acta Psychiatr Scand Suppl. 1989;350:89–90.

29. Dheenan S, Venkatesan J, Grubb BP, et al. Effect of sertraline hydrochloride on dialysis hypotension. Am J Kidney Dis. 1998;31:624–30.

30. Troy SM, Schultz RW, Parker VD, et al. The effect of renal disease on the disposition of venlafaxine. Clin Pharmacol Ther. 1994;56: 14–21.

31. Product information: Effexor ER® extended-release oral capsules, venlafaxine HCl extended-release oral capsules. Philadelphia (PA): Wyeth Pharmaceuticals; 2008.

32. Product information: Pristiq® oral extended-release tablets, desvenlafaxine oral extended-release tablets. Philadelphia (PA): Wyeth Pharmaceuticals; 2008.

33. Product information: Cymbalta® delayed-release oral capsules, duloxetine HCl delayed-release oral capsules. Indianapolis (IN): Eli Lilly and Company; 2008.

34. Product information: Remeron SolTab® orally disintegrating tablet, mirtazapine orally disintegrating tablet. Roseland (NJ): Organon USA Inc; 2007.

35. Lieberman JA, Cooper TB, Suckow RF, et al. Tricyclic antidepressants and metabolite levels in chronic renal failure. Clin Pharmacol Ther. 1985;37:301–7.

36. Massand PS, Tesar GE. Use of stimulants in the medically ill. Psychiatr Clin North Am. 1996;19:515–47.

37. Crone CC, Gabriel GM. Treatment of anxiety and depression in transplant patients. Clin Pharmacokinet. 2004;43: 361–94.

38. Tossani E, Cassano P, Fava M. Depression and renal disease. Semin Dial. 2005;18: 73–81.

39. Hener T, Weisenberg M, Har-Even D. Supportive versus cognitive behavioral intervention programs in achieving adjustment to home peritoneal kidney dialysis. J Consult Clin Psychol. 1996;64: 731–41.

40. Friend R, Singletary Y, Mendell NR, et al. Group participation and survival among patients with end-stage renal disease. Am J Public Health. 1986;76:670–2.

41. Kouidi E, Iacovides A, Iordanidis P, et al. Exercise renal rehabilitation program: psychosocial effects. Nephron. 1997;77: 152–8.

42. Belasco AG, Sesso R. Burden and quality of life of caregivers for hemodialysis patients. Am J Kidney Dis. 2002;39:805–12.

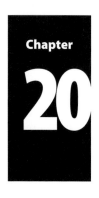

Management of psychiatric syndromes due to endocrine and metabolic diseases

James J. Amos and Jaspreet Chahal

Typical consult question

"Please treat this middle-aged woman with schizoaffective disorder and newly diagnosed pro-lactinoma; please suggest antipsychotic treatment that would not interfere with bromocriptine."

Background

The consultation question above occasionally bedevils psychiatric consultants. It illustrates the challenges inherent in managing patients who happen to suffer both a complex medical illness and a complex psychiatric illness. It's also an example of how important it is to realize that psychiatric disturbances are frequently seen during the course of endocrine disorders. The behavioral effects of endocrinopathies suggest many different psychiatric illnesses, and the neuropsychiatric effects can be among the first manifestations of endocrine disease.

Hypothyroidism

Thyroid hormones are important regulators of metabolism and play an important role in protein synthesis and oxygen consumption. Two main thyroid hormones are thyroxine (T4) and triiodothyronine (T3). T4 is the main hormone secreted; T3 is derived mainly from the extrathyroidal conversion of T4 to T3. T3 then acts at the T3 nuclear receptor to exert its physiologic effects (1).

Hypothyroidism is divided into

- Primary hypothyroidism, which is caused by thyroid failure
- Secondary hypothyroidism, which results from a deficiency in thyroid-stimulating hormone (TSH) production by the pituitary
- Tertiary hypothyroidism, which is due to hypothalamic deficiency of thyroid-releasing hormone (TRH)

Primary hypothyroidism is responsible for most hypothyroid cases. Hashimoto's thyroiditis is the most common cause of primary hypothyroidism in iodine-sufficient areas. It is an autoimmune disorder that can present as an asymptomatic diffuse goiter and may lead to the development of hypothyroidism (2).

Another classification based on measurement of serum levels is as follows:

- Overt hypothyroidism in which patients show classic signs and symptoms of hypothyroidism. It is identified by elevated TSH with reduced serum T4 levels.

Psychosomatic Medicine: An Introduction to Consultation-Liaison Psychiatry, eds. James J. Amos and Robert G. Robinson. Published by Cambridge University Press. © Cambridge University Press 2010.

- Subclinical hypothyroidism is marked by biochemical evidence of mild thyroid hormone deficiency. It is identified by high TSH but normal serum T4 and T3 (2). The patient may have few or no apparent clinical features of hypothyroidism.

Subclinical hypothyroidism affects about 5% of the general population and 15% of elderly women. Common physical manifestations of hypothyroidism include fatigue, weight gain, edema of the face and hands, paresthesias, cold intolerance, constipation, excessive sleepiness, metromenorrhagia, anemia, and hoarseness. Signs may include bradycardia, dry skin, and slowed reflexes. Psychiatric features include depression, dementia, mania, and hallucinations. Before the advent of effective treatment, many patients presented with myxedema madness, marked by paranoid delusions and marked cognitive impairment. Nowadays, between 5% and 15% present with psychosis (3). Hypothyroidism frequently appears in patients presenting with rapid cycling bipolar disorder. Lithium is known to cause clinical hypothyroidism, but one study found it in far fewer non–rapid cycling bipolar patients with hypothyroidism in the context of lithium treatment than in rapid cyclers (3).

Hyperthyroidism

Hyperthyroidism is marked by low TSH and high serum T4 or T3; the subclinical form is defined by low TSH but normal T4 and T3. Major causes of hyperthyroidism include Graves' disease, toxic multi-nodular goiter, and toxic adenomas. However hyperthyroidism can also be caused by ingestion of high levels of thyroid hormone or secretion of thyroid hormone from an ectopic site.

Graves' disease is an autoimmune disorder that presents with diffuse goiter, hyperthyroidism, ophthalmopathy, and psychiatric symptoms. Its prevalence rate is about 1%, and it is the most common cause of hyperthyroidism. It affects women 5- to 10-fold more often than men (4). The role of stress in the origin of Graves' disease is still uncertain.

The most common clinical manifestations of hyperthyroidism are irritability, emotional lability, restlessness, fatigue, tremor, weight loss, palpitations, insomnia, and anxiety. Typical signs include eye stare, lid lag, warm smooth skin, goiter, tachycardia, fine tremor, atrial fibrillation, and brisk reflexes (5). Untreated, the patient can progress to suffer from psychosis and cognitive impairment. Although anxiety disorders dominate the psychiatric presentation, apathetic hyperthyroidism presents with depression, apathy, somnolence, and pseudodementia in the absence of the usual signs and symptoms of hyperthyroidism. Apathetic hyperthyroidism is more common in the elderly, although it has been described in younger patients (4). An acute delirium called Hashimoto's encephalopathy (chronic autoimmune thyroiditis) can occur. True mania, marked by grandiosity, racing thoughts, and pressured speech, is much less commonly observed.

The pathophysiology of the psychiatric manifestations may owe much to the enhancement of beta-adrenergic receptor–mediated effects of catecholamines caused by increasing the density and sensitivity of receptors in the peripheral and central nervous system tissues. Although this may explain the symptoms of anxiety or manic-like presentations, the relationship between hyperthyroidism and depression is more likely due to prolonged subclinical hyperthyroidism exhausting noradrenergic transmission, which is postulated to contribute to depression (4).

Hyperparathyroidism

Parathyroid hormone (PTH) is produced by four parathyroid glands closely apposed to the posterior capsule of four poles of the thyroid gland. PTH regulates serum calcium levels. PTH secretion is regulated by negative feedback of plasma calcium concentrations. When serum calcium is low, PTH is released; at high calcium concentrations, PTH is inhibited. PTH increases serum calcium by promoting bone resorption and calcium retention by kidneys, and by increasing intestinal absorption of calcium (3).

Parathyroid adenomas can cause primary hyperparathyroidism leading to hypersecretion of PTH. Serum calcium levels rise as they fail to inhibit PTH release by the usual negative feedback loop. Hyperparathyroidism increases after age 60 and is two to three times more prevalent in women than in men. Although primary hyperparathyroidism is a frequent cause of asymptomatic hypercalcemia, it could be the earliest manifestation of malignancy. Numerous causes of hypercalcemia have been identified, but hyperparathyroidism and cancer account for 90% of cases. Other causes of hypercalcemia include granulomatous disease, vitamin D intoxication, hyperthyroidism, and hypercortisolism. Lithium causes hypercalcemia in 10% of treated patients.

About 25% of cases are marked by depressed or anxious mood. Lethargy, apathy, poor memory, and decreased attention can be the first signs of this disorder. Delirium and psychosis may appear as well. The normal range of serum calcium varies with the laboratory but generally runs between 8.9 and 10.1 mg/dl. Some authors believe that psychiatric symptoms correlate with calcium blood levels, but others think that no such relationship consistently exists. Mood symptoms, fatigue, apathy, and decreased concentration can occur at levels of 12 to 16 mg/dl. Psychotic symptoms tend to occur at levels of 16 to 19 mg/dl. Coma typically develops when levels exceed 19 mg/dl.

Hypoparathyroidism

Primary hypoparathyroidism is most commonly caused by injury to the parathyroid area during surgery. Other causes are familial, autoimmune, or idiopathic. Lack of PTH, vitamin D deficiency, or non-responsiveness of the body to normal levels of PTH or vitamin D can lead to low serum calcium.

Hypocalcemia presents as neuromuscular excitability including tetany, paresthesias, and seizures. Latent tetany can be observed as Chvostek's or Trousseau's sign. Neuropsychiatric presentations are less common than in hyperparathyroidism but may include intellectual impairment, neurosis, and psychosis (3).

Adrenal disorders

Hypercortisolism in the form of the textbook case of Cushing's syndrome is marked by central weight gain, facial plethora, skin striae, acne, hirsutism, hypertension, osteoporosis, decreased libido, impotence, menstrual dysfunction, and psychiatric symptoms including emotional lability, increased irritability, anxiety, and depression. Adrenocorticotropic hormone (ACTH)-dependent Cushing's syndrome accounts for 70% to 90% of cases and can occur as a pituitary adenoma (known as Cushing's disease) or may result from ectopic ACTH release from a non-pituitary neoplasm. ACTH-independent Cushing's syndrome is due to an adrenal tumor or adrenal hyperplasia secreting cortisol and suppressing ACTH.

Up to 85% of patients with Cushing's syndrome present with psychiatric symptoms. Affective disturbance, including suicidality, is common; psychosis is relatively rare. The depressive disorder tends to be intermittent and associated with marked irritability. Stressful events may play a causal role in the development of Cushing's disease, although not in other forms of Cushing's syndrome (6).

Glucocorticoid excess that results from prescribed corticosteroids is a well-described phenomenon. Mild to moderate psychiatric adverse effects occur in about 28% of patients; severe reactions occur in about 6%. Euphoria and hypomania are the most frequently reported side effects of short-term therapy. Symptoms can range from subtle mood changes to frank psychosis or delirium. The most important risk factor is the corticosteroid dose, with doses above 40 mg a day carrying higher risk for inducing psychiatric symptoms. Neither previous corticosteroid-induced psychiatric disturbances nor previous treatments free of such disturbances predict future responses. A history of psychiatric illness does not predict occurrence, and age does not seem to be a factor (7).

Hypocortisolism

Primary adrenocortical insufficiency results from destruction or dysfunction of the adrenal cortex, which results in increased ACTH in response to decreasing levels of corticosteroid. Autoimmune destruction of the adrenal gland is the most common cause of Addison's disease. Secondary adrenocortical insufficiency arises from pituitary or hypothalamic dysfunction, resulting in decreased corticotropin-releasing hormone (CRH) or ACTH levels, which in turn result in reduced glucocorticoid production. The most common cause of secondary adrenocortical insufficiency is abrupt withdrawal of exogenous long-term glucocorticoid therapy. This occurs because of prolonged pituitary-hypothalamic suppression and adrenal atrophy secondary to the loss of endogenous ACTH (3).

Typical clinical manifestations are weakness, fatigue, hyperpigmentation, anorexia, nausea and vomiting, hypotension, and hypoglycemia. Hyperpigmentation is the most consistent sign of Addison's disease. It is caused by increased action of the melanocyte-stimulating hormone, which is co-secreted with ACTH in response to low circulating cortisol (8). One theory about the pathophysiology of neuropsychiatric symptoms in Addison's disease involves glucocorticoid deficiency. Glucocorticoids probably play important role in memory because the hippocampus has more receptors for them than any other part of the brain. A decrease in glucocorticoids may lead to neural excitability, leading to enhanced ability to detect sensory input, and possibly reducing the threshold for induction of hallucinations. The timing of the arrival of signals from the periphery to the CNS may be disrupted as well, leading to impaired integration of sensory inputs (8).

One can see affective syndromes, apathy, irritability, negativism, poverty of thought, psychosis, delirium, and coma. Psychiatric symptoms can precede the development of physical findings.

Diabetes mellitus

Diabetes mellitus is the most common endocrine condition. Although all forms of diabetes mellitus are characterized by hyperglycemia, the pathogenesis varies. The two broad categories of diabetes mellitus are type 1 and type 2. Type 1 diabetes is characterized by insulin deficiency and results from autoimmune destruction of insulin-producing beta cells of the pancreas (6). The hallmark of type 2 diabetes is insulin resistance in which the body needs increasingly higher levels of insulin to achieve normal glycemia. Type 2 diabetes accounts for 90% to 95% of all people with diabetes mellitus in the United States. Obesity and sedentary lifestyle are the risk factors for type 2 diabetes; usually, weight loss and regular exercise are first-line interventions, although insulin injections are needed for type 1 diabetes.

The most common psychiatric syndrome described in patients with diabetes is depression; its prevalence is two to three times higher than that found in the general population. Depression and hyperglycemia may have a reciprocal relationship in which hyperglycemia is provoked by depression and may, in turn, independently contribute to exacerbating depression.

Other common psychiatric disturbances found in patients with diabetes are schizophrenia, bipolar disorder, and eating disorder. The important health issue in all three groups is weight, although in opposite directions.

Weight gain is commonly observed in patients with schizophrenia, and the most relevant current issue is the added gain due to the use of antipsychotics in this population. Patients with schizophrenia tend to have three times as much intra-abdominal fat as controls matched for age, gender, and lifestyle. Obesity has increased by about 10% in this group since the arrival of atypical antipsychotics, and this has contributed to excess cases of metabolic syndrome, diabetic ketoacidosis, cardiovascular disease, and stroke. Several definitions exist for metabolic syndrome. Current Adult Treatment Panel III (ATP III) criteria define the metabolic syndrome as the presence of any three of the following five traits:

- Abdominal obesity, defined as a waist circumference in men >102 cm (40 in) and in women >88 cm (35 in)
- Serum triglycerides ≥150 mg/dl (1.7 mmol/L) or drug treatment for elevated triglycerides
- Serum high-density lipoprotein (HDL) cholesterol <40 mg/dl (1 mmol/L) in men and <50 mg/dl (1.3 mmol/L) in women, or drug treatment for low HDL cholesterol (HDL-C)
- Blood pressure ≥130/85 mmHg or drug treatment for elevated blood pressure
- Fasting plasma glucose (FPG) ≥100 mg/dl (5.6 mmol/L), or drug treatment for elevated blood glucose (9)

Olanzapine and clozapine are the atypical antipsychotics most commonly associated with weight gain of around 4 to 4.5 kg, respectively, over 10 weeks (8). The weight gain is thought to be associated with clinical improvement in psychopathology. However, even though one study concluded that the known antisuicidal effect of clozapine would prevent 492 deaths by suicide in patients with schizophrenia over a ten-year period, this would be offset by 416 deaths due to clozapine-induced weight gain of 10 kg.

Obesity and overweight have been associated with bipolar disorder as well. Increasing evidence suggests an association with metabolic syndrome. Impaired glucose tolerance and insulin resistance appear more frequently in people with bipolar disorder than in the general population. Connections may be mediated by abnormalities in cortisol regulation that may be triggered by psychological and physiologic stress, activating the hypothalamic-pituitary axis (HPA). Weight gain is also a consequence of psychotropic medications, including lithium and the atypical antipsychotics (10).

It is believed that antagonism of serotonin 2C ($5\text{-}HT_{2C}$) receptors centrally by antipsychotics increases food intake despite the sensation of satiety. Histamine receptor antagonism also stimulates appetite. A genetic factor is involved because a common $5\text{-}HT_{2C}$ receptor promoter region polymorphism has strong associations with weight gain and increased risk of metabolic syndrome in those taking antipsychotics. A differential weight gain potential has been noted among the atypical antipsychotics, with clozapine and olanzapine causing the greatest gains and ziprasidone and aripiprazole showing the least (11).

Intensive management of diabetes itself ironically tends to cause weight gain, which patients with eating disorder try to avoid, sometimes by misusing insulin. The co-existence of type I diabetes and an eating disorder such as anorexia nervosa or bulimia nervosa is estimated to be as high as 16% (12). Women with type 1 diabetes may administer reduced insulin or may omit doses altogether as a means of caloric purging. This practice has been linked to higher hemoglobin A1c levels, higher rates of hospital and emergency room visits, and higher rates of retinopathy and neuropathy than in women who did not report insulin omission (6). A review of more than 500 females showed that concurrence of diabetes and anorexia nervosa resulted in a mortality rate of 34.6 per 1000 person-years, compared with 2.2 per 1000 person-years for those with diabetes alone (12).

Hyperprolactinemia

The most common cause of elevated prolactin in patients with severe mental illness is associated with antipsychotics. Typical antipsychotics in the phenothiazine, butyrophenone, and thioxanthene categories can increase prolactin levels in more than 50% of cases. The atypical agents are less liable to produce this effect, with the exception of risperidone (13). In general, medication-induced hyperprolactinemia causes elevation in the range of 25 to 100 mcg/L (14). The primary action of prolactin is to stimulate lactation. So physiologically, prolactin levels increase during pregnancy and lactation. Pathological causes include prolactin-secreting pituitary adenomas, chronic renal failure, primary hypothyroidism, and lesions of the pituitary stalk and hypothalamus (15).

Prolactinomas account for 40% of all pituitary tumors; 90% are small, intrasellar tumors that rarely increase in size. Hyperprolactinemia in women is linked to small tumors, amenorrhea, infertility, galactorrhea, and osteoporosis. In men, it has been associated with larger tumors than in women, headaches, visual loss, hypopituitarism, infertility, decreased libido, and osteoporosis, while galactorrhea and gynecomastia tend to be less common. The secretion and release of prolactin are mediated by dopamine. Hence, anything that disrupts dopamine secretion interferes with delivery of dopamine to the portal vessels and may cause hyperprolactinemia (14):

- Phenothiazines, butyrophenones, metoclopramide, and risperidone antagonize lactotroph dopamine receptors.
- Monoamine oxidase inhibitors and tricyclic antidepressants disrupt delivery of dopamine to portal vessels.
- Selective serotonin reuptake inhibitors also raise prolactin but rarely exceed normal range.

The link between hyperprolactinemia and psychiatric symptoms is debatable. Some have found increased hostility, depression, anxiety, and feelings of inadequacy (1). However, case reports continue to surface that document concerns about the possibility that dopamine antagonists and dopamine agonists (which are used to treat prolactinomas in an effort to shrink the tumors) "can cancel out each other's effects" (16). These reports typically detail the efforts of clinicians to prevent psychotic episodes in patients who have prolactinomas and are being treated with dopaminergic agents such as bromocriptine or cabergoline.

One of the more recent reports indicated that bromocriptine might cause worsening of psychosis; this was supported by citation of a single, brief paper entitled "Bromocriptine-Induced Schizophrenia" (17). The writer of the latter report described a patient who had no previous history of psychosis who developed "schizophrenia" four days after starting low-dose bromocriptine for a macroprolactinoma (18). The author was an internist, but the patient was evaluated by a psychiatrist, who diagnosed the man with "paranoid schizophrenia." The patient had auditory hallucinations, had the idea that he was being poisoned, and refused to eat or take medications. The refusal to take medications evidently included the bromocriptine, because the patient was pronounced to have "a completely normal mental status" only days later...by the same psychiatrist.

Aside from the low likelihood nowadays that the patient would have been called schizophrenic at all, very little evidence consistently justifies the kind of worry clinicians have about the group of patients with severe mental illness taking antipsychotics and having hyperprolactinemia. Molitch calls the risk of inducing exacerbations of underlying psychosis by using dopamine agonists "small" and cites five case series totaling 45 patients that show no worsening of psychiatric status under these conditions in the great majority of patients treated (13).

Work-up

The biochemical diagnosis of thyroid, parathyroid, and adrenal disorders as well as disorders of prolactin is based on laboratory tests.

Clinical diagnosis of hypothyroidism or hyperthyroidism can be suspected in patients who have typical signs and symptoms of hypothyroidism or hyperthyroidism, as described earlier. For biochemical diagnosis of thyroid disorders, TSH, free T4, and T3 are measured. Positive thyroid peroxidase antibodies may indicate underlying Hashimoto's thyroiditis.

The diagnosis of hypercalcemia is marked by elevated serum calcium and PTH, and by mental status changes, cardiac abnormalities, weakness, lethargy, abdominal pain, and severe dehydration. Hypocalcemia can be marked by latent tetany, as described earlier.

In early 2004, a consensus development conference convened by four organizations, including the American Diabetes Association (ADA), the American Psychiatric Association (APA), the American Association of Clinical Endocrinologists, and the North American Association for the Study of Obesity, recommended that all patients receiving second-generation antipsychotics, regardless of diagnosis, "should receive appropriate baseline screening and ongoing monitoring" (19). Haupt and colleagues concluded from their own retrospective study and from a review of a similar study in the Medicaid population that generally there is low concordance with the specific conference recommendation to measure fasting lipids and glucose at baseline and after 12 weeks of treatment (19).

Assessment of patients with anorexia and diabetes can be difficult. Typical clues include rapid weight gain or loss, insulin omission, elevated glycosylated hemoglobin (HbA1c), and recurrent diabetic ketoacidosis. A single measurement of prolactin in a blood sample obtained at any time of day most often is adequate to establish hyperprolactinemia (14).

Clinical decision-making and treatment

Hypothyroidism is treated by thyroid replacement. Acute Hashimoto's encephalopathy can be treated with glucocorticoids (4). Antidepressants can be combined with thyroid hormone for depression that does not respond to thyroid replacement alone.

Hyperthyroidism is treated by antithyroid drugs such as methimazole and propylthiouracil or by radioiodine or thyroidectomy. Psychotropic medications are usually unnecessary. Treatment of thyroid storm, which consists of extremely exaggerated signs of hyperthyroidism, including psychiatric manifestations, involves beta-blockers (preferably propranolol), an antithyroid drug, and symptomatic management (4).

In most cases, psychiatric symptoms are resolved when hyperparathyroidism is treated and serum calcium levels return to normal. Primary hyperparathyroidism is treated by surgical resection of the adenoma or parathyroidectomy.

Psychiatric symptoms typically remit on successful treatment of Cushing's syndrome. Some patients resistant to antidepressants while in the active phase of Cushing's syndrome become responsive after reduction in corticosteroid level (3). Glucocorticoid replacement alone may not provide adequate relief from hypocortisolism.

Suitable replacement antipsychotics can be found for patients at higher risk with schizophrenia and bipolar disorder with propensity to weight gain and metabolic syndrome. Ziprasidone and aripiprazole tend to carry less risk. A more concerted effort should be made by psychiatrists to develop new approaches to enhance screening and safety monitoring for cardiometabolic risk in this population. This could include referring patients to primary care colleagues for glucose and lipid monitoring.

Evidence suggests that treatment of depression can lead to improvement in diabetes management and improved glycemic control. Although tricyclics may be effective in treating depression, they may worsen blood sugar control. The selective serotonin reuptake inhibitors may be associated with improvement in both blood sugar control and depression. Cognitive-behavioral therapy is also effective for depression and improves hemoglobin A1c levels (6).

Treatment of patients with combined eating disorder and diabetes should reflect a collaborative effort between diabetes specialists and a multi-disciplinary mental health team. Intense diabetes management, especially early on in the nutritional rehabilitation phase, may increase the potential for disordered eating because the patient must think constantly about the effects of food, insulin, and exercise on blood glucose levels. It is unlikely that diabetes management will improve until the eating disorder is treated (12).

Most experts do not recommend treating hyperprolactinemia that arises from psychotropic drugs by using dopamine agonists. In situations in which a reasonable choice of an alternative atypical antipsychotic can be made, a substitution is reasonable as long as patient preference, response, tolerance, and close monitoring are kept in mind.

References

1. Joffe RT, Brasch JS, MacQueen GM. Psychiatric aspects of endocrine disorders in women. Psychiatr Clin North Am. 2003;26(3):683–91.

2. Devdhar M, Ousman YH, Burman KD. Hypothyroidism. Endocrinol Metab Clin North Am. 2007;36(3):595–615.

3. GeffkenGR WardHE, Staab JP, et al. Psychiatric morbidity in endocrine disorders. Psychiatr Clin North Am. 1998;21(2):473–89.

4. Bunevicius R, Prange AJ Jr. Psychiatric manifestations of Graves' hyperthyroidism: pathophysiology and treatment options. CNS Drugs. 2006;20(11):897–909.

5. Manu P, Suarez RE, Barnett BJ. Handbook of medicine in psychiatry. 1st ed. Washington (DC): American Psychiatric Publishing, Inc; 2006. p. xxvii, 605.

6. Goebel-Fabbri A, Musen G, Sparks CR, et al. Endocrine and metabolic disorders. In: Levenson JL, editor. Textbook of

psychosomatic medicine. Washington (DC): American Psychiatric Publishing, Inc; 2005. p. 495–515.

7. Warrington TP, Bostwick JM. Psychiatric adverse effects of corticosteroids. Mayo Clin Proc. 2006;81(10):1361–7.

8. Anglin RE, Rosebush PI, Mazurek MF. The neuropsychiatric profile of Addison's disease: revisiting a forgotten phenomenon. J Neuropsychiatry Clin Neurosci. 2006;18(4):450–9.

9. Grundy SM, Cleeman JI, Daniels SR, et al. Diagnosis and management of the metabolic syndrome: an American Heart Association/National Heart, Lung, and Blood Institute scientific statement. Circulation. 2005;112(17):2735–52.

10. Fagiolini A, Chengappa KN, Soreca I, Chang J. Bipolar disorder and the metabolic syndrome: causal factors, psychiatric outcomes and economic burden. CNS Drugs. 2008;22(8): 655–69.

11. Rege S. Antipsychotic induced weight gain in schizophrenia:mechanisms and management. Aust N Z J Psychiatry. 2008;42(5):369–81.

12. Kelly SD, Howe CJ, Hendler JP, Lipman TH. Disordered eating behaviors in youth with type 1 diabetes. Diabetes Educ. 2005; 31(4):572–83.

13. Molitch ME. Drugs and prolactin. Pituitary. 2008;11(2):209–18.

14. Chahal J, Schlechte J. Hyperprolactinemia. Pituitary. 2008;11(2):141–6.

15. Schlechte JA. Clinical practice: prolactinoma. N Engl J Med. 2003;349(21):2035–41.

16. Melkersson K, Hulting AL. Prolactin-secreting pituitary adenoma in neuroleptic treated patients with psychotic disorder. Eur Arch Psychiatry Clin Neurosci. 2000; 250(1):6–10.

17. Konopelska S, Quinkler M, Strasburger CJ, Ventz M. Difficulties in the medical treatment of prolactinoma in a patient with schizophrenia – a case report with a review of the literature. J Clin Psychopharmacol. 2008;28(1):120–2.

18. Peter SA, Autz A, Jean-Simon ML. Bromocriptine-induced schizophrenia. J Natl Med Assoc. 1993;85(9):700–1.

19. Haupt DW, Rosenblatt LC, Kim E, et al. Prevalence and predictors of lipid and glucose monitoring in commercially insured patients treated with second-generation antipsychotic agents. Am J Psychiatry. 2009;166(3):345–53.

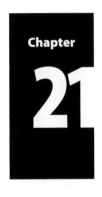

Management of alcohol withdrawal and other selected substance withdrawal issues

Philip A. Bialer and Anthony C. Miller

Typical consult question

"The patient has a history of substance abuse. Please evaluate and help manage detox."

Differential Diagnosis: Alcohol/sedative/hypnotic withdrawal vs. opioid vs. other or no withdrawal

Alcohol withdrawal

Background

The national prevalence of alcohol use is very high, and the prevalence of alcohol use disorders, specifically abuse and dependence, is also very high. Approximately 20% to 25% of patients admitted to the hospital may have an underlying alcohol use disorder (1), and healthcare workers often feel uncomfortable addressing this problem when it is uncovered during the admission process. Some hospitals maintain pre-printed alcohol "detox" order forms, and patients thought to be alcohol abusers are automatically put on these regimens. Most will end up doing well, probably because they ultimately would not have gone through withdrawal. More problematic are patients who have not been adequately screened for an alcohol problem and who start exhibiting signs of alcohol withdrawal, as well as patients whose withdrawal is not being adequately covered by the pre-printed detox sheet.

It is estimated that approximately 51% of persons in the United States drink alcohol, and about 7% are considered to be heavy drinkers (2). By *Diagnostic and Statistical Manual (DSM)-IV* standards, however, not all of these people should be considered alcohol abusers (3). To meet criteria for alcohol abuse, the patient must demonstrate failure to meet obligations such as work duties, recurrent use of alcohol in hazardous situations, such as driving, use of alcohol despite the legal consequences, such as being arrested for driving while intoxicated, or use of alcohol despite interpersonal or social problems. A diagnosis of alcohol dependence requires at least three of the following: the presence of tolerance, withdrawal, drinking more than intended, unsuccessful efforts at cutting down, excessive time spent obtaining and using alcohol, giving up important activities, and continuing to drink despite significant medical problems such as cirrhosis. Alcohol dependence can be seen as a cluster of cognitive, behavioral, and physiologic symptoms indicating that a person continues to use alcohol despite adverse medical, social, and legal consequences.

Alcohol is rapidly absorbed from the duodenum, and peak blood alcohol concentration (BAC) depends on the rate of drinking, the amount of alcohol in the beverage being

Psychosomatic Medicine: An Introduction to Consultation-Liaison Psychiatry, eds. James J. Amos and Robert G. Robinson. Published by Cambridge University Press. © Cambridge University Press 2010.

consumed, the amount and type of food present in the stomach, and the rate of gastric emptying and metabolism. In individuals without alcohol tolerance, a BAC of 100 to 200 mg% leads to significant motor function impairment and BACs between 200 and 400 mg% usually lead to stupor and coma. Alcohol is metabolized by alcohol dehydrogenase and then aldehyde dehydrogenase at a steady rate of 100 mg/kg/hr. Alcohol is a gamma-aminobutyric acid (GABA) agonist and an N-methyl-D-aspartate (NMDA) antagonist. Medical complications of prolonged alcohol use include gastritis and peptic ulcer, cirrhosis and liver failure, anemia, peripheral neuropathy, malnutrition, cardiomyopathy, dementia, and Wernicke-Korsakoff syndrome (4).

Alcohol withdrawal signs and symptoms may begin 6 to 24 hours after the last drink, peaking within 24 to 48 hours. Early signs of withdrawal include increased heart rate and blood pressure, tremors or shakes, diaphoresis, anxiety, insomnia, nausea and vomiting, and occasionally mild fever. Withdrawal may be mild and may dissipate without additional treatment in some patients. In others, however, the symptoms may worsen if left untreated and sometimes may progress to a condition known as delirium tremens (DTs), which usually begins 48 to 72 hours after the last drink. DTs is manifested by autonomic instability, hallucinations, confusion and agitated behavior alternating with lethargy, and sometimes seizures. This is a medical and psychiatric emergency that will be addressed in the management section.

Work-up

Evaluation of suspected alcohol withdrawal should start by obtaining a complete alcohol use history. This includes date of first use, pattern of use (is this person a binge drinker?), amount and type of alcohol consumed (be as specific as possible – cans of beer come in different sizes), and, of particular importance, the time of last use. An alcohol use review of symptoms should include GI, neurological, cardiac, and psychiatric symptoms. It is very important to ask about past treatment for alcohol dependence, especially previous episodes of seizures or DTs. Labs that may be helpful include BAC (a negative result may be consistent with the last drink being longer than 24 hours ago), urine toxicology, liver function tests including gamma-glutamyltransferase (GGT), as elevated levels are consistent with prolonged alcohol use, and erythrocyte indices, particularly mean corpuscular volume (MCV), which may become elevated in people with alcohol dependence (5). Collateral information, if available, may be helpful. Although family members or friends may give a more accurate picture of how much a person is really drinking, some patients may be very adept at hiding the extent of their alcohol use.

The CAGE (acronym of its four questions) questionnaire (6) has often been used to screen individuals for alcohol problems:

- Have you ever

    1. Felt you should cut down on your drinking?
    2. Felt annoyed when criticized about your drinking?
    3. Felt guilty about your drinking?
    4. Taken an eye-opener when you wake up in the morning to steady your nerves?

A positive answer to one or two of the questions should alert the clinician to the potential for alcohol-related problems. Answering yes to three of the questions indicates a very likely diagnosis of abuse or dependence, and answering yes to all four questions is pathognomonic

Table 21.1 Symptom-triggered therapy using CIWA-Ar

- Medication q 1 hour for a score ≥10
- Chlordiazepoxide 50–100 mg
- Diazepam 10–20 mg
- Lorazepam 2–4 mg
- Determine total 24-hour dose
- Taper 20% per day

Key
CIWA-Ar = Clinical Institute Withdrawal Assessment for Alcohol, Revised

for alcohol dependence. Another screening instrument, called the Audit C, has been found useful for identifying a patient at risk for alcohol withdrawal (7).

Once the patient is determined to be in alcohol withdrawal, the most widely used scale to monitor the severity of the withdrawal is the Clinical Institute Withdrawal Assessment for Alcohol, Revised (CIWA-Ar) (8), which is available in the public domain (9). The CIWA-Ar consists of ten domains to be evaluated: nausea/vomiting, tremor, paroxysmal sweats, anxiety, agitation, tactile disturbances, auditory disturbances, visual disturbances, headache/fullness in head, and orientation/clouding of consciousness. Although the patient's vital signs are not included in the scale, they must be monitored and followed. Sustained elevations in blood pressure and pulse should be considered signs of alcohol withdrawal until proven otherwise.

Clinical decision-making and treatment

Evidence-based practice guidelines from the American Society of Addiction Medicine state in no uncertain terms that benzodiazepines are the treatment of choice for alcohol withdrawal (10). Because of toxicity concerns, the use of intravenous or oral ethyl alcohol is discouraged. In general, agents with longer elimination half-lives are preferred because they may be more effective in preventing seizures and may contribute to a smoother alcohol withdrawal. Conversely, shorter-acting benzodiazepines may cause less over-sedation and may be safer in the elderly or in patients with severe liver disease.

Symptom-triggered treatment of alcohol withdrawal using assessment scales such as the CIWA-Ar is the preferred method. A score of less than ten indicates the need for continued monitoring of the patient. A score of 10 to 15 indicates mild withdrawal, 16 to 20 moderate withdrawal, and greater than 20 severe withdrawal. Table 21.1 illustrates medications to be given according to the CIWA-Ar score. After the 24-hour dosage is determined, a detox schedule can be devised by tapering the overall dosage by 20% per day. All patients being treated for alcohol withdrawal should also immediately receive thiamine 100 mg IM/IV for three days to prevent the Wernicke-Korsakoff syndrome, plus folate 1 mg daily.

Although symptom-triggered treatment may minimize the amount of medication used, it also requires that the staff administering the CIWA-Ar be adequately trained, and that the patient's medical team actually review the medication being given and order a detox schedule, rather than just continuing CIWA-Ar monitoring for several days. In many settings, a fixed-schedule regimen, as shown in Table 21.2, may be more practical. Such regimens may

Table 21.2 Fixed schedule regimens for alcohol withdrawal

- Chlordiazepoxide 50 mg q 6 hours for 4 doses, then 25 mg q 6 hours for 8 doses
- Diazepam 10 mg q 6 hours for 4 doses, then 5 mg q 6 hours for 8 doses
- Lorazepam 2 mg q 6 hours for 4 doses, then 1 mg q 6 hours for 8 doses
- Monitor vital signs and other symptoms and give additional medication prn.
- Continue tapering over the next one to two days.

work for most patients, although many may have required no treatment for withdrawal. For other patients experiencing a more severe withdrawal, the fixed regimen may not be adequate. In addition, in medically complicated patients with delirium, there may be multiple causes, which should be thoroughly evaluated and treated.

Although benzodiazepines remain the treatment of choice, some evidence supports using anticonvulsants such as carbamazepine or valproate to treat alcohol withdrawal (11).

Sedative/hypnotic withdrawal

Sedative/hypnotic (benzodiazepine, barbiturate, and related drug) withdrawal is managed by the same principles used to treat alcohol withdrawal. The onset of withdrawal symptoms will depend upon the elimination half-life of the particular substance being used. Pills are more commonly abused in the context of poly-substance dependence, necessitating a more comprehensive evaluation and monitoring for multiple types of withdrawal symptoms. Because withdrawal from alcohol and sedative/hypnotics can be life-threatening in severe cases, treatment of these symptoms takes priority.

Opioid withdrawal

Background

The consultant may be called upon to assist in managing opioid withdrawal related to illicit use, problems with prescription analgesics, or ongoing opioid agonist therapy (OAT) for addiction. Opioids include opiates isolated from opium poppy (codeine and morphine), semi-synthetic opiates (e.g., heroin, hydrocodone, oxycodone, buprenorphine), and non-opiates that act upon the same receptors (e.g., fentanyl, methadone, propoxyphene, tramadol). Central nervous system mu-opiate receptors mediate their analgesic properties as well as euphoria and reinforcement of drug administration. Tolerance and physical dependence develop in sustained therapeutic use or abuse of opioids. Withdrawal symptoms upon cessation strongly motivate individuals with opioid addiction (*DSM-IV* "opioid dependence") and therapeutic users alike to continue taking opioids.

Although opioid withdrawal is rarely dangerous in otherwise healthy adults, it is extremely unpleasant and unnecessary when safe, effective treatments are available. Treatment options involve three basic approaches: opioid-assisted detoxification, symptomatic detoxification, and maintenance OAT. In opioid addiction, 80% or more relapse after detoxification (12, 13). OAT using methadone is markedly more effective at eliminating illicit opioid use and reducing associated morbidity, mortality, criminality, and treatment dropouts (13, 14). Buprenorphine demonstrates similar benefits (13).

U.S. federal restrictions limit opioid use in addiction treatment to three scenarios:

1. Patients hospitalized for a different medical problem can be treated with any opioid to prevent withdrawal symptoms that could complicate the primary medical problem (15).

Table 21.3 Signs and symptoms of acute opioid withdrawal

elevated pulse	muscle spasms	abdominal cramping
elevated blood pressure	myalgia	diarrhea
pupil dilation	arthralgia	vomiting
lacrimation	sweating	anxiety
rhinorrhea	chills	irritability
yawning	piloerection	insomnia

2. Federally accredited opioid treatment programs (OTPs) can administer methadone or buprenorphine for detoxification or maintenance as part of a comprehensive treatment program (16).
3. Qualified physicians may obtain a waiver to prescribe buprenorphine for detoxification or maintenance (17).

Work-up

Withdrawal symptoms begin hours after short-acting opioids (like heroin or morphine) are stopped and last until days after methadone is stopped, which is longer acting. Acute withdrawal abates within days, but sub-acute symptoms of drug craving, irritability, restlessness, sleep disturbance, and increased pain sensitivity can persist for months (13, 18).

Table 21.3 lists signs and symptoms of acute opioid withdrawal.

Colorful terms refer to various aspects of withdrawal: "kicking" (muscle spasm), "cold turkey" (gooseflesh), and "jonesing" (exquisitely described by John Jones in 1701) (19).

Clinical decision-making and treatment

Opioid agonist therapy for patients in the hospital

Managing opioid medications for hospitalized patients already receiving OAT can be straightforward, but obstacles frequently arise. Patients may be afraid to disclose that they use OAT. Clinicians may believe that OAT can be electively discontinued, or that maintenance opioids provide sufficient analgesia for painful conditions or procedures. In reality, OAT must be continued to avoid complicating a medical crisis with opioid withdrawal, and OAT patients usually require *higher* analgesic doses because of tolerance.

Early communication between the inpatient team and the OAT prescriber is critical in determining the usual dosage, when it was last given, and other pertinent medical and social information. The usual maintenance dosage of methadone or buprenorphine should be administered during hospitalization. If the patient is NPO, methadone can be administered intramuscularly at half the usual oral dose divided BID. Buprenorphine can be given by the usual sublingual route to NPO patients if they expectorate the residua. It is available intramuscularly, but the dose equivalence is not well established (20).

Methadone-maintained patients with acutely painful medical or surgical conditions should receive short-acting opioids (e.g., morphine, oxycodone), as would other patients with the same condition, with recognition that dose requirements will likely be higher. If analgesics will be needed after hospitalization, it is important to confer with the OAT prescriber about post-hospital opioid management.

Analgesia in buprenorphine-maintained patients can be more complex. Buprenorphine, a partial opioid receptor agonist with very high receptor affinity, effectively blocks the effects of other opioids. In moderate pain, analgesia sometimes can be achieved by administering buprenorphine more often (every 4 to 6 hours) and increasing the daily total to a maximum of 32 mg/d. With more severe pain, it may be necessary to temporarily convert from buprenorphine to methadone (typically 30 to 40 mg/d) and use short-acting opioids (e.g., morphine, oxycodone) for analgesia (20). Careful planning with the OAT prescriber will be necessary in the latter case, as post-hospital care may be complicated by lack of access to methadone maintenance. To avoid precipitating acute withdrawal from methadone, it is best to hold methadone until mild withdrawal symptoms emerge before restarting buprenorphine. Pain may recur during the transition; short-acting opioids may be needed as a "bridge" during the transition.

Opioid-assisted detoxification in the hospital

Hospitalized patients with active opioid addiction who are not on OAT, do not want it, or cannot access it often require opioid withdrawal treatment to avoid medical complications. Acute opioid withdrawal can complicate medical problems by increasing blood pressure and pulse, via fluid loss from vomiting and diarrhea, or by interfering with treatment adherence.

The most effective way to rapidly control opioid withdrawal is to administer an opioid. Methadone is often chosen because its long half-life allows for less frequent dosing and fewer intradose withdrawal symptoms. Methadone is given in small, frequent doses as needed for withdrawal symptoms, with effective titration to control withdrawal symptoms within one to two days, while avoiding over-sedation. Each day's dose begins with the previous day's total given as a single morning dose, with additional doses given as needed until withdrawal symptoms are stabilized.

Buprenorphine can be used as an alternative to methadone. As a partial agonist, the "ceiling effect" of buprenorphine limits its utility in individuals with high opioid tolerance. If buprenorphine precipitates worsened withdrawal symptoms, or if withdrawal symptoms fail to stabilize on buprenorphine at 16 mg/d, switching to methadone should be considered. A validated withdrawal rating scale such as the Clinical Opiate Withdrawal Scale (COWS) is useful in identifying precipitated withdrawal and in verifying the effectiveness of treatment (21). The COWS is in the public domain and is available on-line (22).

After withdrawal symptoms are stabilized, the opioid is usually tapered gradually, unless transition to maintenance OAT is planned. If a patient has no intention of stopping illicit use, it is legally permissible to maintain the patient on an opioid while hospitalized. Clinicians generally avoid this approach, which can be viewed as facilitating addiction, but it may merit consideration in select situations.

Tapering the opioid slowly enough to avoid recurring withdrawal symptoms is seldom accomplished in fewer than 10 days. It is reasonable to begin tapering by 10% per day as tolerated. Hospital stays are often too brief to complete such a taper, but patients often do not have access to an OTP or a qualified buprenorphine prescriber to continue the taper after discharge. Alternatives include accelerating the taper, switching to non-opioid treatment for withdrawal, abruptly stopping the medication upon hospital discharge, or lengthening the hospitalization. An additional option – prescribing a buprenorphine taper to be completed after discharge – is available to waivered physicians (17).

See Table 21.4 for sample detoxification regimens.

Table 21.4 Sample opioid withdrawal protocols

	Methadone	Buprenorphine	Clonidine
Day 1	5–10 mg PO every 4–6 hours as needed to a maximum of 40 mg	4 mg SL every 4–6 hours to a maximum of 16 mg	0.1–0.2 mg PO every 4–6 hours as needed to a maximum of 1.2 mg
Day 2	Day 1 total as a single morning dose AND 5–10 mg PO every 4–6 hours as needed	Day 1 total as a single morning dose AND 4 mg SL every 4–6 hours as needed to a maximum of 16 mg	0.1–0.2 mg PO every 4–6 hours as needed to a maximum of 1.2 mg
Subsequent days until stabilized	Previous day total as a single morning dose AND 5–10 mg PO every 4–6 hours as needed	If not stabilizing at 16 mg/d for 2 days, consider switch to methadone.	Day 2 total divided into three equal doses
Tapering days	Once-daily dosing, decreasing by 10% per day	Once-daily dosing, decreasing by 1–2 mg per day	TID dosing, decreasing daily total by 0.2 mg per day

Methadone and buprenorphine drug interactions

A few key drug interactions need to be kept in mind with regard to methadone and buprenorphine:

1. All opioids cause respiratory depression, which can be exacerbated by benzodiazepines, barbiturates, alcohol, and other opioids.
2. Methadone and buprenorphine are both chiefly metabolized by cytochrome P450 3A4 (CYP3A4). Their effects are exaggerated by CYP3A4 inhibitors (e.g., erythromycin, fluconazole, fluvoxamine) and are attenuated by CYP3A4 inducers (e.g., carbamazepine, phenytoin, rifampin.)
3. Methadone can cause repolarization delay (QT interval prolongation) (16). EKG monitoring is warranted when methadone is used with other drugs or conditions that can cause repolarization delay (e.g., many antiarrhythmic, antidepressant, and antipsychotic drugs; hypokalemia; hypomagnesemia).
4. Buprenorphine blocks or attenuates the effects of other opioids (including methadone) and should not be used in combination with them.
5. The effects of methadone are attenuated by partial or mixed opioid agonists (e.g., buprenorphine, butorphanol, nalbuphine, pentazocine). If other opioid analgesics are needed with methadone, they should be full agonists.

Symptomatic detoxification

Occasionally, it may not be desirable to treat withdrawal with an opioid because of legal, medical, or patient preference issues. Non-opioid treatments can ameliorate withdrawal symptoms, but often do not eliminate them. The most studied treatments are the alpha-2-adrenergic agonists clonidine and lofexidine (23, 24). Clonidine can be given at 0.1 to 0.2 mg orally every 4 hours as needed for opioid withdrawal until no additional reduction in symptoms is achieved, or the patient is on the highest dose that he can tolerate (up to a maximum of 1.2 mg/d is reached). The dosage is tapered and discontinued over 3 to 5 days. See Table 21.4 for a sample regimen. Hypotension – especially orthostatic – is the major limiting side effect. Vital signs should be monitored closely during initiation, with doses omitted for hypotension (systolic blood pressure less than 90 mmHg), bradycardia (pulse less than

60 bpm), or sedation. Lofexidine is less likely to cause hypotension, but is not approved in the United States (23, 24). Adjunct medications for opioid withdrawal symptoms can include non-steroidal anti-inflammatory drugs for myalgias and arthralgias, dicyclomine for abdominal cramping, antiemetics for nausea and vomiting, and benzodiazepines for insomnia and anxiety.

Accelerated methods

"Rapid" detoxification using opioid antagonists such as naltrexone or naloxone to accelerate withdrawal does not consistently improve outcomes and increases problems with vomiting, diarrhea, and delirium. Detoxification under general anesthesia entails even further risk and is not recommended (24, 25).

Pregnancy

Opioid withdrawal in pregnancy increases risk of fetal distress, miscarriage, and preterm labor, and should be quickly stabilized with an opioid. Methadone maintenance is the standard of care for opioid addiction in pregnancy. Many OTPs offer priority admission to pregnant women (16). However, methadone is not given without risk to the fetus, which likely will experience withdrawal symptoms postpartum. Early involvement of addiction medicine and maternal-fetal medicine specialists is advisable.

References

1. Lohr RH. Treatment of alcohol withdrawal in hospitalized patients. Mayo Clin Proc. 1995;70:777–82.

2. Substance Abuse and Mental Health Administration. Results from the 2007 National Survey on Drug Use and Health: national findings. Rockville (MD): Office of Applied Studies; 2008. NSDUH Series H-34. DHHS Publication No. SMA 08-4343.

3. American Psychiatric Association: Diagnostic and statistical manual of mental disorders. 4th ed. Washington (DC): American Psychiatric Association; 1994.

4. Mannelli P, Pae CU. Medical comorbidity and alcohol dependence. Curr Psychiatr. 2007;9:217–24.

5. Miller PM, Spies C, Neumann T, et al. Alcohol biomarker screening in medical and surgical settings. Alcohol Clin Exp Res. 2006;30:185–93.

6. Ewing JA. Detecting alcoholism: the CAGE questionnaire. JAMA. 1984;252:1905–7.

7. Bush K, Kivlahan DR, McDonell MB, et al. The AUDIT alcohol consumption questions (AUDIT-C): an effective brief screening test for problem drinking. Arch Intern Med. 1998;158:1789–95.

8. Sullivan JT, Sykora K, Schneiderman J, et al. Assessment of alcohol withdrawal: the revised clinical institute withdrawal assessment for alcohol scale (CIWA-Ar). Br J Addict. 1989;84:1353–7.

9. Available at: http://www.ncbi.nlm.nih.gov/books/bv.fcgi?rid=hstat5.table.40602. Accessed May 26, 2009.

10. Mayo-Smith MF. Pharmacological management of alcohol withdrawal: a meta-analysis and evidence-based practice guideline. American Society of Addiction Medicine Working Group on Pharmacological Management of Alcohol Withdrawal. JAMA. 1997;278:144–51.

11. Leggio L, Kenna GA, Swift RM. New developments for the pharmacological treatment of alcohol withdrawal syndrome: a focus on non-benzodiazepine GABAergic medications. Prog Neuropsychopharmacol Biol Psychiatry. 2008;32:1106–17.

12. Kakko J, Svanborg KD, Kreek MJ, Heilig M. 1-year retention and social function after buprenorphine-assisted relapse prevention treatment for heroin dependence in

Sweden: a randomised, placebo-controlled trial. Lancet. 2003;361:662–8.

13. Kreek MJ. Rationale for maintenance pharmacotherapy of opiate dependence. In: O'Brien CP, Jaffe JH, editors. Addictive states. New York (NY): Raven Press; 1992. p. 205–30.

14. Joseph H, Stancliff S, Langrod J. Methadone maintenance treatment (MMT): a review of historical and clinical issues. Mt Sinai J Med. 2000;67:347–64.

15. Substance Abuse and Mental Health Services Administration. Frequently asked questions about buprenorphine and the Drug Addiction Treatment Act of 2000. Available at: http://buprenorphine. samhsa.gov/faq.html#A14. Accessed May 6, 2009.

16. Center for Substance Abuse Treatment. Medication-assisted treatment for opioid addiction in opioid treatment programs. Rockville, MD: Substance Abuse and Mental Health Services Administration, 2005. Treatment Improvement Protocol (TIP) Series 43. DHHS Publication No. (SMA) 05-4048.

17. Substance Abuse and Mental Health Services Administration. Physician waiver qualifications. Available at: http://buprenorphine.samhsa.gov/./ waiver_qualifications.html Accessed May 6, 2009.

18. Himmelsbach CK. Studies on the relation of drug addiction to the autonomic nervous system: results of cold pressor tests. J Pharmacol Exp Ther 1941; 73: 91–98.

19. Jones J. The mysteries of opium reveal'd. London: Richard Smith; 1701.

20. Alford DP, Compton P, Samet JH. Acute pain management for patients receiving maintenance methadone or buprenorphine therapy. Ann Intern Med. 2006;144:127–34.

21. Wesson DR, Ling W. The Clinical Opiate Withdrawal Scale (COWS). J Psychoactive Drugs. 2003;35:253–9.

22. California Society of Addiction Medicine. Clinical Opiate Withdrawal Scale. Available at: http://www.csam-asam.org/ pdf/misc/COWS.doc. Accessed May 6, 2009.

23. Gowing L, Farrell M, Ali R, White JM. Alpha2-adrenergic agonists for the management of opioid withdrawal. Cochrane Database Syst Rev. 2009;(2):CD002024. DOI: 10.1002/14651858.CD002024.pub3.

24. Van Den Brink W, Haasen C. Evidenced-based treatment of opioid-dependent patients. Can J Psychiatry. 2006;51:635–46.

25. Gowing L, Ali R, White JM. Opioid antagonists under heavy sedation or anaesthesia for opioid withdrawal. Cochrane Database Syst Rev. 2006;(2):CD002022. DOI: 10.1002/14651858.CD002022.pub2.

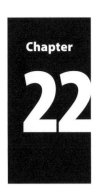

Managing depression in pregnancy

Robin C. Kopelman

Typical consult question

"Please evaluate and treat this twenty-five year old pregnant female with a history of depression, currently in the second trimester of an unplanned pregnancy, who stopped her antidepressant medication at the time of a positive pregnancy test."

Depression is a significant public health problem that disproportionately affects women, often during the childbearing years. Perinatal depression, which refers to depression during both pregnancy and the post-partum period, is common, particularly in low-income and ethnic minority populations. It is associated with adverse consequences for the mother, infant, and other family members and often goes undetected and untreated. Depression during the perinatal period is associated with assessment and treatment challenges requiring unique collaboration between patient and maternal and child health and mental healthcare providers.

Background

Epidemiology of depression during pregnancy and the post-partum period

Although many women and their providers still believe that pregnancy "protects" women from experiencing depression, research studies show that it is widespread. In the obstetric clinic setting, nearly 40% of women are identified with a mental health disorder, most commonly depression (1, 2). The prevalence of antenatal depression in the community is approximately 10% (3), but may be as high as 27.6% among women in poor urban communities (4). Post-partum depression is also common, with around 13% of women meeting criteria for major or minor depression (5).

Although depression during pregnancy and during the post-partum period is not necessarily due to the same causes, the two types are inextricably linked by the process of childbirth and the context in which they occur. Antenatal depression and post-natal depression share risk factors including poor social support, particularly from the partner (5, 6), and a family or personal history of depression (5). Women with a history of one or more episodes of post-partum depression have a 25% risk of recurrence (7). The presence of depressive symptoms during pregnancy is also a significant risk factor for post-partum depression (8).

Other mood concerns during the post-partum period include post-partum blues and post-partum psychosis. Post-partum depression must be distinguished from each of these. "The blues" are quite common, and practitioners should not consider this a disorder, with up to 75% of women experiencing symptoms such as mood lability, sensitivity, and tearfulness

Psychosomatic Medicine: An Introduction to Consultation-Liaison Psychiatry, eds. James J. Amos and Robert G. Robinson. Published by Cambridge University Press. © Cambridge University Press 2010.

(9). Post-partum psychosis is estimated to occur in 1 to 2 women per 1000 deliveries (10), with onset within the first couple weeks after delivery (11).

Consequences of depressive disorders in the perinatal period

Perinatal depression has a number of adverse outcomes for the whole family. Depression in pregnancy is associated with an increased risk for pre-eclampsia (12), preterm delivery (13), and fetal growth retardation (14). Depressed pregnant women obtain less adequate prenatal care (15) and have more negative health behaviors (e.g., tobacco use) (16), which negatively impact outcomes.

Partners of women with post-partum depression may experience elevated levels of depression (17). Children of women with post-partum depression are at increased risk for developmental, cognitive, and emotional problems (18, 19). Post-partum depression in mothers (and their partners) is associated with fewer positive parent-infant interactions (20).

Work-up

Not unlike the medical conditions described in other chapters, assessment of depression during the perinatal period is a challenge because of the overlap of depressive symptoms with the normal experiences of pregnancy and childbirth. Fatigue, sleep changes, changes in libido, and changes in appetite or weight can be attributed to the perinatal period. Using a depression rating scale facilitates identification of mood disorders when it is used in addition to a standard interview. In fact, many women are referred following completion of such a tool, as screening in the obstetric setting is recommended (21). The Edinburgh Postnatal Depression Scale (EPDS) (22) is a commonly used screening measure. It focuses on psychological symptoms rather than on the somatic symptoms associated with new parenthood and has been validated for use in pregnancy (23). Clinicians also need to verify duration of the perinatal woman's symptoms. A period of two weeks of symptoms is necessary to diagnose depression, whereas the EPDS, for example, assesses a woman's experience over the previous seven days. Similarly, the blues typically arises and resolves in the first 7 to 14 days post-partum (24).

Assessment of suicidal, homicidal, and infanticidal ideation is critical. Women with perinatal depression do have thoughts of harming themselves or the infant (25), and the increased risk for suicide is a particular concern for these women (26, 27). Thyroid disorders are commonly associated with both pregnancy and the post partum period (28), making it important to evaluate thyroid functioning. Assessment of tobacco use and substance use, as always, remains important.

The majority of cases of depression identified in the obstetric setting will be unipolar depression, but do screen for bipolar depression to identify women at risk for or who have developed post-partum psychosis. Research data suggest that post-partum psychosis is often a manifestation of bipolar disorder. Symptoms include mood lability, delusions that are often focused on childbirth themes, hallucinations, and, in particular, marked cognitive disturbance (29). Carefully assess women with post-partum psychosis for suicidal and homicidal/infanticidal ideation. Although infanticide is quite rare, women with post-partum psychosis are more likely to experience thoughts of harming their infants than are women with non-psychotic post-partum depression and are at risk for neglecting their infant (30, 31). The cognitive disturbance associated with post partum psychosis makes thorough evaluation for delirium essential (29).

Clinical decision-making and treatment

Following evaluation for perinatal mood disorder, follow-up or intervention may be indicated for some women who are not currently depressed. For example, women who are experiencing severe blues symptoms are more likely to go on to develop a depressive episode (32). Likewise, women who are not symptomatic in pregnancy or the post-partum period, but who have a history of depression, especially post-partum depression, may benefit from a preventive intervention with psychotherapy or antidepressant medication, although research data are limited at this time. A woman might elect to initiate prophylactic treatment with a selective serotonin reuptake inhibitor approximately 48 hours after delivery, or may start a preventive intervention spanning pregnancy and the post-partum period, such as a group based on the principles of interpersonal psychotherapy (IPT) (33, 34).

Nonpharmacologic treatments

Psychotherapy may be an effective option for some women with perinatal depression. For women with milder symptoms who prefer psychosocial treatment, it should be considered first-line. Psychological treatments, like IPT, are efficacious for antenatal depression (35). At present, no efficacy studies have demonstrated the benefit of cognitive-behavioral therapy (CBT) for antenatal depression. For post-partum women with milder symptoms, various psychosocial treatments delivered by non–mental health or mental health professionals have been shown to improve depressive symptoms. For more severe depression, benefit has been shown only in studies with well-defined treatments, such as IPT or CBT, delivered by highly trained professionals (36).

Pharmacologic treatments

Psychotropic medication will be the first choice for many women, particularly those with more severe illness, or for whom other treatments are inaccessible. Psychotropic medications, however, do cross the placenta and are present in amniotic fluid (37, 38). In addition to the specific medication concerns outlined below, good general guidelines for treatment include (1) using the least number of medications, (2) using the lowest possible dose, and (3) selecting a previously effective medication or medication that has been effective for a genetically related family member. Because of changes in blood volume and possible changes in medication metabolism, however, upward dose adjustments may be clinically indicated (39).

Overall, most research on antidepressants during pregnancy has focused on the selective serotonin reuptake inhibitors (SSRIs), and they are undoubtedly the most commonly prescribed. Some studies have demonstrated an increased risk of select anomalies (e.g., omphalocele) with SSRI exposure (40, 41). Concern has been raised about paroxetine in particular, as two studies suggest it confers an increased risk of cardiac defects with first-trimester exposure. The manufacturer subsequently changed product warning labels (42). Findings remain controversial (43), but at present, avoid initiating new treatment with paroxetine in women of childbearing age, and consider fetal echocardiography in women exposed during early pregnancy (44).

An association between SSRIs and premature delivery and low birth weight has been demonstrated (13, 45). Timing of exposure (third trimester) and duration of exposure may be factors (45). First-trimester exposures historically have been of greatest concern, but third-trimester exposure also may be of concern because of "neonatal abstinence syndrome." Neonatal complications associated with third-trimester exposure to SSRIs and serotonin-norepinephrine reuptake inhibitors (SNRIs) may include tremors, feeding difficulties, irritability, increased muscle tone, respiratory problems, hyperreflexia, increased crying, and sleep changes (46). Symptoms usually start within hours of delivery and go away within 1 to 2 weeks, often requiring no intervention. Third-trimester exposure to SSRIs has also been associated with a possible increased risk for persistent pulmonary hypertension of the newborn (PPHN) (47). These issues reinforce the potential benefit of using the lowest effective dose for the shortest duration, but discuss with the pregnant patient the potential for relapse when making a decision to reduce or temporarily discontinue medication.

Studies examining mirtazapine (48), bupropion (49), venlafaxine (50), trazodone, and nefazodone (51), as well as the tricyclic antidepressants (TCAs) (52), do not suggest an increased risk of fetal anomalies. Monoamine oxidase inhibitors (MAOIs) generally are not recommended for use in the perinatal period because of the lack of data and the potential for hypertensive crisis (53). Few longitudinal studies have examined outcomes for children exposed to antidepressants or depression during pregnancy (54).

Antidepressants and lactation

Current research indicates that serum levels of antidepressant drugs in infants of breast-feeding mothers are typically undetectable or very low (55). Despite the low levels found in breastfeeding infants, providers should advise mothers to monitor infants for medication effects including irritability, sedation, or feeding changes (54). In a pooled analysis, levels were particularly low for sertraline, paroxetine, and nortriptyline, making these medications preferred. Elevated infant levels occurred with fluoxetine and citalopram (56). Several cases of adverse events have been reported with use of all types of antidepressants. Most reports involve fluoxetine, probably because of its long half-life (54). Again, few long-term studies have been conducted, and clear evidence of developmental problems has not been described (57).

Alternative options for depression treatment in the perinatal period

Many women are interested in avoiding medication during the perinatal period but may not find psychotherapy accessible or acceptable. Treatment with omega-3 fatty acids (58, 59) and light therapy (60) may be beneficial for depression during pregnancy. Women should understand that the data on these treatments are limited.

Women with severe depressive symptoms that do not respond to pharmacotherapy and women with psychosis may benefit from electroconvulsive therapy, which has been used in pregnancy and the post-partum period. Maternal and fetal precautions are indicated (61).

Treatment with mood stabilizers and antipsychotics in the perinatal period

Other psychotropic medications sometimes are used adjunctively for women with unipolar depression and commonly for women with bipolar disorder or post-partum psychosis. Both carbamazepine and valproate are considered human teratogens and should be avoided in pregnancy when possible. Each is associated with increased risk for neural tube defects and other fetal malformations (62). Lamotrigine may be another option for treatment, with a more favorable safety profile than the other anticonvulsant mood stabilizers (63).

Lithium use is of concern in pregnancy because of the increased risk for Ebstein's anomaly and neonatal toxicity (62). Monitor blood levels closely during pregnancy. Current guidelines recommend stopping lithium 24 to 48 hours before delivery and restarting after delivery at pre-pregnancy dosing (64). Lithium is not commonly prescribed for breastfeeding women.

Reproductive safety data for atypical antipsychotics are extremely limited. No evidence currently indicates that these medications are associated with negative consequences in the perinatal period, but mixed reports have been published (44, 54). Typical antipsychotic drugs, especially haloperidol, have a larger amount of reproductive safety data available. Their use might be preferable to use of an atypical drug or anticonvulsant (44).

Role of healthcare providers

Despite the potential consequences, less than one-third of depressed perinatal women receive treatment (65, 66). Financial issues and concerns about safety of medications during pregnancy may play a significant role (67). Often, women discontinue medication as a direct result of conception (68). Relapse rates for those women who discontinue antidepressants during pregnancy are high, with higher relapse rates reported in women with depression for longer than 5 years, with more than four episodes, and of younger age (69).

For perinatal women with depression, healthcare providers have significant responsibility in the decision-making phase, particularly in framing treatment choices and guiding women through the process. Assess the contextual and clinical factors that impact women's preferences, including their ability to access treatment and the personal risks associated with illness (70, 71). Document the discussion of risks associated with treatment and non-treatment and alternative treatment options that were discussed. Ensure that your patient is able to provide informed consent, and involve the partner whenever possible. Maternal healthcare providers, when specialty mental healthcare is involved, should be supported and collaborated with. It is essential that women who present in the perinatal period are identified and treated to achieve better outcomes for women and their families.

References

1. Smith MV, Rosenheck RA, Cavaleri MA, et al. Screening for and detection of depression, panic disorder, and PTSD in public-sector obstetric clinics. Psychiatr Serv. 2004;55(4):407–14.

2. Kelly R, Zatzick D, Anders T. The detection and treatment of psychiatric disorders and substance use among pregnant women cared for in obstetrics. Am J Psychiatry. 2001;158(2):213–9.

3. O'Hara MW. Social support, life events, and depression during pregnancy and the puerperium. Arch Gen Psychiatry. 1986; 43:569–73.

4. Hobfoll SE, Ritter C, Lavin J, et al. Depression prevalence and incidence among inner-city pregnant and postpartum women. J Consult Clin Psychol. 1995;63(3):445–53.

5. O'Hara MW, Swain AM. Rates and risk of postpartum depression – a meta-analysis. Int Rev Psychiatry. 1996;8(1):37–54.

6. Gjerdingen DK, Froberg DG, Fontaine P. The effects of social support on women's health during pregnancy, labor and delivery, and the postpartum period. Fam Med. 1991;23:370–5.

7. Wisner KL, Perel JM, Peindl KS, et al. Prevention of recurrent postpartum depression: a randomized clinical trial. J Clin Psychiatry. 2001;62:82–6.

8. O'Hara MW, Zekoski EM, Philipps LH, Wright EJ. Controlled prospective study of postpartum mood disorders: comparison

of childbearing and nonchildbearing women. J Abnorm Psychol. 1990;99(1): 3–15.

9. Flynn HA. Epidemiology and phenomenology of postpartum mood disorders. Psychiatr Ann. 2005;35:544–651.

10. Kendell RE, Chalmers JC, Platz C. Epidemiology of puerperal psychoses. Br J Psychiatry. 1987;150:662–73.

11. Attia E, Downey J, Oberman M. Postpartum psychoses. In: Miller L, editor. Postpartum mood disorders. Washington (DC): American Psychiatric Publishing, Inc; 1999. p. 99–117.

12. Kurki T, Hiilesmaa V, Raitasalo R, et al. Depression and anxiety in early pregnancy and risk for preeclampsia. Obstet Gynecol. 2002;95:487–90.

13. Wisner KL, Sit DKY, Hanusa BH, et al. Major depression and antidepressant treatment: impact on pregnancy and neonatal outcomes. Am J Psychiatry. 2009;166(5):557–66.

14. Hofman S, Hatch MC. Depressive symptomatology during pregnancy: evidence for an association with decreased fetal growth in pregnancies of lower social class women. Health Psychol. 2000;19: 535–43.

15. Kelly RH, Danielsen BH, Golding JM, et al. Adequacy of prenatal care among women with psychiatric diagnoses giving birth in California in 1994 and 1995. Psychiatr Serv. 1999;5(12):1584–90.

16. Zuckerman B, Amaro H, Bauchner H, Cabral H. Depressive symptoms during pregnancy: relationship to poor health behaviors. Am J Obstet Gynecol. 1989;160: 1107–11.

17. Soliday E, McCluskey-Fawcett K, O'Brien M. Postpartum affect and depressive symptoms in mothers and fathers. Am J Orthopsychiatry. 1999;6(1):30–8.

18. Murray L, Fiori-Cowley A, Hooper R, Cooper P. The impact of postnatal depression and associated adversity on early mother-infant interactions and later infant outcome. Child Dev. 1996;67(5): 2512–26.

19. Phillipps LH, O'Hara MW. Prospective study of postpartum depression: 4$\frac{1}{2}$ year follow-up of women and children. J Abnorm Psychol. 1991;100: 151–5.

20. Paulson JF, Dauber S, Leiferman JA. Individual and combined effects of postpartum depression in mothers and fathers on parenting behavior. Pediatrics. 2006;118(2):659–68.

21. Gaynes BN, Gavin N, Meltzer-Brody S, Lohr KN, et al. Perinatal depression: prevalence, screening accuracy, and screening outcomes. Rockville (MD): AHRQ; 2005.

22. Cox JL, Holden JM, Sagovsky R. Detection of postnatal depression: development of the 10-item Edinburgh Postnatal Depression Scale. Br J Psychiatry. 1987;150: 782–6.

23. Murray L, Cox J. Identifying depression during pregnancy with the Edinburgh Postnatal Depression Scale (EPDS). J Reprod Infant Psychol. 1990;8:99–107.

24. O'Hara MW, Schlechte JA, Lewis DA, Varner MW. Controlled prospective study of postpartum mood disorders: psychological, environmental, and hormonal variables. J Abnorm Psychol. 1991;100(1):63–73.

25. Berggren-Clive K. Out of the darkness and into the light: women's experiences with depression after childbirth. Can J Commun Ment Health. 1998;17(1):103–20.

26. Appleby L. Suicide during pregnancy and in the first postnatal year. Br Med J. 1991; 302:137–40.

27. Oates M. Deaths from suicide and other psychiatric causes: why mothers die. Report on confidential enquiries into maternal deaths in the United Kingdom. Confidential Enquiry into Maternal and Child Health (CEMACH). 2004 [cited 2005 April 26, 2005]. Available from: www.cemach.org.uk/publications/ WMD2000_2002/content.htm.

28. Lazarus JH, Kokandi A. Thyroid disease in relation to pregnancy: a decade of change. Clin Endocrinol. 2000;53(3):265–78.

29. Sit D, Rothschild AJ, Wisner KL. A review of postpartum psychosis. J, Womens Health (Larchmt). 2006;15(4):352–68.

30. Kumar R, Marks M, Platz C, Yoshida K. Clinical survey of a psychiatric mother and baby unit: characteristics of 100 consecutive admissions. J Affect Disord. 1995;3(1):11–22.

31. Wisner KL, Peindl K, Hanusa BH. Symptomatology of affective and psychotic illnesses related to childbearing. J Affect Disord. 1994;30:77–87.

32. Henshaw C, Foreman D, Cox J. Postnatal blues: a risk factor for postnatal depression. J Psychosom Obstet Gynaecol. 2004; 25(3–4):267–72.

33. Wisner KL, Perel JM, Peindl KS, et al. Prevention of postpartum depression: a pilot randomized clinical trial. Am J Psychiatry. 2004;161(7):1290–2.

34. Zlotnick C, Miller IW, Pearlstein T, et al. A preventive intervention for pregnant women on public assistance at risk for postpartum depression. Am J Psychiatry. 2006;163(8):1443–5.

35. Stuart S, O'Hara MW. Psychosocial treatments for mood disorders in women. In: Steiner M, Yonkers KA, Eriksson E, editors. Mood disorders in women. London: Martin Dunitz, Ltd; 2000. p. 521–42.

36. Kopelman R, Stuart S. Psychological treatments for postpartum depression. Psychiatr Ann. 2005;35:556–65.

37. Doering P, Stewart RB. The extent and character of drug consumption during pregnancy. JAMA. 1978;239:843–6.

38. Hostetter A, Ritchie JC, Stowe ZN. Amniotic fluid and umbilical cord blood concentrations of antidepressants in three women. Biol Psychiatry. 2000;4(10): 1032–4.

39. Sit D, Perel JM, Helsel JC, Wisner KL. Changes in antidepressant metabolism and dosing across pregnancy and early postpartum. J Clin Psychiatry. 2008;69(4): 652–8.

40. Alwan S, Reefhuis J, Rasmussen SA, et al. Use of selective serotonin-reuptake

41. Louik C, Lin AE, Werler MM, et al. First-trimester use of selective serotonin-reuptake inhibitors and the risk of birth defects. N Engl J Med. 2007;356(26): 2675–83.

42. GlaxoSmithKline. Use of Paxil or Paxil CR during pregnancy. [cited 2009 June 9]. Available from: http://us.gsk.com/docs-pdf/media-news/mi_letter_paroxetine_pregnancy.pdf

43. Einarson A, Pistelli A, DeSantis M, et al. Evaluation of the risk of congenital cardiovascular defects associated with use of paroxetine during pregnancy. Am J Psychiatry. 2008;165(6):749–52.

44. ACOG Committee on Practice Bulletins – Obstetrics. ACOG Practice Bulletin: Clinical management guidelines for obstetrician-gynecologists, number 92, 2008. Use of psychiatric medications during pregnancy and lactation. Obstet Gynecol. 2008;111(4):1001–20.

45. Chambers CD, Johnson KA, Dick LM, et al. Birth outcomes in pregnant women taking fluoxetine. N Engl J Med. 1996;335: 1010–5.

46. Moses-Kolko EL, Bogen D, Perel J, et al. Neonatal signs after late in utero exposure to serotonin reuptake inhibitors: literature review and implications for clinical applications. JAMA. 2005;293(19): 2372–83.

47. Chambers CD, Hernandez-Diaz S, Van Marter LJ, et al. Selective serotonin-reuptake inhibitors and risk of persistent pulmonary hypertension of the newborn. N Engl J Med. 2006;354(6):579–87.

48. Djulus J, Koren G, Einarson TR, et al. Exposure to mirtazapine during pregnancy: a prospective, comparative study of birth outcomes. J Clin Psychiatry. 2006;67(8):1280–4.

49. Chun-Fai-Chan B, Koren G, Fayez I, et al. Pregnancy outcome of women exposed to bupropion during pregnancy: a prospective comparative study. Am J Obstet Gynecol. 2005;192(3):932–6.

50. Einarson A Fatoye B, Sarkar M, et al. Pregnancy outcome following gestational exposure to venlafaxine: a multicenter prospective controlled study. Am J Psychiatry. 2001;158(10):1728–30.

51. Einarson A, Bonari L, Voyer-Lavigne S, et al. A multicentre prospective study to determine the safety of trazodone and nefazodone use during pregnancy. Can J Psychiatry. 2003;48(2):106.

52. Simon GE, Cunninghma ML, Davis RL. Outcomes of prenatal antidepressant exposure. Arch Gen Psychiatry. 2002;159: 2055–61.

53. Gracious BL. Phenelzine use throughout pregnancy and the puerperium: case report, review of the literature, and management recommendations. Depress Anxiety. 1997;6(3):124–8.

54. Pearlstein T. Perinatal depression: treatment options and dilemmas. J Psychiatry Neurosci. 2008;33(4):302–18.

55. Gjerdingen D. The effectiveness of various postpartum depression treatments and the impact of antidepressant drugs on nursing infants. J Am Board Fam Pract. 2003;16(5): 372–82.

56. Weissman AM, Levy BT, Hartz AJ, et al. Pooled analysis of antidepressant levels in lactating mothers, breast milk, and nursing infants. Am J Psychiatry. 2004;161(6): 1066–78.

57. Gentile S. SSRIs in pregnancy and lactation: emphasis on neurodevelopmental outcome. CNS Drugs. 2005;19(7): 623–33.

58. Freeman MP, Davis M, Sinha P, et al. Omega-3 fatty acids and supportive psychotherapy for perinatal depression: a randomized placebo-controlled study. J Affect Disord. 2008;110(1–2):142–8.

59. Su K-P, Huang S-Y, Chiu C-C, Shen WW. Omega-3 fatty acids in major depressive disorder: a preliminary double-blind, placebo-controlled trial. Eur Neuropsychopharmacol. 2003;13(4):267–71.

60. Epperson C, Terman M, Terman J, et al. Randomized clinical trial of bright light therapy for antepartum depression: preliminary findings. J Clin Psychiatry. 2004;65(3):421–5.

61. Pinnette M, Santarpio C, Wax J, Blackstone J. Electroconvulsive therapy in pregnancy. Obstet Gynecol. 2007;110:465–6.

62. Yonkers KA, Wisner KL, Stowe Z, et al. Management of bipolar disorder during pregnancy and the postpartum period. Am J Psychiatry. 2004;161(4):608–20.

63. Cunnington M, Tennis P, the International Lamotrigine Pregnancy Registry Scientific Advisory C. Lamotrigine and the risk of malformations in pregnancy. Neurology. 2005;64(6):955–60.

64. Newport DJ, Viguera AC, Beach AJ, et al. Lithium placental passage and obstetrical outcome: implications for clinical management during late pregnancy. Am J Psychiatry. 2005;162(11):2162–70.

65. Flynn HA, Blow FC, Marcus SM. Rates and predictors of depression treatment among pregnant women in hospital-affiliated obstetrics practices. Gen Hosp Psychiatry. 2006;28(4):289–95.

66. Smith MV, Rosenheck RA, Cavaleri MA, et al. Screening for and detection of depression, panic disorder and PTSD in public sector obstetric clinics. Psychiatr Serv. 2004;55:407–14.

67. Kopelman RC, Moel J, Mertens C, et al. Barriers to care for antenatal depression. Psychiatr Serv. 2008;59(4):429–32.

68. Marcus SM, Flynn HA, Blow F, Barry K. A screening study of antidepressant treatment rates and mood symptoms in pregnancy. Arch Womens Ment Health. 2005;8(1):25–7.

69. Cohen LS, Altshuler LL, Harlow BL, et al. Relapse of major depression during pregnancy in women who maintain or discontinue antidepressant treatment. JAMA. 2006;295(5):499–507.

70. Wisner K, Zarin D, Holmboe E, et al. Risk-benefit decision making for treatment of depression during pregnancy. Am J Psychiatry. 2000;157:1933–40.

71. Sit DKY, Wisner KL. Decision making for postpartum depression treatment. Psychiatr Ann. 2005;35(7):577–85.

209

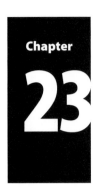

Psychiatric aspects of organ transplantation

Michael Marcangelo and Catherine Crone

Typical consult question

"Evaluate the patient for possible organ transplantation."

Background

Transplantation has become a standard procedure for end-stage organ disease. In 2008, 27,961 organ transplants were performed in the United States, with 6217 of those transplants coming from living donors (1). Organ transplantation has been demonstrated to extend survival and improve quality of life for the majority of recipients. Under ideal circumstances, a psychosocial evaluation would consist of a multi-disciplinary, multi-visit assessment that would provide the transplant team with an accurate picture of the patient's psychiatric and social history. More often, psychosocial evaluations involve single visits, particularly when patients present acutely ill and in need of transplantation. Depending on the severity of their condition, they may have a difficult time answering questions or providing adequate history (e.g., intubation, encephalopathy, pain); therefore ancillary sources of information (i.e., family members, healthcare providers) must be included. Although the request to see the patient may be related primarily to concerns about a specific psychiatric disorder, the consultant should attempt to evaluate all relevant aspects of the case. Ultimately, the goals of the psychosocial evaluation are to identify potential problems or risk factors that may interfere with successful post-transplant outcomes, and then to help the team actively address these issues.

Patients who face transplantation often are quite disabled as a result of their underlying illness. Depending on the availability of an organ, patients may wait for transplantation over extended periods of time, requiring repeated hospital stays for re-stabilization or prolonged hospital stays as their health deteriorates. At times, patients may be quite ill, yet not ill enough to qualify for advancement on the transplant waiting list. While waiting for an organ, patients may have to stop working, may alter their important relationships, and ultimately may lose their sense of identity as breadwinner or caregiver because of their illness. These stressors combined with declining health place them at increased risk for psychiatric disorders. One advantage of patients' severe and possibly protracted illness is that it provides a window into their health-related behavior, their attendance at physician appointments, their ability to take medications as prescribed, and their psychological responses to illness.

Psychosomatic Medicine: An Introduction to Consultation-Liaison Psychiatry, eds. James J. Amos and Robert G. Robinson. Published by Cambridge University Press. © Cambridge University Press 2010.

These factors all are likely to influence their behavior after transplant and thus their overall survival.

Work-up

a. Pre-transplant period

Evaluation of patients for organ transplantation requires examination of both medical and psychosocial factors. Medical considerations include the patient's physiologic need for transplant, as well as co-morbid medical conditions (e.g., renal impairment, diabetes mellitus) that may complicate recovery and successful outcomes. Psychosocial factors include the patient's psychological preparedness for transplantation, informed consent, and social support. Psychosocial evaluations are performed on all candidates for transplantation, although social workers provide the majority. Depending on the transplant team and the individual patient circumstances, psychiatrists often are asked to provide psychosocial evaluations as well. Although patients sometimes can be seen as scheduled outpatients, severity of illness may require inpatient consultation.

Psychosocial evaluation of transplant candidates should be as comprehensive as time and circumstances allow. A complete psychiatric diagnostic assessment is the cornerstone of this evaluation, with a special focus on issues that may adversely impact transplant outcome. One of these issues is substance abuse, as this may have contributed to the condition necessitating transplant (e.g., alcoholic cirrhosis, cocaine-induced cardiomyopathy, tobacco-related emphysema). Continued use of these substances or relapse post transplantation can increase the risk of graft loss and death (2). Current and past psychiatric history, severity of psychiatric illness, receptiveness to treatment, response to treatment, and self-destructive behaviors all should be assessed. Social support is particularly important for successful outcomes as patients require considerable assistance when they are first discharged to home (3). The availability of persons to provide day-to-day care, organize medications, assist with ambulation and rehabilitation, and provide transportation to clinic visits needs to be established. Evaluation of candidates should include questions aimed at assessing their understanding of the risks and benefits of transplantation, their expectations of transplant, and their acceptance of the long-term commitment to their health. Questions regarding adherence to their medical care, including medications, attendance at scheduled appointments or treatments (e.g., dialysis), use of supplemental oxygen, completion of pulmonary rehabilitation, dietary changes, and abstinence from harmful substances should be included. Last, a bedside cognitive exam, such as the Mini-Mental Status Examination, should be administered to assess patients' current level of cognitive functioning.

In addition to assessing the patient directly, evaluation should include a review of medical and psychiatric records when possible. Records can provide information that supports or refutes the patient's claims and that may be helpful in determining whether the patient is being honest. Because patients may be anxious or desperate for transplant, distortion or minimization of information may occur during the interview. If a patient is suffering significant cognitive impairment, examination of records along with discussion with family members and other healthcare providers may provide a more accurate history.

When transplant teams ask for a psychosocial evaluation, they often want a definitive answer about the patient's ability to accept a transplant and provide stewardship for the organ. Giving a definitive Yes-No answer about such a major decision – if the patient does not receive the transplant, he or she is almost certain to die in the near future – is impossible to do with perfect accuracy. Instead, the team should be informed about the risk factors the patient presents with – psychiatric, social, adherence – and should be given the chance to make a decision based on input from all team members. The psychiatric input should help the team prepare to meet the needs of each individual patient as well as provide them with guidance about how to best work with the patient.

Generally, a few circumstances suggest absolute contraindications to transplant. These include active suicide ideation, active psychosis, recent suicide attempts, and chronic self-destructive behavior. Even though many centers will refrain from listing patients with these conditions, the decision to list varies from center to center and from patient to patient. Special mention must be made in cases involving fulminant hepatic failure from intentional acetaminophen overdose. Patients are often young and lack a history of prior suicide attempts. For these patients, their willingness to receive ongoing psychiatric care, their ability to understand the need for transplant, and the presence of adequate family support can make them acceptable candidates. They must be assessed urgently as hepatic encephalopathy leading to coma may occur within 48 to 72 hours after the overdose. If patients are unable to be interviewed directly for transplantation, assessment must involve discussion with family members, significant others, close friends, and healthcare providers. Active substance use is another contraindication, particularly if patients were previously informed of their end-organ disease but did not pursue abstinence (4). Added concerns are raised when patients have repeatedly failed attempts to achieve abstinence or sobriety. Last, patients who consistently demonstrate an inability to collaborate with the transplant team or other healthcare providers and adhere to their medical regimen should not be considered for transplantation. An example of this is the hemodialysis patient who repeatedly misses scheduled dialysis, skips medications, and does not adhere to diet and fluid restrictions. If social factors such as lack of financial resources or transportation have been ruled out as factors compromising the patient's ability to cooperate with care, this behavior should be considered evidence of non-adherence.

Psychosocial rating scales are also used. The Psychosocial Assessment of Candidates for Transplantation (PACT) is an example. It was developed in the 1980s, and the results of a study on its reliability were published in 1989 (5). The scale was never really intended to be used as a tool for candidate selection. Its original purposes included studying the pre-transplant psychosocial evaluation process itself and learning how different programs weight various factors in patient selection.

The Transplant Evaluation Rating Scale (TERS) is another psychosocial rating scale that was developed as a research instrument, although it was used as a selection tool. The TERS showed good interrater reliability but was thought to be more cumbersome to use than the PACT (6, 7).

The newest rating scale is the Stanford Integrated Psychosocial Assessment for Transplantation (SIPAT). It was developed by Jose Maldonado, MD, FAPM, and colleagues at Stanford. The group determined minimal listing criteria, and the scale is obviously intended to be used as a selection tool. This 18-item scale is being validated against the PACT, and an interrater reliability study is under way (8).

Clinical decision-making and treatment

a. Pre-transplant period

The most common psychiatric disorders encountered in the pre-transplant population are depression, anxiety, adjustment disorders, and substance use disorders. Once detected, these disorders can be treated with psychotherapy and medications. Rates of depression prior to transplant for heart, lung, and liver patients average about 20%, and anxiety disorders are present in as many as 33% of patients (9). Care must be taken to use medications with a minimum of drug-drug interactions when treating these patients. Among the selective serotonin reuptake inhibitors (SSRIs), citalopram and sertraline have the fewest drug-drug interactions and are likely the safest to use. Dosing of medications also should take into account the presence of altered pharmacokinetics due to end-stage organ disease. In general, this will require starting patients at smaller dosages and titrating medications on a more gradual basis until clinical response is achieved.

If the patient is medically stable and has an active substance use disorder, he or she should be referred for treatment before receiving a transplant. Many centers require patients to demonstrate a six-month period of abstinence before they are placed on the waiting list; however, studies have not consistently demonstrated the predictive value of this length of abstinence. Rather than emphasize abstinence, recommendations should focus on having patients develop an understanding of their addiction, their triggers, and their coping styles. Referral to 12-step programs and formal rehabilitation programs can help patients to develop greater insight into their substance abuse and to begin to develop healthier coping techniques.

Behavioral contracts can prove useful by clearly outlining expectations for patients and the consequences, should they fail to adhere to treatment recommendations. The psychiatrist can play an important role in helping the team adhere to these contracts if the patient breaks the terms that have been set forth. One of the advantages of treatments that bridge the patient to transplant, such as hemodialysis or ventricular assist devices, is that they provide the team with time to address the patient's compliance problems and social issues. Treatment of any underlying psychiatric illness can help. Repeated visits with members of the team can provide patients with a level of support that they didn't previously experience. If a patient continues to demonstrate adherence difficulties during the bridge to transplant period, this suggests that they are poor candidates.

Delirium is a common complicating factor in end-stage organ failure and may mimic other psychiatric disorders such as depression. Correct detection and diagnosis are necessary, as addition of psychotropic agents such as anxiolytics and antidepressants can worsen behavior and cognitive function. Hepatic encephalopathy often presents with obvious impairment of consciousness, but deficits can be subtle and may be detected only by bedside cognitive testing (e.g., trailmaking, digit symbol, line tracing). If patients are delirious, careful review of medications with the goal of minimizing psychoactive medications that may be exacerbating the problem is essential. Anticholinergic medications, hypnotics, and pain medications all can contribute to delirium and should be minimized when possible. Correction of electrolyte disturbances, acid-base balance, anemia/blood loss, underlying infection, and oxygenation levels is needed. For hepatic encephalopathy, medications that reduce ammonia, such as lactulose and rifaximin, can produce significant improvement. If the patient's delirium is impacting his or her safety, low doses of scheduled antipsychotics can be used.

b. Perioperative period

Patients who have just received transplants often develop post-operative delirium. Typical causes, such as hypoxia, metabolic disturbance, and polypharmacy, are the most common, but transplant-specific causes must be considered as well. Immunosuppressive medications, necessary after transplant to prevent rejection, cause neuropsychiatric side effects including delirium. These can occur even at therapeutic drug levels. Cyclosporine, tacrolimus, and prednisone all can cause increased levels of anxiety or decreased levels of consciousness. If patients have elevated levels of cyclosporine or tacrolimus, lower doses can lead to resolution of symptoms, but for some patients complete discontinuation of the medication is necessary. Tacrolimus, a first-line agent for many transplant programs, can cause posterior reversible encephalopathy syndrome, a severe delirium that can feature visual hallucinations, seizures, and MRI changes suggestive of damage to the occipital and parietal lobes. This syndrome reverses once the medication is withdrawn and is of particular interest in the liver transplant population, where higher rates of neurological complications following transplant are reported (10). In these patients, posterior hyperintensities on T2-weighted MRI images supports the diagnosis and reverses with withdrawal of the medication.

c. Post-transplant period

In patients who have already been transplanted, depression and anxiety disorders remain the most common diagnoses. Evidence suggests that patients develop these disorders during the first post-transplant year at rates that exceed those seen before transplant, so patients need continued monitoring (11). Medications that had to be specially dosed before transplant to account for organ dysfunction now may have to be dosed at higher levels because patients have functioning organs again. If patients have returned to substance use after transplant, they should be referred for intensive treatment and followed closely. Although slip-ups do not predict graft loss, a return to heavy alcohol or drug use is associated with adverse outcomes including graft loss and death (12).

A number of patients will suffer setbacks or complications after transplant and fail to make a full recovery; a smaller number will die soon after transplant. Early bad outcomes are difficult for transplant teams because of the effort and hope that typically are invested in a transplant patient. As a member of the team, the psychiatrist can facilitate discussion, help the team move forward, and continue to work effectively with new candidates. Assisting patients with the realities of life after transplant, particularly those patients who make less than a full recovery, is just as important as providing support before transplant. Psychotherapy can assist patients with this adjustment and help complete the process that began with candidate selection.

References

1. United Network of Organ Sharing (UNOS) Web site. Available from: http://www. OPTN.org. Accessed May 28, 2009.

2. Gedaly R, McHugh PP, Johnston TD, et al. Predictors of relapse to alcohol and illicit drugs after liver transplantation for alcoholic liver disease. Transplantation. 2008;86:1090–5.

3. Dobbels F, Vanhaecke J, Dupont L, et al. Pretransplant predictors of posttransplant adherence and clinical outcome: an evidence base for pretransplant psychosocial screening. Transplantation. 2009;87: 1497–504.

4. Webb K, Shepherd L, Neuberger J. Illicit drug use and liver transplantation: is there

a problem and what is the solution?
Transpl Int. 2008;21(10):923–9.

5. Olbrisch ME, Levenson JL, Hamer R. The
    PACT: a rating scale for the study of
    clinical decision-making in psychosocial
    screening of organ transplant candidates.
    Clin Transpl. 1989;3:164–9.

6. Presberg BA, Levenson JL, Olbrisch ME,
    Best AM. Rating scales for the psychosocial
    evaluation of organ transplant candidates:
    comparison of the PACT and TERS with
    bone marrow transplant patients.
    Psychosomatics. 1995;36(5):458–61.

7. Twillman RK, Manetto C, Wellisch DK,
    Wolcott DL. The Transplant Evaluation
    Rating Scale: a revision of the psychosocial
    levels system for evaluating organ
    transplant candidates. Psychosomatics.
    1993;34(2):144–53.

8. Maldonado J, Plante, R, David E. The
    Stanford Integrated Psychosocial
    Assessment for Transplantation (SIPAT).

    Academy of Psychosomatic Medicine:
    integrating clinical neuroscience in
    psychosomatic medicine across the
    lifespan. Presented in Miami, FL;
    November 2008; p. 45.

9. Spaderna H, Smits JMA, Rahmal AO,
    Weidner G. Psychosocial and behavioural
    factors in heart transplant candidates – an
    overview. Transpl Int. 2007;20(11):909–20.

10. Marco S, Celcilia F, Patrizia B. Neurologic
    complications after solid organ transplanta-
    tion. Transpl Int. 2009;22(3):269–78.

11. Dew MA, DiMartini AF. Psychological
    disorders and distress after adult
    cardiothoracic transplantation.
    J Cardiovasc Nurs. 2005;20(5 Suppl):
    S51–S66.

12. Pfitzmann R, Schwenzer J, Rayes N, et al.
    Long-term survival and predictors of
    relapse after orthotopic liver transplan-
    tation for alcoholic liver disease. Liver
    Transpl. 2007;13:197–205.

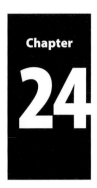

Chapter 24

Preoperative psychiatric evaluation for bariatric surgery

Kathy Coffman

Typical consult question

"The patient, a thirty-nine year old female with history of binge eating, depression, and sexual abuse in childhood, was referred for evaluation for gastric bypass and Roux-en-Y. The questions posed were whether this patient would be able to adhere to the post-operative exercise and nutritional regimen."

Background

Obesity is a disease with a multi-factorial origin including behavioral, environmental, genetic, metabolic, neuroendocrine, and psychological factors, as described by Fobi in a masterful review on surgical treatments of obesity. Mortality related to obesity has risen to more than 300,000 deaths per year, second to smoking as a preventable cause of death in the United States.

Medical co-morbidity of morbid obesity includes the following:

- Coronary artery disease
- Cancer of the breast, uterus, and prostate
- Diabetes
- NASH (non-alcoholic steatotic hepatitis) cirrhosis
- Dyslipemia
- Gastroesophageal reflux disease
- Hypertension
- Low back pain
- Osteoarthritis of the hips, knees, and ankles
- Sleep apnea

Other consequences may include the following:

- Depression
- Eating disorders
- Job discrimination
- Discrimination in dating
- Problems with transportation
- High health insurance premiums (1)

Psychosomatic Medicine: An Introduction to Consultation-Liaison Psychiatry, eds. James J. Amos and Robert G. Robinson. Published by Cambridge University Press. © Cambridge University Press 2010.

Bariatric surgery has become mainstream over the past 10 years, with more than 177,000 bariatric surgeries done in the United States in 2006 alone (2). The practice of psychiatric evaluation for bariatric candidates originated from a consensus development conference in 1991 sponsored by the National Institutes of Health (NIH) (3). At the time, there were no psychiatric contraindications for surgery.

The goals of evaluation then were to

- Select motivated patients
- Discuss options other than surgery
- Discuss the risks and benefits of surgery, and success rates of available bariatric procedures
- Provide education about vitamin and mineral deficiencies if patients did not adhere to the post-operative regimen

Inclusion of mental health professionals in bariatric evaluations was due to the high prevalence of psychiatric and behavioral complications in the morbidly obese. Anxiety disorders, such as social phobia (18%) and obsessive-compulsive disorder (OCD) (13.6%), are common in bariatric candidates and may require treatment (4). Up to half of bariatric candidates may have major depression (5). Major depression in patients with a body mass index (BMI) >40 kg/m^2 was five times more likely within the past year than in normal weight individuals (6). Personality disorders may exist in as many as 72% of candidates (7). Because psychiatric problems tend to normalize after bariatric surgery, some have concluded that these problems did not cause obesity, but were the result of morbid obesity (8).

Most patients who are seeking bariatric surgery have been dieting since adolescence – an average of 4.7 attempts – without stopping the progressive weight gain (9). Bariatric candidates reported significantly more emotional eating and greater impact of weight on quality of life than did patients who elected a residential cognitive-behavioral weight control program (10). Most morbidly obese patients (73.4%) stated that medical co-morbidity was the reason for weight loss surgery, followed by psychological reasons and quality of life (11). Body self-esteem improves after bariatric surgery, as measured with the Body-Esteem Scale for Adolescents and Adults (BESAA) (12).

Rea et al. showed that Short-Form Survey Instrument (SF-36) scores at one year post Roux-en-Y gastric bypass (RNYGBP) were better than those at baseline and in normal weight controls, regardless of complications (13). Tsuda et al. noted that around 30% of patients referred for bariatric surgery were rejected for surgery, most commonly because of lack of insurance (47.8%). Other reasons cited included BMI below the criterion of 35 kg/m^2 with co-morbid conditions, or BMI <40, or being medically, psychologically, or socially unsuitable (14). Walfish et al. noted that 15% of candidates were delayed or were turned down for psychiatric causes, most commonly because of psychotic disorders (51%), inadequately treated depression (39%), or lack of understanding of the surgical risks and postoperative regimen (30%) (15).

Silecchia et al. reported that 13% of 498 consecutive gastric banding patients required major reoperation. Ten patients underwent band removal and 10 had revision surgery (16). Causes for reoperation included the following:

- Erosion (20%)
- Psychological issues (15%)

- Inadequate weight loss (20%)
- Dilatation of the pouch (37%)

Younger patients, women, and divorced patients were more likely to want plastic surgery after bariatric surgery, but more than half needed a payment plan (17). Predictors of better outcomes with bariatric surgery include adherence to the routine and attendance at follow-up visits. Narcissistic personality showed a negative correlation with weight loss up to 36 months after surgery (18). Kalarchian et al. found that a lifetime Axis I mood or anxiety disorder correlated with less weight loss at 6 months post surgery ($p < .001$), but those with a past history of substance abuse lost more weight (19).

Four major systematic reviews concluded that pre-operative occurrence of binge eating, depression, or vomiting did not predict sub-optimal weight loss (7, 20–22). Sallet showed that 90% of those with binge eating disorders (BEDs) or sub-clinical binge eating disorders had satisfactory weight loss after bariatric surgery (23).

The frequency of eating disorders, including BED, night eating syndrome (NES), and uncontrolled eating, was significantly reduced after surgery ($p = .05$). Grazing increased post-operatively from 26.3% to 38%, as did BED changed habits. Both grazing and uncontrolled eating affected weight loss postoperatively (24). Although some programs have mandated pre-operative treatment for binge eating disorder, only one study has explored the efficacy of any intervention on BED. A brief, four-session cognitive-behavioral group intervention was shown to significantly reduce binge eating cognition and behavior. Efficacy did not vary with ethnicity or gender (25).

Outcomes in bariatric patients with history of sexual abuse are satisfactory. Only one study found that those with history of sexual abuse had differences in expected weight loss (EWL) of 57.7% versus 66.3% in controls at 12 and 24 months ($p < .05$) (26).

Two studies showed that gastric banding candidates with childhood sexual abuse, non-sexual abuse, or neglect showed no difference in outcomes versus those with no childhood mistreatment (27, 28). Despite severe sexual abuse resulting in multiple personality disorder, a Hispanic female lost 45 kg after gastroplasty, although psychological issues created difficulties (29). No significant difference in success with RNYGBP was noted between African American, Caucasian, and Hispanic patients (30, 31).

Bariatric candidates from the adolescent and geriatric age groups are being evaluated, with a few considerations to keep in mind. Up to 25% of children have a BMI higher than the 85th percentile for age and sex. Two studies included adequate numbers of teens. Outcomes in 50 teens undergoing laparoscopic banding showed a mean EWL of 61.4%, with mean BMI decreasing from 45.2 to 32.6 at mean follow-up of 34 months. All pre-operative co-morbidities were resolved. Only one minor complication was reported (32). To be eligible for surgery, teens must attain Tanner Stage IV sexual maturity and 95% of axial growth (33). A retrospective review on 40 adolescents seen for laparoscopic adjustable gastric banding (LAGB) rated quality of life of obese adolescents as similar to children with cancer. With a Beck Depression Inventory (BDI) cutoff of 16, 32% of the teens met the criteria for depression, and 25% had harmed themselves (cutting, burning, scratching) – almost double the rate in a normal teenage control sample. These teens may require support and careful follow-up if bariatric surgery is elected (34).

Bariatric surgery in geriatric adults refers to those 60 years of age and older. Evaluation of cognitive functioning is key, as the obese have double the likelihood of dementia as those of normal weight. Cognitive functioning affects capacity for informed consent, adherence with post-operative nutrition guidelines to avoid vitamin and mineral deficiencies, and learning of new behaviors. Screening using the Mini-Mental State Examination was recommended, with referral for neuropsychological evaluation if scores were more than one standard deviation from the mean for age and educational level (35).

Gender differences in bariatric surgery are being investigated. Males present with significantly higher BMIs, but females show more anxiety, depression, and social anxiety and have tried more diets (2). Predictors of long-term post-operative weight loss included lower baseline BMI, higher educational level, and male sex. Only one personality variable, egoism, was associated with lower long-term weight loss (36). Women of reproductive age (18 to 45 years old) make up 49% of all patients having bariatric surgery (37). Female bariatric candidates report more sexual dysfunction than controls matched for age, education, and marital status (38).

Health risks for obese parturients include the following:

- Hypertension
- Pre-eclampsia
- Gestational diabetes
- More frequent pre-term labor
- Higher perioperative morbidity
- Higher risks of cesarean section (39)

All these risks were lower after LABG, including half the cesarean section rate of obese controls – 15.3% versus 34.4% (p < .01) (40). Patel et al. recommend waiting two years after bariatric surgery before pregnancy to avoid nutritional complications. Improvement in fertility may be noted after bariatric surgery (41).

Few long-term studies of maintenance of weight loss after bariatric surgery have been conducted. Only one study compared sustained weight loss over one year with surgical versus non-surgical methods. Both groups gained small, statistically significant amounts, but no difference was noted in the amount of weight re-gained.

Surgical subjects were less active, consumed more fatty food, and had higher depression scores (42). Another study of patients with RNYGBP showed that all improved on binge eating, emotional status, and physical health, regardless of the amount of weight loss or preoperative psychological distress. Although professional and non-romantic relationships improved, romantic relationships were unaffected (43). Two large meta-analytic comparisons listed excess weight loss with gastric banding ranging from 40.7% to 56.4%, and with gastric bypass ranging from 61.5% to 74.8%. Mortality at 30 days was 0.1% for gastric banding and 0.5% for gastric bypass (44, 45). However, early mortality for Medicare beneficiaries at 30 days was 1.5% for women and 3.7% for men, and it was fivefold higher for those over 75 years than for those aged 65 to 74 years (46).

Work-up

Generally, bariatric patients are referred for evaluation for clearance for insurance requirements. Patients may need re-assurance that the purposes of the evaluation are to help them understand the options for weight loss and to identify areas that may need to be addressed to maximize the chances for success in losing weight.

Several strategies have been proposed to develop a standardized bariatric psychiatric evaluation, including the Boston Interview for Gastric Bypass (47, 48) and another proposal by Wadden and Sarwer (49). A useful outline for guidance that combines the best of both approaches is as follows:

A. Chief complaint – reason for referral can clarify the purpose of the interview
B. History of present illness

   1. Bariatric surgery

      a. First consideration of surgical weight loss
      b. Motivation for surgery now
   2. Knowledge of success rates, and risks of lap band versus lap RYGBP (surgeon's note)
   3. Adherence to pre-operative bariatric program (nutritionist's note)
   4. Understanding of post-operative program (nutritionist's note)

      a. Liquid diet four weeks post-operatively, then small portions
      b. Eating slowly to avoid vomiting
      c. Avoiding fatty food, high-calorie liquids, and concentrated sweets to avoid dumping syndrome
      d. Support group for peer interaction
      e. Vitamin and mineral supplementation
      f. Follow-up visits with surgeon and nutritionist
   5. Age of onset of obesity and impact on quality of life
   6. History of diets and maximum weight loss with each (nutrition's note)
   7. Eating patterns – highest and lowest weights since teens, current BMI

      a. Eating disorders – anorexia, binging, bulimia, grazing, night eating
      b. History of diet pills, diuretics, herbal or OTC remedies, laxatives
   8. Stressors – i.e., life events, employment, financial, foreclosure, marital – help determine optimal timing for bariatric surgery.
   9. Support system – family, friends, caregiver, insurance, and transportation
  10. Coping skills employed during difficult times in life
  11. Goals of weight loss and expectations – generally most want to be more active and healthy

      a. Time course of expected weight loss, and odds of regain
      b. Body image – weight or dress/suit size that would mean success
        i. Extreme concern over appearance raises red flags.
      c. Physical abilities
        i. No driving, lifting >10 lb post-operatively
        ii. Daily exercise regimen after bariatric surgery
      d. Effects of weight loss on professional and romantic relationships
        i. Men may expect to be more successful with romance, but if social phobia is present may need psychotherapy
        ii. Women may have to contend with more attention; no longer viewed as asexual because of being overweight
  12. Role models for bariatric surgery – family, friends, support group members

C. Past medical history

1. Medical co-morbidity – back pain, diabetes, dyslipidemia, hypertension, joint problems, sleep apnea
2. Past problems with surgery

D. Past psychiatric history – psychiatric admission, harm to self or others

1. Screening for disorders that may need treatment

E. Medications
F. Social history – employment history, alcohol and substance abuse history
G. Family psychiatric history – depression, eating disorders, psychosis, substance abuse
H. Family medical history – relatives with obesity and co-morbid conditions
I. Laboratory – thyroid functions, cholesterol and lipid profile, EKG
J. Mental status examination including Mini-Mental Status Examination

1. May include screening 15 minutes before appointment

   a. Beck Depression Inventory
   b. SF-36 or the World Health Organization (WHO) Quality of Life Instrument (WHOQOL-BREF)

Screening may have utility other than excluding candidates, such as

- Decreasing the low risk of suicide after bariatric surgery
- Identifying high-risk eating disorders such as bulimia for treatment
- Identifying psychiatric disorders requiring treatment for better long-term success
- Providing referrals for smoking or substance abuse rehabilitation before surgery

Medical criteria for bariatric surgery include the following:

- BMI >40 kg/m², or >35 kg/m² with medical co-morbidity
- Acceptable operative risk
- Failed multiple weight loss programs

Contraindications to bariatric surgery include the following:

- Active psychosis
- Active bulimia nervosa
- Severe personality disorders
- Active substance abuse or dependence
- Mental retardation without adequate social support
- Suicide attempts or psychiatric admissions within the past year

Psychometric evaluation of bariatric surgery candidates

Many of the instruments used in evaluation of bariatric surgery candidates, such as the Eating Disorder Examination Questionnaire (EDE-Q) (50) and the Millon Behavioral Medicine Diagnostic (MBMD), do not have proven utility or psychometric validity (51). The Minnesota Multi-Phasic Personality Inventory, 2nd edition (MMPI-2), has been investigated and Kinder et al. found that many bariatric candidates have elevated MMPI profiles, considered to be "invalid" profiles probably because of image management (52).

Items that reflect physical symptoms may confound the Beck Depression Inventory because of consequences of obesity, such as chronic pain, sleep problems, and sexual dysfunction. Total BDI score and the cognitive-affect subscale do discriminate between those with and without depression. The optimal cut point was set at 12 for the BDI, and 7 for the cognitive-affective subscale. Those with chronic pain had higher mean total BDI scores (12.5 vs. 9.0, p < .01) (53).

The Night Eating Questionnaire (NEQ) has convergent validity with other measures of disordered eating, night eating, mood, sleep, and stress. This instrument was found to have good discriminant validity in diagnosing NES (54). Health-related quality of life in bariatric patients has been measured using the WHOQOL-BREF. Obese subjects had lower scores for physical, psychological, and social domains, but not for environmental domain, particularly those with BMI greater than 32 kg/m². Bariatric candidates had BMI of 32 to 40 kg/m² with medical co-morbidity or BMI >40 kg/m² (55).

Pre-operative and post-operative adherence

One study showed that only 56% of patients given behavioral treatment recommendations before surgery were adherent, and 44% were not. Adherence was not related to age, anxiety, BMI, depression, eating disorders, education, marital status, or race. However, 69% of men were non-adherent versus 38% of women (56). Bariatric surgery can result in the following:

- Dehydration
- Lactose intolerance
- Protein-calorie malnutrition
- Altered absorption of bile salts and electrolytes
- Altered absorption of calcium, iron, and other vitamins and minerals causing osteopenia and osteoporosis

Roughly one-third to two-thirds of bariatric patients are non-adherent to nutritional regimens after surgery. This non-compliance is attributed to pre-existing psychological co-morbidity of bariatric patients, including one-third who have a history of substance abuse disorders (57). One study on 100 consecutive RNYGBP patients showed that one year post bariatric surgery, more than 50% did not adhere in some area, particularly with exercise (41%) and snacking (37%). Concerns expressed included depression (12%), medical complications related to surgery (9%), sexual concerns (4%), and relationship problems (2%) (58).

References

1. Fobi MAI. Surgical treatment of obesity: a review. J Natl Med Assoc. 2004;96:61–75.

2. Mahony D. Psychological gender differences in bariatric surgery candidates. Obes Surg. 2008;18:607–10.

3. NIH Conference. Gastrointestinal surgery for severe obesity. Consensus Development Conference Panel. Ann Intern Med. 1991; 115:956–61.

4. Rosik CH. Psychiatric symptoms among prospective bariatric surgery patients: rates of prevalence and their relation to social desirability, pursuit of surgery and follow-up attendance. Obes Surg. 2005;15:677–83.

5. Hsu LKG, Benotti PN, Dwyer J, et al. Nonsurgical factors that influence the outcome of bariatric surgery: a review. Psychosom Med. 1998;60:338–46.

6. Wadden TA, Sarwer DB. Behavioral assessment of candidates for bariatric surgery: a patient-oriented approach. Surg Obes Relat Dis. 2006;2:171–9.

7. Sawrer DB, Wadden TA, Fabricatore AN. Psychosocial and behavioral aspects of bariatric surgery. Obes Res. 2005;12: 639–48.

8. Vallis TM, Butler GS, Perey B, et al. The role of psychological functioning in morbid obesity and its treatment with gastroplasty. Obes Surg. 2001;11:716–25.

9. Gibbons LM, Sarwer DB, Crerand CE, et al. Previous weight loss experiences of bariatric surgery candidates: how much have patients dieted prior to surgery? Obesity (Silver Spring). 2006;14(Suppl 2): 70S–76S.

10. Stout AL, Applegate KL, Friedman KE, et al. Psychological correlates of obese patients seeking surgical or residential behavioral weight loss treatment. Surg Obes Relat Dis. 2007;3:369–75.

11. Munoz DJ, Lal M, Chen EY, et al. Why patients seek bariatric surgery: a qualitative and quantitative analysis of patient motivation. Obes Surg. 2007;17: 1487–91.

12. Madan AK, Beech BM, Tichansky DX. Body esteem improves after bariatric surgery. Surg Innov. 2008;15:32–7. Epub 2008 Apr 2.

13. Rea JD, Yarbrough DE, Leeth RR, et al. Influence of complications and extent of weight loss on quality of life after laparoscopic Roux-en-Y gastric bypass. Surg Endosc. 2007;21:1095–1100. Epub 2007 Mar 13.

14. Tsuda S, Barrios L, Schneider B, et al. Factors affecting rejection of bariatric patients from an academic weight loss program. Surg Obes Relat Dis. 2009;5:199–202. Epub 2008 Oct 1.

15. Walfish S, Vance D, Fabricatore AN. Psychological evaluation of bariatric surgery applicants: procedures and reasons for delay or denial of surgery. Obes Surg. 2007;17:1578–83. Epub 2007 Nov 14.

16. Silecchia G, Bacci V, Bacci S, et al. Reoperation after laparoscopic adjustable gastric banding: analysis of a cohort of 500 patients with long-term follow-up. Surg Obes Relat Dis. 2008;4:430–6. Epub 2008.

17. Gusenoff JA, Messing S, O'Malley W, et al. Temporal and demographic factors influencing the desire for plastic surgery after gastric bypass surgery. J Am Soc Plast Recon Surg. 2007;121:2120–6.

18. Pontiroli AE, Fossati A, Vedani P, et al. Post-surgery adherence to scheduled visits and compliance, more than personality disorder, predict outcome of bariatric restrictive surgery in morbidly obese patients. Obes Surg. 2007;17:1492–7.

19. Kalarchian MA, Marcus MD, Levine MD, et al. Relationship of psychiatric disorders to 6-month outcomes after gastric bypass. Surg Obes Relat Dis. 2008;4:544–9. Epub 2008.

20. Herpertz S, Kielmann R, Wolf AM, et al. Do psychosocial variables predict weight loss or mental health after obesity surgery? A systematic review. Obes Res. 2004;12: 1554–69.

21. van Hout GCM, Verschure SKM, van Heck GL. Psychosocial predictors of success following bariatric surgery. Obes Surg. 2005;15:552–60.

22. Wadden TA, Sarwer DB, Fabricatore AN, et al. Psychosocial and behavioral status of patients undergoing bariatric surgery: what to expect before and after surgery. Med Clin North Am. 2007;91:451–69.

23. Sallet PC, Sallet JA, Dixon JB, et al. Eating behavior as a prognostic factor for weight loss after gastric bypass. Obes Surg. 2007; 17:445–51.

24. Colles SL, Dixon JB, O'Brien PE. Grazing and loss of control related to eating: two high-risk factors following bariatric surgery. Obesity (Silver Spring). 2008; 16:615–22. Epub 2008.

25. Ashton K, Drerup M, Windover A, et al. Brief, four-session group CBT reduces binge eating behaviors among bariatric surgery candidates. Surg Obes Relat Dis. 2009;5:257–62. Epub 2009 Jan 18.

26. Fujioka K, Yan E, Wang HJ, et al. Evaluating preoperative weight loss, binge eating disorder, and sexual abuse history on Roux-en-Y gastric bypass outcome. Surg Obes Relat Dis. 2008;4: 137–43.

27. Larsen JK, Geenan R. Childhood sexual abuse is not associated with a poor outcome after gastric banding for severe obesity. Obes Surg. 2005;15:534–47.

28. Grilo CM, White MA, Masheb RM, et al. Relation of childhood sexual abuse and other forms of maltreatment to 12-month postoperative outcomes in extremely obese gastric bypass patients. Obes Surg. 2006; 16:454–60.

29. Bloomston M, Zervos EE, Powers PS, et al. Bariatric surgery and multiple personality disorder: complexities and nuances of care. Obes Surg. 1997;7:363–6.

30. Madan AK, Whitfield JD, Fain JN, et al. Are African-Americans as successful as Caucasians after laparoscopic gastric bypass? Obes Surg. 2007;17:460–4.

31. Guajardo-Salinas GE, Hilmy A, Martinez-Ugarte ML. Predictors of weight loss and effectiveness of Roux-en-Y gastric bypass in the morbidly obese Hispano-American population. Obes Surg. 2008;18:1369–75. Epub 2008 Mar 7.

32. Silberhumer GR, Miller K, Kriwanek S, et al. Laparoscopic adjustable gastric banding in adolescents: the Austrian experience. Obes Surg. 2006;16:1062–7.

33. Dufour F, Champault G. Is bariatric surgery in adolescents appropriate? J Chir (Paris). 2009;146:24–9. Epub 2009 Apr 22.

34. Duffecy J, Bleil ME, Labott SM, et al. Psychopathology in adolescents presenting for laparoscopic banding. J Adol Health. 2008;43:623–5.

35. Henrickson HC, Ashton KR, Windover AK, et al. Psychological considerations for bariatric surgery. Obes Surg. 2009;19: 211–6.

36. Larsen JK, Geenen R, Maas C, et al. Personality as a predictor of weight loss maintenance after surgery for morbid obesity. Obes Res. 2004;12:1828–34.

37. Maggard MA, Yermilov I, Li Z, et al. Pregnancy and fertility following bariatric surgery: a systematic review. JAMA. 2008; 300:2286–96.

38. Assimakopoulos K, Panayiotopoulos S, Iconomou G, et al. Assessing sexual function in obese women preparing for bariatric surgery. Obes Surg. 2006;16: 1087–91.

39. Abodeely A, Roye GD, Harrington DT, et al. Pregnancy outcomes after bariatric surgery: maternal, fetal and infant implications. Surg Obes Relat Dis. 2008;4:464–71. Epub 2007 Nov 5.

40. Ducarme G, Revaux A, Rodrigues A, et al. Obstetric outcome following laparoscopic adjustable gastric banding. Int J Gynaecol Obstet. 2007;8:244–7. Epub 2007 Apr 16.

41. Patel JA, Colella JJ, Esaka E, et al. Improvement in infertility and pregnancy outcomes after weight loss surgery. Med Clin North Am. 2007;91:515–28, xiii.

42. Bond DS, Phelan S, Leahy TM, et al. Weight-loss maintenance in successful weight losers: surgical vs non-surgical methods. Int J Obes (London). 2009;33:173–80. Epub 2008 Dec 2.

43. Wolfe BL, Terry ML. Expectations and outcomes with gastric bypass surgery. Obes Surg. 2006;16:1622–9.

44. Buchwald H, Avigdor Y, Braunwald E, et al. Bariatric surgery: a systematic review and meta-analysis. JAMA. 2004; 292:1724–37.

45. Cunneen SA. Review of meta-analytic comparisons of bariatric surgery with a focus on laparoscopic adjustable banding. Surg Obes Relat Dis. 2008;4:S47–S55.

46. Flum DR, Salem L, Elrod JA, et al. Early mortality among Medicare beneficiaries undergoing bariatric surgical procedures. JAMA. 2005;294:1903–8.

47. Sogg S, Mori D. The Boston interview for gastric bypass: determining the psychological suitability of surgical candidates. Obes Surg. 2004;14:370–80.

48. Sogg S, Mori DL. Revising the Boston interview: incorporating new knowledge and experience. Surg Obes Relat Dis. 2008;4:455–63. Epub 2008 Apr 23.

49. Wadden TA, Sarwer DB. Behavioral assessment of candidates for bariatric surgery: a patient-oriented approach. Obesity (Silver Spring). 2006;14(Suppl 2): 53S–62S.

50. Hrabosky JI, White MA, Masheb RM, et al. Psychometric evaluation of the eating disorder examination-questionnaire for bariatric surgery candidates. Obesity (Silver Spring). 2008;16:763–9. Epub 2008.

51. Walfish S, Wise EA, Streiner DL. Limitations of the Millon Behavioral Medicine Diagnostic (MBMD) with bariatric surgical candidates. Obes Surg. 2008;18:1318–22. Epub 2008 May 10.

52. Kinder BN, Walfish S, Scott Young M, et al. MMPI-2 profiles of bariatric surgery patients: a replication and extension. Obes Surg. 2008;18:1170–9. Epub 2008 May 20.

53. Krukowski RA, Friedman KE, Applegate KL. The utility of the Beck Depression Inventory in a bariatric surgery population. Obes Surg. 2008 Oct 8. Epub ahead of print.

54. Allison KC, Lundgren JD, O'Reardon JP, et al. The Night Eating Questionnaire (NEQ): psychometric properties of a measure of severity of the night eating syndrome. Eat Behav. 2008;9:62–72. Epub 2007 Mar 28.

55. Chang CY, Hung CK, Chang YY, et al. Health-related quality of life in adult patients with morbid obesity coming for bariatric surgery. Obes Surg. 2009;19:820.

56. Friedman KE, Ashmore JA, Applegate KL. Recent experiences of weight-based stigmatization in a weight loss surgery population: psychological and behavioral correlates. Obesity (Silver Spring). 2008;16(Suppl 2):S69–S74.

57. Song A, Fernstrom MH. Nutritional and psychological considerations after bariatric surgery. Aesthet Surg J. 2008;28:195–9.

58. Elkins G, Whitfield P, Marcus J, et al. Noncompliance with behavioral recommendations following bariatric surgery. Obes Surg. 2005;15:546–51.

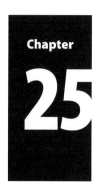

25

Psychiatric care at the end of life: hospice and palliative medicine

Michelle Weckmann

Typical consult question

"Please see this 82-year-old male with severe COPD and chronic pain who was admitted for a respiratory infection. He has a past history of anxiety treated with Paroxetine. After we brought up the idea of hospice, he's been sleeping more and does not want to participate in rehab, telling us that it hurts too much and it's too hard to breathe. We think that he might be depressed."

Background

Patients nearing death face tremendous psychological challenges. Dying patients experience various symptoms as death draws closer, making it difficult to distinguish between psychological distress and somatic distress, because the usual diagnostic clues are confounded by co-existing medical symptoms and sometimes by the dying process itself (1). The prevalence of certain mental illnesses (depression, anxiety, delirium) increases when a patient is diagnosed with a terminal illness. As many as 50% of these patients suffer from mental illness at the end of life, with the most common diagnoses being depression, anxiety and delirium. Other psychiatric disorders such as schizophrenia and bipolar disorder do not show an increased prevalence, but symptoms may worsen as a patient struggles with the knowledge that he has a terminal illness (2).

Although depression is common at the end of life, it is not a normative response to a terminal diagnosis. The prevalence of depression has been estimated to be as high as 75% in patients with advanced and life-threatening conditions (3). Depression at the end of life has been shown to decrease the quality of life, increase reports of pain and other symptoms (4), increase requests for hastened death, and increase the risk of suicide (1, 5). In advanced cancer, depression is associated with increased mortality (5).

Anxiety disorders are commonly seen at the end of life, and anxiety has a frequency of 14% to 28% in cancer patients, with the most common diagnoses being generalized anxiety disorder (6) and post-traumatic stress disorder (PTSD) (2). Anxiety is even higher in patients with chronic obstructive pulmonary disease (COPD), approaching 34% (7).

Substance abuse is becoming increasingly widespread among the general population; this is leading to an increase in the number of patients at the end of life who have used illicit substances, making it essential to screen for illicit drug use, because adverse drug interactions can be dangerous and active substance abuse can weaken already tenuous social supports associated with advanced disease and its treatment (8). Substance abuse can also interfere with a patient's compliance with treatment. Alcohol remains the most common substance

Psychosomatic Medicine: An Introduction to Consultation-Liaison Psychiatry, eds. James J. Amos and Robert G. Robinson. Published by Cambridge University Press. © Cambridge University Press 2010.

abused at the end of life, with a prevalence of 7% to 27% (9); abuse of other substances ranges from 0.4% to 15% (benzodiazepines 0.7%, opioids 2.1%, amphetamines 0.4%, cocaine 2.1%, marijuana 14.4%) (10).

The prevalence of delirium varies greatly but may approach levels as high as 85% during the final stages of a terminal illness (11, 12). It is also worth mentioning that the issue of decision-making capacity comes up with great frequency as a patient nears the end of life (often secondary to delirium). This issue is discussed in greater detail in Chapter 4.

To work with dying patients, a psychiatrist must have a basic understanding of both palliative care and hospice. The World Health Organization says that palliative care is "… *the active total care of patients whose disease is not responsive to curative treatment. Control of pain, of other symptoms, and of psychological, social, and spiritual problems is paramount. The goal of palliative care is achievement of the best quality of life for patients and their families. Many aspects of palliative care are also applicable earlier in the course of the illness in conjunction with anticancer treatment.*" With this definition, a psychiatrist who is engaging in end-of-life discussions or is treating a psychiatric disorder in a terminal patient is providing palliative care. However, good palliative care depends upon the involvement of an interdisciplinary team so that all aspects of a patient's and a family's suffering are evaluated and addressed. It is perfectly reasonable to suggest a palliative care consult to a primary team if you believe that a patient with a terminal illness is suffering. Learners often find it difficult to delineate the differences between palliative care and hospice. All of hospice is palliative care, but not all of palliative care is hospice.

Hospice provides care with a palliative approach (management of symptoms) for patients in the last six months of life. Although palliative medicine can be provided at any point in a disease trajectory, the patient does not have to have a life expectancy of less than six months.

It is also essential that all physicians have a basic understanding of hospice services and know when referral to hospice is appropriate. Hospice is a philosophy of care built around the concept that the dying patient has physical, psychological, social and spiritual aspects of suffering. Hospice care can be provided in any setting but typically occurs in the patient's home (13). The core structure of hospice includes an interdisciplinary team which consists of multiple disciplines including medical directors, nursing, hospice health aides, social work, chaplain, volunteers, and bereavement. The interdisciplinary team provides access to a wide range of services to support the primary caregiver, who is responsible for the majority of the patient care. To be eligible for hospice, a patient must have a terminal illness and an estimated prognosis of six months or less. Most hospice agencies and hospice patients utilize the medicare hospice benefit.

To be eligible for the Medicare hospice benefit, four criteria must be met (14):

- Eligibility for Medicare part A (hospital insurance)
- Enrollment in a Medicare-approved hospice
- The patient must sign a statement choosing hospice
- The patient's personal physician and the hospice medical director both must certify that the patient has a terminal illness with an estimated life expectancy of less than six months

Hospice can be a tremendous financial benefit to patients because the hospice benefit covers all expenses related to the terminal illness, including medication, skilled nursing, nursing aides, and hospital equipment. In general, most hospice referrals come from physicians, despite the fact that anyone including social workers, nurses, or family can make a hospice referral (15). The trend in the United States has been to refer patients in their last days of life. Nationwide, the median length of stay is 26 days (16). When given the option, 83% of terminal patients choose hospice (15, 17). Unfortunately, most referrals are precipitated by a crisis immediately before death. This is often a consequence of patients living with a chronic condition that they may not understand is terminal, combined with the reluctance of a physician to give a terminal diagnosis and prognosis (18, 19). Late referrals are detrimental to both the patient and the hospice because of the costs related to initiating services and the limited time allowed to form a therapeutic relationship (15, 20). Research has shown that caregiver satisfaction with hospice increased when the patient was enrolled longer than 30 days (21), and that patients who spend at least two months in hospice show the greatest benefit (22, 23). The psychiatric diagnosis most often associated with hospice admission is dementia. In general, a patient with dementia is eligible for hospice services if she needs assistance with all activities of daily living (ADLs), cannot communicate her needs effectively, and shows a medical decline such as weight loss or infection (24, 25).

Work-up

The cornerstone of a good evaluation in a patient with a terminal illness is as always a thorough psychiatric evaluation based on *DSM-IV* criteria, with a high index of suspicion for depression and delirium. However, patients may not be able to undergo an extensive interview because of their poor health status, and the use of screening tools can be beneficial. Simply asking "Are you depressed?" and "Have you lost interest in activities?" is both sensitive and specific in screening for depression in terminally ill patients (1). Positive answers should be followed up with a focus on the cognitive aspects of depression because somatic symptoms can sometimes result from the underlying illness. Evidence of hopelessness, helplessness, worthlessness, guilt, or suicide ideation is a better indicator of depression in patients with a terminal illness than are neurovegetative symptoms. Risk factors for depression are listed in Table 25.1.

It is also important to differentiate grief from depression (Table 25.2). Grief is a normal expression of loss (often anticipatory in these patients) and can have psychological, social, and somatic manifestations. Grief is often experienced in waves which may be severe, but the intensity should diminish with time. Self-image is typically preserved with grief, as is the ability to feel pleasure and hope (26).

Terminally ill patients with anxiety often present with prominent somatic manifestations which may overshadow the cognitive symptoms. It is important to look for the source of anxiety because it may be related to the terminal condition (fear of death, medication side effects, under-treated symptoms such as pain or dyspnea) and not simply to an actual underlying anxiety disorder (1, 27). Medications which are common at the end of life such as bronchodilators, beta-adrenergic receptor stimulants, corticosteroids, metoclopramide, and neuroleptic drugs all can cause anxiety, and their use should be evaluated during the work-up (28). It is also important to be on the lookout for withdrawal states (alcohol, opioids, benzodiazepines) and rebound anxiety from inadequate dosing regimens.

Substance abuse is believed to be less common at the end of life, but "drug-seeking" behavior must be differentiated from pseudoaddiction. Pseudoaddiction is an iatrogenic syndrome wherein patients "act out" from distress due to unrelieved pain, anxiety, or insomnia, and it can be confused with drug-seeking behavior (29). In pseudoaddiction, "acting out and drug-seeking" behaviors resolve when the pain is adequately treated. It is essential to ensure that

Table 25.1 Risk factors for depression in palliative care patients (3)

Having a terminal diagnosis
Certain types of cancer: pancreatic cancer, brain tumors
Co-morbidities: hypothyroidism, coronary artery disease, macular degeneration, diabetes mellitus, Alzheimer's disease, Parkinson's disease, multiple sclerosis, stroke, Huntington's disease
Physical disability
Poor pain and symptom control
Metabolic abnormalities: hypercalcemia, tumor-generated toxins, uremia, abnormal liver function
Medications: amphotericin, centrally acting antihypertensive agents, H_2-blockers, metoclopramide, cytotoxic drugs, corticosteroids, interferon, interleukin
Radiation therapy
Malnutrition
Cognitive loss
Previous personal history of depression
Family history of depression
Age of the patient (more common in younger patients)
Request to withhold or withdraw from treatment
Requests for assisted suicide
Substance abuse
Poor social support
Lack of close confiding relationships
Financial strains

Table 25.2 Grief compared with depression in terminally ill patients (4)

Characteristics of Grief	Characteristics of Depression
Patients experience feelings, emotions and behaviors that result from a particular loss.	Patients experience feelings, emotions and behaviors that fulfill criteria for a major psychiatric disorder; distress is usually generalized to all facets of life.
Almost all terminally ill patients experience grief, but only a minority develop full-blown affective disorders requiring treatment.	Major depression occurs in 1% to 53% of terminally ill patients.
Patients usually cope with distress on their own.	Medical or psychiatric intervention is usually necessary.
Patients experience somatic distress, loss of usual patterns of behavior, agitation, sleep and appetite disturbances, decreased concentration, social withdrawal.	Patients experience similar symptoms plus hopelessness, helplessness, worthlessness, guilt and suicidal ideation.
Grief is associated with disease progression.	Depression has an increased prevalence (up to 77%) in patients with advanced cancer; pain is a major risk factor.
Patients retain the capacity for pleasure.	Patients enjoy nothing.
Grief comes in waves.	Depression is constant and unremitting.
Patients express passive wishes for death to come quickly.	Patients express intense and persistent suicide ideation.
Patients are able to look forward to the future.	Patients have no sense of a positive future.

these patients are provided with adequate pain relief because a history of substance abuse is a tremendous risk factor for under-treatment (8) and can prompt maladaptive drug-seeking behaviors. It is important to note that pseudoaddiction is seen in patients both with and without a previous history of substance abuse.

Delirium is common in medically ill patients and has a significant impact on the lives of both the patient and caregivers. Delirium at the end of life can be reversed about 50% of the time, and consideration should be given to an appropriate medical evaluation only if it is consistent with patient and family goals. Delirium in this population is more likely to be reversed if it is related to medication, hypoxia, dehydration, or hypercalcemia (30). The work-up and treatment of delirium are fully discussed in Chapter 4, but some attention will be given to what has been described as terminal delirium. This is an agitated delirium which occurs in some patients during the few days preceding death and is the most frequent reason cited for initiating palliative sedation. The diagnosis of terminal delirium is often made retrospectively. In general, terminal delirium is incredibly distressing to patients and their caregivers.

Clinical decision-making and treatment

Depression responds as well to treatment in medically ill patients as in healthy individuals, and effective treatment can result in improvement in the symptoms of the underlying terminal condition. In patients with COPD, depression treatment improved respiratory symptoms, in addition to improving depression symptoms (31). The first step in assessing and treating depression at the end of life should be ensuring that the patient has adequate pain control. Uncontrolled pain is a major risk factor for depression and suicide among patients with cancer (5). Once pain and other uncontrolled symptoms are addressed, psychopharmacology is the most frequent choice for treating clinical depression in this patient population, in part because of the limited time available for treatment. Psychostimulants, selective serotonin reuptake inhibitors (SSRIs), and tricyclic antidepressants are the mainstay of treatment for depressed terminally ill patients (Table 25.3). For patients with a longer life expectancy, an SSRI is a good initial choice, specifically, citalopram and sertraline, because they have fewer active metabolites which can accumulate and cause toxicity (4, 32). For patients with severe depression and an expected life span of more than 4 weeks, it is often useful to begin treatment concurrently with a psychostimulant and an antidepressant. Psychostimulants take effect quickly; however, they are not the initial drug of choice for patients who have a prognosis of longer than 6 to 8 weeks (32, 33). For patients with a life expectancy of less than 8 weeks, depression can be successfully controlled with a psychostimulant alone; in addition, methylphenidate has been shown to improve appetite, increase energy, and decrease cancer-related fatigue (32). Caution does have to be used when one is prescribing a psychostimulant because it can worsen anxiety and interfere with sleep. Mirtazapine deserves special consideration because it has the added benefit of treating depression, as well as improving insomnia, nausea, and pain in patients with cancer (34, 35).

The mainstay of treatment for anxiety at the end of life is benzodiazepines. It is important to initiate psychological support and behavioral interventions, but these are rarely effective without pharmacotherapy (1). Unfortunately, no comprehensive, evidence-based randomized control trials have looked at the treatment of anxiety at the end of life; however, the standard of care involves the utilization of short-acting benzodiazepines (typically, alprazolam and lorazepam) to control symptoms quickly. Lorazepam has the added benefit of

Table 25.3 Recommended medications for psychiatric disorders in terminally ill patients (adapted in part from a table by Block (4)

Agent	Advantages	Disadvantages	Onset of Action	Starting Dose	Usual Daily dose	Side Effects
Depression						
Methylphenidate	Rapid acting, well tolerated, counters opioid-induced fatigue, effective in 70%–82% of patients, may improve appetite, energy, and cognitive functioning	Cardiac decompensation, can cause/worsen confusion	<24 hr	2.5–5 mg qam	10–20 mg	A mean of 11% of patients experience restlessness, dizziness, nightmares, insomnia, palpitations, arrhythmia, tremor, dry mouth or Rare psychosis
Sertraline	Safe and effective, few side effects, easy to titrate	Inhibits cytochrome P450D2 and has interactions with other drugs	2–4 weeks	12.5–25 mg	50–100 mg	Nausea, GI distress, insomnia, headache, sexual dysfunction, anorexia
Nortriptyline	Can help with neuropathic pain, can be given orally and rectally, can monitor drug levels	Can cause sedation and hypotension	2–4 weeks	10–25 mg	25–75 mg	Anticholinergic side effects (delirium, dry mouth, constipation)
Mirtazapine	May improve sleep, anxiety, nausea, and appetite	Can cause excessive sedation and hypotension	2–4 weeks	7.5–15 mg qhs	15–30 mg	Anticholinergic side effects (delirium, dry mouth, constipation)
Anxiety						
Lorazepam	Can improve nausea, dyspnea, and anxiety, safer in hepatic dysfunction	Can cause sedation, confusion, falls, decreased respiration	30–60 min	0.5–1 mg prn q 4 hr	0.5–1 mg qid	Sedation (15%) as well as dizziness and unsteadiness
Delirium						
Haloperidol	Can decrease nausea, available in oral elixir, can be given subcutaneously	May cause restlessness or extrapyramidal symptoms	30–60 min (oral) 5–15 min IV/SQ	0.5–1 mg q 1 hr prn	1–5 mg over 24 hr	Increased risk of death in elderly patients from cardiac causes or infections. QTc prolongation, NMS
Chlorpromazine	Can decrease nausea and treat hiccups	Can cause sedation, confusion, falls, dry mouth, hypotension	30–60 min oral 15–30 min IV/SQ	25–50 mg TID prn PO 5–10 mg/hr SQ	50 mg tid PO 5–50 mg/hr SQ	Hypotension, constipation and dry mouth more common; NMS and prolonged QTc rare
Olanzapine	May improve nausea, pain, and appetite, available in an oral dissolving tablet	Can cause sedation, confusion and hypotension	30–60 min	2.5–5 mg	5 mg BID	Increased risk of sudden cardiac death, dizziness and insomnia; NMS

decreasing (anticipatory) nausea and is safer in patients who have compromised hepatic function because it is has no active metabolites. If life expectancy is greater than 6 to 8 weeks, a trial of SSRIs can be started concurrently, but their usefulness is limited given their relatively long latency to effect. Neuroleptics such as haloperidol and chlorpromazine are useful when benzodiazepines are contraindicated or ineffective and can be beneficial in decreasing nausea as well. Opioid analgesics are particularly effective for anxiety which accompanies pain and dyspnea.

It is important to mention psychotherapy as treatment for the terminally ill. In general, it is more effective when combined with pharmacotherapy. Typically the goals are more finite. The focus should be placed more on providing a nurturing supportive relationship and less on patient insight, and the therapist may have to take a more active role as a patient advocate. Although cognitive and interpersonal approaches may be most effective because of the limited time often available, providing psychoeducation and normalizing emotional responses can be particularly beneficial.

Substance abuse at the end of life should not be ignored, but the goal of treatment often is not abstinence. It is important to address and manage substance abuse in a patient with a terminal illness because it tends to worsen psychiatric conditions and make palliative care interventions less effective. Additionally, to medications patients with addiction may need large amounts of opioids and benzodiazepines to relieve distress secondary to tolerance and low tolerance for distress. Active treatment of substance abuse through counseling is indicated, but treatment with medications such as acamprosate calcium (Campral) or disulfiram (Antabuse) is not recommended because of side-effect profiles and lack of evidence of efficacy in this patient population. It is completely appropriate to use tools to ensure compliance, such as implementing medication contracts, dispensing limited supplies, maintaining pill counts, and conducting urine toxicology, with the goal of safe substance use while physical symptoms such as pain are controlled.

Delirium treatment at the end of life is similar to delirium treatment at any other time, but treatment should be entered into with patient and family goals firmly in mind. The goal is not always to cure the delirium. Initial treatment may involve a limited medical work-up (if indicated) and correction of simple metabolic disturbances if desired. If a patient is dehydrated, a fluid bolus using hypodermoclysis, wherein fluid is infused into the subcutaneous tissue, can often improve delirium, is well tolerated, and can easily be given at home. Non-pharmacologic measures should also be implemented. No agents have been approved by the U.S. Food and Drug Administration (FDA) to treat delirium at the end of life, but haloperidol and chlorpromazine are commonly used and have the added benefit of improving nausea. Haloperidol is commercially available in a liquid form (2 mg/ml) and can be given sublingually in a patient who does not swallow well. Chlorpromazine can be given rectally. Both can be given parentally or subcutaneously by continuous infusion, but care should be taken if chlorpromazine IV is given, because of the risk of hypotension. Although benzodiazepines are commonly given for the treatment of delirium at the end of life, the literature shows that they can worsen outcome (5). They are better reserved for the treatment of an agitated delirium when neuroleptics have failed. This author has found that terminal delirium often responds to a continuous subcutaneous chlorpromazine infusion (starting dose 5 to 10 mg/hr) with the dose being titrated upward until the patient is calm. If neuroleptics have failed and the patient has a very distressing terminal delirium, a continuous infusion of midazolam is usually effective; however, if the goal of the patient and family is sedation, a palliative care (or ethics) consult should be obtained.

In summary, mental illness is common at the end of life, but it is not universal and should never be considered normal just because someone has received bad news and has a terminal illness. It is important to differentiate depression and anxiety from normal anticipatory grief and to treat aggressively. Treatment of patients with a terminal illness is similar to treatment at other times of life, except that use of augmenting agents such as methylphenidate and benzodiazepines earlier in the treatment plan is emphasized. Palliative care and hospice referrals can be valuable tools in your treatment arsenal and should be considered. We can't stop people from dying, but we can help relieve the suffering associated with mental illness at the end of life.

References

1. Chochinov HM. Psychiatry and terminal illness. Can J Psychiatry. 2000;45(2):143–50.

2. Miovic M, Block S. Psychiatric disorders in advanced cancer. Cancer. 2007;110(8):1665–76.

3. Noorani NH, Montagnini M. Recognizing depression in palliative care patients. J Palliat Med. 2007;10(2):458–64.

4. Block SD. Assessing and managing depression in the terminally ill patient. ACP-ASIM End-of-Life Care Consensus Panel. American College of Physicians – American Society of Internal Medicine. Ann Intern Med. 2000;132(3):209–18.

5. Breitbart W, Rosenfeld B, Pessin H, et al. Depression, hopelessness, and desire for hastened death in terminally ill patients with cancer. JAMA. 2000;284(22):2907–11.

6. Chochinov HM, Wilson KG, Enns M, et al. Desire for death in the terminally ill. Am J Psychiatry. 1995;152(8):1185–91.

7. Breitbart W, Bruera E, Chochinov H, et al. Neuropsychiatric syndromes and psychological symptoms in patients with advanced cancer. J Pain Symptom Manage. 1995;10(2):131–41.

8. Goy E, Ganzini L. End-of-life care in geriatric psychiatry. Clin Geriatr Med. 2003;19(4):841–56, vii–viii.

9. Brenes GA. Anxiety and chronic obstructive pulmonary disease: prevalence, impact, and treatment. Psychosom Med. 2003;65(6):963–70.

10. Kirsh KL, Passik SD. Palliative care of the terminally ill drug addict. Cancer Invest. 2006;24(4):425–31.

11. Bruera E, Neumann C, Brenneis C, et al. Frequency of symptom distress and poor prognostic indicators in palliative cancer patients admitted to a tertiary palliative care unit, hospices, and acute care hospitals. J Palliat Care. 2000;16(3):16–21.

12. SAMHSA: Results from the 2007 National Survey on Drug Use and Health: national findings. Washington (DC): U.S. Department of Health and Human Services; 2007.

13. Gagnon B: Delirium in terminal cancer; a prospective study using daily screening, early diagnosis, and continuous monitoring. J Pain Symptom Manage. 2000;19(6):412–26.

14. Lawlor PG, Gagnon B, Mancini IL, et al. Occurrence, causes, and outcome of delirium in patients with advanced cancer: a prospective study. Arch Intern Med. 2000;160(6):786–94.

15. Miller S. The emergence of Medicare hospice care in US nursing homes. Palliat Care. 2001;15:471–80.

16. Weckmann MT. The role of the family physician in the referral and management of hospice patients. Am Fam Physician. 2008;77(6):807–12.

17. McGorty EK, Bornstein BH. Barriers to physicians' decisions to discuss hospice: insights gained from the United States hospice model. J Eval Clin Pract. 2003;9(3):363–72.

18. National Hospice and Palliative Care Organization. NHPCO's facts and figures – 2005 findings. Alexandria (VA): National Hospice and Palliative Care Organization; 2006.

19. Weggel JM. Barriers to the physician decision to offer hospice as an option for terminal care. World Med J. 1999;98(3): 49–53.

20. Brickner L, Scannell K, Marquet S, et al. Barriers to hospice care and referrals: survey of physicians' knowledge, attitudes, and perceptions in a health maintenance organization. J Palliat Med. 2004;7(3): 411–8.

21. Sanders BS, Burkett TL, Dickinson GE, et al. Hospice referral decisions: the role of physicians. Am J Hosp Palliat Care. 2004; 21(3):196–202.

22. Stillman MJ. Differences in physician access patterns to hospice care. J Pain Symptom Manage. 1999;17:157–63.

23. Teno J. Family perspectives on end-of-life care at the last place of care. JAMA. 2004; 291(1):88–93.

24. Lynn J. Perspectives on care at the close of life: serving patients who may die soon and their families: the role of hospice and other services. JAMA. 2001;285(7):925–32.

25. Christakis N. Survival of Medicare patients enrolled in hospice programs. Presented at: Annual American Academy of Hospice and Palliative Medicine; Chicago; 1997.

26. Aupperle PM, MacPhee ER, Strozeski JE, et al. Hospice use for the patient with advanced Alzheimer's disease: the role of the geriatric psychiatrist. Am J Alzheimers Dis Other Demen. 2004;19(2): 94–104.

27. Medical guidelines for determining prognosis in selected non-cancer diseases. 2nd ed. Arlington (VA): National Hospice Organization; 1996.

28. Chochinov HM, Wilson KG, Enns M, et al. "Are you depressed?" Screening for depression in the terminally ill. Am J Psychiatry. 1997;154(5):674–6.

29. Periyakoil VS, Hallenbeck J. Identifying and managing preparatory grief and depression at the end of life. Am Fam Physician. 2002;65(5):883–90.

30. Lyness JM. End-of-life care: issues relevant to the geriatric psychiatrist. Am J Geriatr Psychiatry. 2004;12(5):457–72.

31. Roth AJ, Massie MJ. Anxiety and its management in advanced cancer. Curr Opin Support Palliat Care. 2007;1(1):50–6.

32. Weissman DE. Understanding pseudoaddiction. J Pain Symptom Manage. 1994; 9(2):74.

33. Morita T. Underlying pathologies and their associations with clinical features in terminal delirium of cancer patients. J Pain Symptom Manage. 2001;22(6):997–1006.

34. Ferrando SJ. Commentary: integrating consultation-liaison psychiatry and palliative care. J Pain Symptom Manage. 2000;20(3):235–6.

35. Breitbart W. Suicide in cancer patients. Oncology (Williston Park). 1987;1(2): 49–55.

36. Rozans M, Dreisbach A, Lertora JJ, et al. Palliative uses of methylphenidate in patients with cancer: a review. J Clin Oncol. 2002;20(1):335–9.

37. Hardy SE. Methylphenidate for the treatment of depressive symptoms, including fatigue and apathy, in medically ill older adults and terminally ill adults. Am J Geriatr Pharmacother. 2009;7(1):34–59.

38. Kim SW, Shin IS, Kim JM, et al. Effectiveness of mirtazapine for nausea and insomnia in cancer patients with depression. Psychiatry Clin Neurosci. 2008;62(1):75–83.

39. Theobald DE, Kirsh KL, Holtsclaw E, Donaghy K, Passik SD: An open-label, crossover trial of mirtazapine (15 and 30 mg) in cancer patients with pain and other distressing symptoms. J Pain Symptom Manage. 2002;23(5):442–7.

40. Breitbart W, Marotta R, Platt MM, et al. A double-blind trial of haloperidol, chlorpromazine, and lorazepam in the treatment of delirium in hospitalized AIDS patients. Am J Psychiatry. 1996;153(2): 231–7.

Chapter

26

Demoralization in the medical setting

Marcus Wellen and Thomas Wise

Typical consult question

"He's depressed . . . . but I don't know what you can do about it."

The patient, Mr. A., is a fifty year old married male with a functional gastroparesis due to a five-year course of high-volume peritoneal dialysis. The current admission was the tenth in the past year for dehydration, as the patient could not maintain adequate fluid intake because of his gastroparesis. The surgeon who requested the consultation noted, "We can't really do much for him except wait and hope he gets better. Of course, he's depressed."

Mr. A. described his struggles with nausea, vomiting, and pain and became tearful when he reflected on how long he had suffered from this disease process. However, his major complaint was the time he spent away from his wife and seven year old daughter. On a follow-up visit, he seemed surprisingly upbeat one afternoon. He gestured to his iPod and told me, "This is my antidepressant. My wife downloaded the video of our daughter's dance recital and I've been watching it all day."

Background

How do we explain the above case? Individuals with physical disorders are often depressed. So why would he be so animated for a protracted time after seeing his daughter's video? The concept of demoralization may offer an answer.

A challenge in identifying demoralized patients is the lack of consensus on how to define demoralization in the medically ill. This is due in part to the fact that the concept of demoralization is not a psychiatric term but rather is a term borrowed from the lay literature long before it was applied to how a person reacts to medical illness. The term *demoralize* is thought to come from the French "demoraliser," a term coined during the French revolution to describe "the lower morale" of an army (10). Compounding matters is the disagreement between leaders in the field regarding whether demoralization is, in fact, a normal or an abnormal reaction (1). However, as Philip Slavney mentioned, the "first step in recognizing demoralization is to think of it" (2). One of the most common diagnosis in a psychiatric consultation service is that of "adjustment disorder," which offers very little to our understanding of the patient or its relationship to affective disorders (21). Thus the concept of demoralization is an important addition to our diagnostic taxonomy.

Consultation psychiatrists often are called to evaluate patients with medical disorders that impact the quality of their lives and limit pre-morbid physical, social, and emotional function. Confounding the assessment is that patients with medical illness often complain of

Psychosomatic Medicine: An Introduction to Consultation-Liaison Psychiatry, eds. James J. Amos and Robert G. Robinson. Published by Cambridge University Press. © Cambridge University Press 2010.

painful effects of depression and concurrent symptoms of sleep difficulties, lowered energy, and diminished interest. One approach has been to consider *demoralization* as a unique clinical entity that captures the essence of such reactions (1–9). A demoralized patient reports no emotional difficulties until disease onset; moreover, the disease and its impact leave the patient worried and frightened. How should this patient be diagnosed? Often demoralized patients do not formally qualify for a designation of major depressive disorder because a number of symptoms and the time frame do not meet those presented in the *Diagnostic and Statistical Manual of Mental Disorders (DSM)* taxonomy (7).

One of the first authors to describe in detail the phenomenon of demoralization was the internist Dr. George Engel, in his classic paper "The Giving Up–Given Up Complex," although he does not use the term *demoralization* (11). Engel describes five aspects of the "giving up–given up" complex that later re-surface in the medical literature as the concept of demoralization:

1. Hopelessness and helplessness
2. Subjective incompetence
3. Less perceived social support or gratification from others
4. Broken sense of connectedness between the past and the future
5. Re-experiencing of earlier failures

Nearly a decade later, Dr. Jerome Frank described demoralization specifically in the setting of medical illness, although he did recognize this concept as being common in patients with other life stressors (12). He described demoralization as "a state of hopelessness, helplessness, and isolation in which the person is preoccupied with merely trying to survive" (13). The development of demoralization results from a "persistent inability to cope" when faced with stressors that separate the individual from what once gave life meaning, such as close relationships with another or one's own values (12). These traditions have shaped much of the current understanding of demoralization as it applies to patients with medical illness.

What remain central to the concept of demoralization are the qualities of helplessness and hopelessness (14). The helplessness experienced by a patient with medical illness has multiple facets which include the limitations of the disease state, a sense of impotence, a sense of incompetence, and poor perceived social support. The practical limitations of certain disease states cannot be ignored or minimized with false assurances by the consultant. For example, it will not benefit the patient with paralysis due to a car accident to hear from a physician that "everything will be all right." Paradoxically, false assurance will increase the patient's sense that there is no help to be had from others, given how misunderstood he is. Alternatively, it behooves the consultant to avoid over-identifying with the patient's plight, as the patient will likely mirror the consultant's own despair. The realities of the disease state or perceived disability will often lead to a sense of impotence or powerlessness, and then, subjective incompetence.

Subjective incompetence is an essential facet of demoralization (14). Subjective incompetence is "the self-perceived incapacity to perform tasks and express feelings deemed appropriate in a stressful situation" (14). Subjective incompetence has roots in catastrophic thinking, as the patient compares past failures and current limitations, arriving at the conclusion that future failure is guaranteed. When a person feels helpless to such a degree, he may feel as if no person can empathize with him, resulting in poor perceived social support. Poor perceived social support has been implicated in poor health outcomes and has become a target of therapy in recent times (15). In this fashion, the patient's ability to cope is overwhelmed, and he is left feeling alone, frightened, and without options.

When faced with such helplessness, the demoralized patient can lose meaning or purpose, otherwise defined as hopelessness (16). The meaning of an event, in this case medical illness, has been described by using this appraisal theory, which describes how events can have attached emotional meaning (17). A medical illness may lose personal meaning if it attacks a person's physical integrity or sense of self. For example, a patient with a severe burn may be physically disfigured, while at the same time suffering a significant amount of pain. In this case, it is difficult for the medical illness to have any positive meaning or purpose. When the medical illness has no ascribed positive meaning, then it becomes difficult for the helpless patient to think about the future in a constructive fashion, because he doubts his ability to effect positive change. Furthermore, it is difficult for the demoralized patient to imagine himself in his current disabled state carried forward as unchanged in the future.

The psychiatrist should evaluate whether the disconnection of meaning is a function of the hospital environment and treatment, or whether it is a result of the illness itself, which can cause pain and suffering as well as the specter of death. The rule-based society of the hospital imposes many restrictions on the patient. First, many hospitals have visiting hours that reduce contact with the patient's support group. Second, the hospital staff tends to prefer that patients remain in their room during their hospital stay, so that staff members can examine and treat the patient at their convenience. This essentially removes from patients many of the active coping mechanisms that they would normally utilize when faced with distress or boredom. Third, many hospitals have a rigid structure that includes vital sign checks and laboratory draws, which serve as constant reminders to patients of the gravity of their illness, thus reinforcing the sick role. However, despite the disconnection of meaning that may take place in the hospital environment, it is not uncommon to find patients who voice a sense of meaninglessness in the outpatient setting. This seems to occur when patients cannot escape from a medical illness that has significantly altered their former role in life. Instead, the sick role has supplanted their identity, thus affecting their social and occupational functioning in a broad way. For example, patients with a history of severe cardiac illness or fibromyalgia often voice that they can no longer work or interact with family members and friends in ways they formerly enjoyed. That which has given their life purpose and meaning has been stripped from them and, to that effect, they can experience anger and a sense of isolation.

Work-up

The question of how to differentiate the phenomenon of demoralization from other depressive states such as an adjustment disorder with depressed mood or a major depressive disorder (MDD) remains important. A recent study attempted to address this issue by applying a recently developed diagnostic criterion for demoralization (18) to determine the percentage of medical outpatients who suffer from demoralization, MDD, or both (7). Results showed that of 245 patients, 30.4% were identified as demoralized and 16.7% were identified as suffering from MDD (7). It is interesting to note that although there appeared to be a significant overlap between the demoralized patients and patients with MDD, 43.7% of patients with MDD were not classified as demoralized, and 69.0% of patients who met the criteria for demoralization did not meet the *DSM-IV* criteria for MDD (7). These results indicate that

Table 26.1

Demoralization

A.
1. Do you feel you have failed to meet your expectations or those of other people (concerning your work, family, social and/or economic status)?
Yes ___   No ___
2. Is there an urgent problem you feel unable to cope with?
Yes ___   No ___
3. Do you experience feelings of helplessness, hopelessness, and/or giving up?
Yes ___   No ___
B. Does your state of feeling exceed a month?
Yes ___   No ___
C. Did this feeling occur before the manifestation of a physical disorder or exacerbate it?
Yes ___   No ___

Diagnosis: A [1 **and/or** 2 **and/or** 3] = yes + B = yes + C = yes

further thought needs to be given to how one can best differentiate between demoralization, MDD, and adjustment disorder with depressed mood.

The difficultly in differentiating demoralization from MDD lies in the fact that the symptoms of hopelessness and helplessness are key features shared between demoralization and MDD as described in the *DSM-IV-TR*. Furthermore, it may be difficult to differentiate between the sense of subjective incompetence found in demoralization and the symptom of worthlessness found in MDD. Finally, the somatic neurovegetative symptoms found in MDD are often obfuscated by the medical illness or by treatment of the medical illness. Although standardized criteria for demoralization have been proposed, none have been fully embraced by psychiatrists or incorporated into the *DSM*, which makes the objective research of demoralization difficult (6, 18). For instance, Porcelli et al. have offered a diagnostic criterion, which is included in Table 26.1 (19).

From a clinical perspective, the method by which to differentiate between demoralization and MDD lies in both anhedonia and nihilism often found in MDD (20). With regards to anhedonic depression, Clark et al. studied 312 medically ill inpatients and found differences between depression and demoralization in coping, and social, family, and physical functioning (20). This may explain the nihilistic thinking, such as "I will never get better," or "no one can help me," observed in MDD. The behavior that the consultant can observe on the medical unit is help-rejecting behavior such as not allowing for nursing care, not participating in physical or occupational therapy, and refusing or restricting eating. Finally, if the patient is fortunate enough to recover from the medical illness implicated in demoralization, then typically the depressive symptoms will also resolve as the patient begins to experience both mastery over the illness and meaning in his life again.

Adjustment disorders, the most frequent psychiatric diagnosis in the medical setting, may have the most in common with demoralization in the medical setting (21). However, adjustment disorders have also been described as "sub-threshold" disorders that are not on the order of the major psychiatric disorders, allowing physicians to identify and treat distressed patients before a major psychiatric disorder develops (22). Despite the ambiguity and overlap, the aforementioned qualities of demoralization, loss of meaning and subjective incompetence appear to differentiate this phenomenon from an adjustment disorder. Furthermore, these particular qualities may serve as targets for therapy.

Clinical decision-making and treatment

To begin to develop a diagnostic framework, the provider should take a consistent approach to the patient with medical illness, especially given the fact that the patient may be in an emotional crisis at the time. A longitudinal history of illness, which includes both the pre-morbid and the morbid state, can tell a provider much about who the patient is. Particular attention should be paid to the patient's social and occupational identity, so the provider can start to understand how the patient's life has changed. During this history, it is also helpful to gain information about patients' experience of illness by learning about how they learned about the diagnosis, their response to the diagnosis, and what the diagnosis means to them.

When initially evaluating a patient with a medical disorder, it is essential for the clinician to understand how the patient has experienced the disease. Patients may view a psychiatric consultation as a suggestion that their suffering is not warranted or their illness is not "real." It is useful to initially ask patients what they think about their physician's request for a psy-chiatric evaluation. Questioning how they currently "feel" would naturally follow. It is then important to take a longitudinal history of their illness, which can validate patients' illness experiences and can begin to foster a therapeutic alliance with the consultant. This may seem counterintuitive given the phenomenologic description of a mental illness in the *DSM-IV-TR*, but the narrative is therapeutic for patients and informative for providers. Essentially, it allows patients to describe in a historical fashion their illness experience; moreover, patients are often able to make connections about how the illness has affected them both function-ally and emotionally during this process. As a part of the longitudinal history, a provider begins to understand the experience of illness, the patient's personality style, and how he or she characteristically copes with new situations or challenges. Central in this process are the observations that the interviewer makes about the patient with regards to appearance, affect, and appropriateness of content. With this general approach, a provider builds the diagnostic framework that forms the foundation of an understanding of the patient's perspective.

In approaching the patient with medical illness, it is often helpful to understand how the patient learned about the diagnosis and subsequent treatment. The longitudinal history of symptoms can serve as a therapeutic bridge and as a way to observe the way in which the patient approaches novel or threatening situations. During this process, a provider can learn to what degree the patient resisted pre-morbidly the idea of morbidity or mortality. This process has been called denial, but this concept should be considered on a spectrum of adaptive versus maladaptive coping. Adaptive denial is a rational weighing of concern about new physical findings or information with a person's known body of knowledge about illness. Maladaptive denial devalues one's own true knowledge of illness. For example, if a patient with chronic lung disease continues to smoke in the face of worsening shortness of breath or hemoptysis, then the individual has devalued what he knows as possible outcomes of long-term smoking. This is done in most cases because the individual is very uncomfortable with thoughts of death or suffering and "denies" that the behavior is harmful.

When patients are overwhelmed by the disease state, they may express a spectrum of anxiety. On one end of the spectrum, patients may appear to be detached as they attempt to isolate the affect, dispassionately presenting their medical history. On the other end of the spectrum are patients who appear so anxious that they can hardly organize their history or chief complaint. These patients may give many circumstantial details, which can try the physician's patience. This can be off-putting to our colleagues, especially in cases of pain or other somatic symptoms of unclear origin, as their approach uses a logarithmic approach to rule out certain diseases in a logical and step-wise fashion. Gentle re-direction can get the interview back on course. When an anxious patient in pain or distress is interviewed with this model, he may feel not listened to, which only serves to increase the overall level of anxiety and distress. Because of this complicated interaction between patient and physician, many patients with the chief complaint of pain or another unexplained somatic complaint will typically relate an experience of perceived abandonment by other providers in the past. By encouraging the patient to relate a history of symptoms, the psychosomatic physician can engender a sense of trust that can be immediately therapeutic, so the provider can more clearly elucidate the patient's personality style.

It is important to ascertain patients' personality style to learn how they characteristically cope with new situations or challenges. Those patients who have high trait neuroticism (i.e., "worriers") will generally worry and feel vulnerable (23). Predictably, when faced with medical illness, those with high neuroticism will have elevated tendencies to ruminate, be pessimistic, and get anxious (24). On the other end of the spectrum are those who try to seek out more information to allay anxiety. This is often denoted as obsessional traits. When such individuals undergo stress, they will tend to ask more questions and seek more data to allay anxiety. This can take the form of seeking multiple opinions or getting information from the Internet. It is important for the physician to take this not as a critique of his or her personal competence but as evidence of a coping style.

Finally, the patient's previous experience with medical illness – for example, those who have experienced illness through friends and family – is a final cornerstone for the clinician in understanding the patient's perspective. When a patient has a pre-conceived idea about illness or treatment, it can become challenging to cause a foundational shift in opinion about the illness or treatment. This certainly is challenging given the fact that both the understanding and the treatment of medical illness progress fairly rapidly. The challenge is further compounded if the patient's experience has affected an individual, especially someone close to him, and if the experience involved a significant amount of pain or disfigurement.

The ultimate goal of treatment of the demoralized patient is the restoration of morale (12). Treatment of demoralization syndromes depends on multiple factors. First, what is the issue that is fostering the dysphoria; how does it impact upon the individual's life trajectory; what is the patient's personality temperament; and what social supports are available? These elements must be identified for the clinician to begin to help restore the morale of demoralized patients. The clinician can then discern whether the patient feels helpless in that the environment is letting him down, or hopeless in that he has let himself down and is inadequate for the challenge facing him. For helpless patients who are "giving up," environmental and social support can often remit the demoralized state, while those who have "given up" require more intensive pharmacotherapy plus psychotherapy. Thus the clinician will utilize both psychotherapeutic interventions and pharmacotherapy depending upon the unique situation of the demoralized patient.

Case discussion

Mr. A. experienced demoralization given the fact that his medical condition, for which there is no particular hope of immediate improvement, had rendered him dependent on the hospital for his basic life-sustaining needs. His own efforts to move forward in his life were constantly rebuffed by frequent relapses of nausea and vomiting. Furthermore, in the effort to sustain his life, he had been separated from his family, that which previously gave him purpose and meaning. Therefore, when reconnected with his family, he no longer felt defined and limited by his medical illness.

References

1. de Figueiredo J. Diagnosing demoralization in consultation psychiatry. Psychosomatics. 2000;41(5):449–50.

2. Slavney PR. Diagnosing demoralization in consultation psychiatry. Psychosomatics. 1999;40(4):325–9.

3. Clarke DM, Kissane DW. Demoralization: its phenomenology and importance. Aust N Z J Psychiatry. 2002;36(6):733–42.

4. Griffith JL, Gaby L. Brief psychotherapy at the bedside: countering demoralization from medical illness. Psychosomatics. 2005;46(2):109–16.

5. Jacobsen JC, Maytal G, Stern TA. Demoralization in medical practice. Prim Care Companion J Clin Psychiatry. 2007; 9(2):139–43.

6. Kissane DW, Wein S, Love A, et al. The Demoralization Scale: a report of its development and preliminary validation. J Palliat Care. 2004;20(4):269–76.

7. Mangelli L, Fava GA, Grandi S, et al. Assessing demoralization and depression in the setting of medical disease. J Clin Psychiatry. 2005;66(3):391–4.

8. Murphy JM. Diagnosis, screening, and 'demoralization': epidemiologic implications. Psychiatr Dev. 1986;4(2): 101–33.

9. Shader RI. Demoralization revisited. J Clin Psychopharmacol. 2005;25(4):291–2.

10. Random House Unabridged Dictionary. 2006.

11. Engel GL. A life setting conducive to illness: the giving-up-given-up complex. Bull Menninger Clin. 1968;32(6):355–65.

12. Frank JD. Psychotherapy: the restoration of morale. Am J Psychiatry. 1974;131(3): 271–4.

13. Frank JD, Frank JB. Persuasion and healing: a comparative study of psychotherapy. Baltimore (MD): John Hopkins University Press;1991. p. 35.

14. de Figueiredo JM, Frank JD. Subjective incompetence, the clinical hallmark of demoralization. Compr Psychiatry. 1982;23(4):353–63.

15. Broadhead E, Kaplan B, James S. The epidemiologic evidence for a relationship between social support and health. Am J Epidemiol. 1983;117(5):521–37.

16. Clarke DM, Kissane DW. Demoralization: its phenomenology and importance. Aust N Z J Psychiatry. 2002;36(6):733–42.

17. Smith CA, Lazarus RS. Emotion and adaptation. Handbook of personality: theory and research. New York: Guilford; 1990. p. 609–37.

18. Fabbri S, Fava GA, Sirri L, et al. Development of a new assessment strategy in psychosomatic medicine: the diagnostic criteria for psychosomatic research. Adv Psychosom Med. 2007;28:1–20.

19. Porcelli P, Sonino N. Psychological factors affecting medical conditions: a new classification for DSM-V. Adv Psychosom Med. 2007;180.

20. Clarke DM, Kissane DW, Trauer T, et al. Demoralization, anhedonia and grief in patients with severe physical illness. World Psychiatry. 2005;4(2):96–105.

21. Strain JJ, Smith GC, Hammer JS, et al. Adjustment disorder: a multisite study of its utilization and interventions in the consultation-liaison psychiatry setting. Gen Hosp Psychiatry. 1998;20(3):139–49.

22. Strain JJ, Diefenbacher A. The adjustment disorders: the conundrums of the diagnoses. Compr Psychiatry. 2008;49(2): 121–30.

23. Watson D, Clark L. Negative affectivity: the disposition to experience aversive emotional states. Psychol Bull. 1984;96: 465–90.

24. Lyness JM, Duberstein PR, King DA, Cox C, Caine ED. Medical illness burden, trait neuroticism, and depression in older primary care patients. Am J Psychiatry. 1998;155(7):969–71.

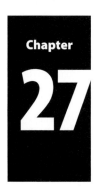

27

Psychotherapy for the hospitalized medically ill patient

Scott Temple and Scott Stuart

Typical consult question

"This nineteen year old male has become uncooperative and aggressive toward staff on the Burn Unit. Please evaluate for depression, and treat."

Medical illness, generally, and hospitalization, in particular, pose significant psychological challenges to the patient and the patient's family. In addition, medical patients at times can pose a challenge to the hospital staff treating them, particularly when mood, anxiety, or personality difficulties disrupt team relationships and interfere with adherence to medically necessary procedures. Often, the role of the consultation-liaison staff is to sort out complex presenting problems and to determine who needs intervention: the patient, the patient's support network, or the hospital staff. This chapter will focus on assessment and intervention strategies.

Background

Hospitalization poses a significant psychological challenge to most people, and it is no surprise that mood and anxiety problems are common among both hospitalized and non-hospitalized medical patients (1). Rates of depressive and anxiety symptoms in newly diagnosed, and early-stage treatment of, breast and gynecologic cancers, for example, approach 50% (2–4). In addition, the patient's social support network is often stressed. Moreover, the patient's inability or unwillingness to cooperate with medical personnel can tax the patience and understanding of the physicians, nurses, and others involved in the patient's care.

The role of the consultation-liaison psychiatrist is to rapidly assess what are often highly complex presenting problems, and to determine what intervention is appropriate for resolution of the particular case. This may include a decision to provide psychiatric medication or psychological therapies (including family therapy), or to intervene with the medical staff. Thus, the ideal consultation-liaison team includes personnel skilled in providing all of the above service components.

Work-up

The system perspective

The first step in sorting out the presenting problem often involves at least a brief meeting with the unit caregivers. It is vital to ascertain the degree to which the presenting problem

Psychosomatic Medicine: An Introduction to Consultation-Liaison Psychiatry, eds. James J. Amos and Robert G. Robinson. Published by Cambridge University Press. © Cambridge University Press 2010.

includes difficulties in obtaining the patient's cooperation with medical treatment, regardless of eventual diagnosis of the patient. Getting at least a quick overview of the patient through the eyes of nursing staff, the attending physician, and other involved providers is often pivotal in developing a formulation for the case, along with an intervention strategy. In addition, as will be described later, on some occasions the intervention must be directed towards the staff on the unit, making medical providers the "patient" as well. Difficult patients, particularly those who are interpersonally offensive or non-adherent to treatment, can elicit reactions from caregivers that may compound the problem.

The patient

Clinical assessment requires astute listening and observation skills. Patients often need to tell their story, and simply exploring patients' understanding of their illness can be of benefit (5). In addition, a host of screening instruments for depression and anxiety can be employed, once adequate rapport has been established to secure patient adherence with paper-and-pencil measures. Such measures may include the Beck Depression Inventory (BDI-II), the Beck Anxiety Inventory (BAI-II), the Brief Symptom Inventory (6), or the Patient Health Questionnaire (PHQ-9) (7). All are well-validated instruments that can be administered relatively easily and briefly. In ideal medical settings, screening instruments will already be completed routinely by all patients.

In addition to establishing the presence of a *DSM-IV* Axis I disorder, the clinician must develop a more refined understanding of the meaning of the illness to the patient, as well as the function served by the presenting symptoms. Two well-validated psychotherapy models, cognitive-behavioral therapy (CBT) (8, 9) and interpersonal psychotherapy (IPT) (10, 11), provide frameworks for formulating and intervening with hospitalized patients.

CBT, in particular, targets maladaptive appraisals and coping strategies for patients with the depressive and anxiety disorders so common in hospitalized patients. CBT has also been adapted for use specifically with medically ill patients (12, 13).

IPT is well suited to the needs of medically ill patients, although it is not perhaps as widely disseminated as CBT. Developed initially as a treatment for depression (14), it taps into domains that are highly relevant to the needs of hospitalized medical patients. Those domains are thought to be pivotal in the formation of depression, although not necessarily causal. They include Role Transitions, Role Disputes, Grief, and Interpersonal Deficits. As will be seen below, all of these content areas are potentially relevant for understanding distress, symptoms, and adaptive difficulties in hospitalized medical patients, as well as for developing intervention strategies. Adjusting, even temporarily, to the role of a "sick person" can be unusually taxing for many. Interpersonal disputes involving family or co-workers may spill over into, or contribute to, interpersonal disputes with medical staff. Unresolved grief over prior losses can trigger symptoms in hospitalized patients, who may face the stress of hospitalization without the social support of a longed for, but deceased, family member. Finally, interpersonal deficits, including communication difficulties, can also contribute to a patient's difficulties in understanding and cooperating with the medical team.

Among the content areas for formulating and intervening are the following:

- *Patient appraisals and illness narratives:* Depressed and/or anxious patients may interpret their illness, their hospitalization, and the motivation of caregivers in idiosyncratic and maladaptive ways. For example, a depressed patient who believes that his newly diagnosed heart disease means "my life is over" may withdraw and become hopeless and non-compliant with staff and family members, just at the time when his or her active engagement is most necessary. Anxious patients may have catastrophic beliefs about upcoming medical procedures that are re-played in their minds as they lie in bed. In addition, health problems may threaten a patient's sense of self (5).

- *Role transitions:* Hospitalization often represents a disruption in roles, not only for the patient, but for the family of the patient. Patients who themselves are accustomed to caring for others may be ill equipped to be the one cared for. Patients who maintain businesses or who have supervisory responsibilities for others may suffer as a consequence of the disruption in their ability to serve these roles. In addition, illness may represent an important life transition for the patient, depending upon the nature of the illness, its impact, and its chronicity. Assessing the nature of role disruptions and possible life transitions, for both the patient and the patient's family, may be key in developing an appropriate intervention strategy, as will be shown below. IPT is particularly well suited for providing the clinician with a framework for conceptualizing and intervening in role and life transitional difficulties.

At the same time, role disruptions and life transitions become intertwined with patient beliefs about these changes. Such changes in patient functioning may well impinge on, and tax the resources of, family members. At times, interventions with family members are central to helping the patient during his or her hospitalization. The consultant's role may include helping the patient access social support not only from family members, but from their broader network of friends and colleagues, or from their religious community. This emphasis on social support in times of crisis is also a hallmark of IPT.

Role disputes and interpersonal deficits

Patients with longstanding interpersonal difficulties can often bring their propensities for conflict into the hospital with them. The astute consultant will help sort out whether a conflictual patient is experiencing a temporary and potentially more easily manageable role dispute, caused by poor matching of expectations between the patient and the treatment team, or whether longstanding interpersonal deficits are making the situation more challenging. Where possible, the consultant will work to reduce role disputes through psychoeducation, and by helping the patient and the treatment team reach agreement about treatment objectives and procedures. When longstanding interpersonal deficits are at work, the consultant works to reduce emotional reactivity and to reduce the social isolation that may be exacerbating patient difficulties.

Clinical decision-making and treatment

Brief, focused individual psychotherapy can be of considerable benefit during times of health crisis. Cognitive-behavioral therapy (CBT) is a well-validated therapy for a wide range of clinical conditions (8). It has also been adapted for the medically ill (1, 5). Targeting maladaptive patient beliefs and coping strategies sometimes can lead to rapid resolution of the presenting problem. In fact, maladaptive beliefs may be more important than the actual severity of the illness in determining adjustment to illness (5).

Problematic patient behavior can rapidly become understandable to the consultant, once these appraisals are elicited during a clinical interview. In fact, sensitive listening to the patient's personal illness narrative is a first and vitally important step in intervening. Understanding the personal meaning that the patient imputes to illness and hospitalization is itself an important intervention. Helping to normalize the patient's feelings of helplessness, fear, despair, and anxiety is a vital intervention. Once the patient experiences the sense that the consultant understands him or her, it becomes easier for the consultant to explore, expose, and change the patient's maladaptive beliefs and coping strategies, in favor of more adaptive and possibly accurate alternatives.

CBT for health problems is based on the assumption that cognition mediates emotional and behavioral responses to medical illness. CBT dovetails with ancient wisdom traditions, which teach that it is not what happens to a person, but his or her interpretation of what happens that is critical. Depressed thinking is often reflected in what Beck described as the cognitive triad, which consists of negative automatic thoughts about the self ("I'm a loser"), the world ("Nobody cares about me"), and the future ("I will never amount to anything") (15). Anxiety chiefly consists of overestimations of threat and an underestimation of one's ability to cope with real and perceived threat, as well as with an uncertain future (16). Anxious cognitions in the medically ill might include the following: "I can't stand getting an operation; I'll go nuts," or "I'm going to die; I just know it," or "I can't cope with injections."

This stream of painful thinking is often unnoticed and unchallenged by the patient. Such thoughts, which Aaron T. Beck, MD, the founder of Cognitive Therapy, described as "automatic thoughts," are accessible to patients, once they are encouraged to tap into the stream of thoughts and visual images that occur in emotionally charged trigger situations, such as occur during hospitalization. Thus, automatic thoughts serve as a form of private communication, are highly believable, and exert a profound influence on emotions and on behavior. By encouraging the patient to share with the consultant the stream of private automatic thoughts, the consultant can sometimes quickly learn to unlock seemingly puzzling symptoms of depression and anxiety.

Common treatment strategies include the use of mood logs and thought records (15, 18). This might involve asking a hospitalized patient to rate mood on an hourly basis, and to chart his mood during the day, to find variations. Such variations may reveal trigger situations for distorted cognitions, or may reveal difficulty coping with painful medical procedures and other stressors present during hospitalization. Patients in CBT are taught to examine their thinking for repeated biases, such as in the cognitive triad, or the cognitive features of anxiety, and to create alternative, more adaptive ways of viewing themselves and their circumstances. Rooted also in behavior therapy, CBT encourages the use of adaptive coping strategies, and may foster the development of new coping skills or communication skills, as deemed necessary for the patient.

The use of guided discovery and Socratic questioning forms the heart of a CBT approach to treatment (15–18). By adopting a non-judgmental, gently curious, and inquisitive style of interviewing, the clinician helps reveal the hidden meanings of the patient's hospitalization. For depressed patients, such beliefs as "I'm as good as dead," "The nurses hate me," "I will never be a decent parent again," or "My career is over; therefore my life is over" become grist for the therapeutic mill. Helping patients develop more flexible appraisals of their life circumstances and more flexible coping strategies can be of considerable benefit.

Instilling hope is vital, whether the patient is facing a brief, resolvable medical crisis or is in the first phase of a lifelong adjustment to devastating illness or injury. In the case of the latter, it is especially important to respect patient defenses. Thus, the newly paraplegic college athlete must be allowed to mourn and grieve when he or she says "My career is over;

therefore my life is over." Without understanding the patient's sense of loss, the clinician will meet nothing but resistance if he or she tries to coax the patient into focusing on all the other avenues of life that remain open.

Helping the patient find adaptive coping responses is also an important part of psychotherapy for the hospitalized patient. Patients may believe that they do not have the resources to cope with the current situation, perhaps because of the presence of depression and anxiety, or perhaps because their lifelong coping style makes them ill equipped to deal with the role disruption and life transitions that they may now be facing. The active, behavioral components of CBT help boost the patient's sense of efficacy, thereby reducing hopelessness and helplessness in hospitalized patients.

Normalizing the patient's emotional response may also provide comfort. Normalizing strategies employed by the consultant help patients recognize that their emotional, behavioral, and cognitive responses make sense in light of their crisis, and that it is normal to experience deep fear and confusion at times of crisis.

Basic psychoeducation regarding hospitalization and its impact on people can also provide considerable relief. In particular, helping patients understand clearly what will be expected of them, and what they can expect of others caring for them, can provide relief to patients in the hospital. Finally, it is important for the consultant to be aware that psychiatric symptoms may not reflect the presence of a severe disorder. Rather, people in hospitals, at times of role and transitional stress, may simply find that their daily coping resources are taxed beyond their limit, thus leaving them symptomatic, although they fundamentally possess an adequate reserve of coping resources for the long haul.

Bringing in family members for brief, focused interventions may be of inestimable value. This includes the same psychoeducational and normalization interventions used in individual therapy. In addition, family problem-solving sessions can be of importance in helping patients accept a sick role, knowing that their role is perhaps being temporarily filled by others in their family or social network.

Finally, brief therapy may involve helping staff and patient cooperate with one another more effectively. Communication style is a key intervention focus in IPT for medical problems, for example (19).

At times, intervention strategies must involve not only the patient and the patient's family, but the unit staff as well.

Case example

Tom S. is a nineteen year old Caucasian male, who was admitted to the burn unit for second-degree burns over 25% of his body. After four days, he suddenly became agitated and verbally hostile and aggressive toward the burn technician who was debriding him in the debridement tank. He has since refused debridement and is increasingly angry and fearful.

Upon entering the unit, the consultant met with staff and discovered that several staff members were angry with the patient after he made racially hostile statements to an African American burn technician, while in the debridement tank. The burn technician was especially insulted and angry with the patient. The patient and the technician were now at loggerheads regarding the patient's debridements.

When the consultant met individually with the patient, on the burn unit, she expected to learn that the patient was agitated because of fear of the pain caused by the debridement procedure. However, by using a gentle, questioning style of interviewing, she learned that the patient had little fear of pain and did not consider the pain in the tank to be excruciating. Rather, as he approached the tank, he began to have vivid visual images of drowning. In particular, he feared that as the gurney swung him up from his bed and into the tank, his head would hit the edge of the tank, rendering him unconscious as he plunged into the water and drowned. He had never verbalized this frightening visual image, and finally, after several days of debridement, he impulsively screamed "You're going to kill me, you n – ."

The consultant took time to explore with the patient the unrealistic nature of his fears, confirming, by having him consult with staff, that no patient had ever drowned during debridement in the many years of the burn unit's existence. The patient's fears and agitation were largely alleviated.

However, there remained the matter of the staff's understandable anger towards Tom, particularly the anger of the African American burn technician who did the debridements. The consultant mediated between Tom and the technician as well as she could, encouraging Tom to apologize to the technician for his behavior, and to explain in detail the terror he felt on his way into the tank's waters. The consultant held a meeting with the burn technician and other staff on the burn unit to talk about Tom, and about the difficulties and challenges he posed for the staff. Although nothing approaching a "friendship" between the two ensued, the patient was able to work collaboratively with the staff, and to successfully complete his course of treatment and be released to outpatient care for his burn injuries.

Conclusion

The role of the consultation-liaison psychiatrist is complex and challenging, and involves the capacity to rapidly assess the patient, key members of the patient's interpersonal network, and, at times, the physician and/or unit calling for the consultation. Interventions may be necessary in any of these areas, including the pharmacologic management of the patient. For this reason, a consultation-liaison team, whose personnel can provide services in any of these areas, is optimal.

References

1. Guthrie E, Sensky T. Psychological interventions in patients with physical symptoms. In: Guthrie E, Lloyd G, editors. Textbook of liaison psychiatry. Cambridge: Cambridge University Press; 2007.

2. Levin T. Mixed anxiety-depression symptoms in a large cancer cohort: prevalence by cancer type. In press.

3. Fowler JM, Carpenter KM, Gupta P, Golden-Kreutz DM, Andersen BL. The gynecologic oncology consult: symptom presentation and concurrent symptoms of depression and anxiety. Obstet Gynecol. 2004;103(6):1211–7.

4. Golden-Kreutz DM, Andersen BL. Depressive symptoms after breast cancer surgery: relationships with global, cancer-related, and life event stress. Psycho-Oncology. 2004;13:211–20.

5. Sensky T. Cognitive therapy with medical patients. In: Wright J, editor. American Psychiatric Association Press review of psychiatry. Vol 23, No 3. Washington (DC): American Psychiatric Publishing; 2004. p. 83–121.

6. Derogatis LR, Melisaratos N. The brief symptom inventory: an introductory report. Psychol Med. 1983;13(3): 595–605.

7. Kroenke K, Spitzer R, Williams J. The PHQ-9: validity of a brief depression severity measure. J Gen Intern Med. 2001;16:606–13.

8. Butler AC, Chapman JE, Forman EM, Beck AT. The empirical status of cognitive-behavioral therapy: a review of meta-analyses. Clin Psychol Rev. 2006; 26(1):17–31.

9. Chambless DL, Ollendick TH. Empirically supported psychological interventions: controversies and evidence. Annu Rev Psychol. 2001;52:685–716.

10. Stuart S, Robertson M. Interpersonal psychotherapy: a clinician's guide. New York: A. Hodder Arnold; 2003.

11. Temple S, Gedde J. Psychotherapy for depression: current empirical status and future directions. In: Tyrer P, Silk K, editors. Cambridge textbook of effective treatments in psychiatry. Cambridge: Cambridge University Press; 2007.

12. Yates WR, Bowers WA. Cognitive therapy for the medical-psychiatric patient. In: Stoudemire A, Fogel BS, Greenberg D, editors. Psychiatric care of the medical patient. 2nd edition. New York: Oxford University Press; 2000. p. 51–60.

13. DiTomasso RA, Martin DM, Kovnat KD. Medical patients in crisis. In: Dattilio FM, Freeman A, editors. Cognitive-behavioral strategies in crisis intervention. 2nd ed. New York: Guilford Press; 2000. p. 409–28.

14. Klerman G, Weissman M, Rouinsaville B, Chevron E. Interpersonal psychotherapy of depression. New York: Basic Books; 1984.

15. Beck AT, Rush J, Shaw B, Emery G. Cognitive therapy of depression. New York: Guilford Press; 1979.

16. Beck A, Emery G. Anxiety disorders and phobias: a cognitive perspective. New York: Basic Books; 1986.

17. Padesky CA. Socratic questioning: changing minds or guided discovery. Keynote address delivered at the European Congress of Behavioural and Cognitive Therapies; September 24, 1993; London, UK.

18. Westbrook D, Kennerley H, Kirk J. An introduction to cognitive behaviour therapy: skills and applications. London: Sage; 2007.

19. Stuart S, Noyes R. Interpersonal psychotherapy for somatizing patients. Psychother Psychosom. 2006;75:209–19.

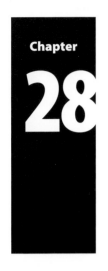

Chapter 28

Children's reactions and consequences of illness and hospitalization and transition of care from pediatric to adult settings

Susan Turkel and Maryland Pao

Typical consult question

"Please evaluate this twelve year old with sickle cell disease who had a bone marrow transplant three weeks ago. He was doing well, but had a seizure last night and now seems confused and says he is seeing spiders crawling on his bed."

Background

Psychiatric consultation for medically ill children and adolescents may be sought for psychological aspects of specific diseases such as anxiety with pulmonary diseases, disorders unique to the medically ill such as delirium, or behavioral problems common in children across disease entities such as non-adherence. The psychological effects of specific medical conditions like asthma or cancer have been the focus of scientific inquiry.

The most common pediatric chronic illness is asthma, which has been associated with psychiatric problems in both children and parents. More than one-third of children with asthma have anxiety disorders. Increased severity of illness is associated with increased psychosocial problems. Family therapy and pharmacologic treatments for anxiety and depression are effective for treating children with asthma.

Pediatric patients with cancer have rates of depression similar to the general population (1), influenced, in part, by avoidant coping styles (2). Cognitive-behavioral techniques, topical anesthetics, and sedation given before and during invasive cancer treatments or procedures such as bone marrow aspirations can decrease anxiety, distress, and pain in pediatric patients with cancer.

Delirium is relatively common and has a similar presentation in pediatric patients as in adults. (See example above.) Disorientation and psychosis appear to be less common or more difficult to assess in young children. The presentation, causes, treatments, and outcomes of pediatric and adult delirium are comparable (3). Treatment begins by identifying and addressing the underlying cause. This includes elimination of medications associated with delirium, frequent re-orientation and re-assurance, and pharmacologic treatment with antipsychotic medication (4).

Psychosomatic Medicine: An Introduction to Consultation-Liaison Psychiatry, eds. James J. Amos and Robert G. Robinson. Published by Cambridge University Press. © Cambridge University Press 2010.

Table 28.1 Factors affecting adherence to treatment

- Age and cognitive development
- Extended illness and multiple medications
- Culture and family characteristics
- Disruptive and oppositional behaviors

Table 28.2 Factors determining a child's response to illness

- Age
- Developmental level
- Cognitive level
- Previous experiences
- Coping skills
- Family response
- Family's support
- Nature of the illness
- Physical consequences of illness

Non-adherence with treatment, another common consultation request, ranges from 11% to 93% in children and adolescents. It influences treatment response, leads to additional prescriptions, and extends the course of illness (5). Both patient-specific and system variables affect pediatric adherence (Table 28.1).

Chronically ill children are at risk for depression, anxiety, somatization, and illness falsification. Assessing psychiatric illness is often difficult because of physical symptoms which may mimic psychiatric symptoms or interfere with diagnostic measures. Depression appears to be similarly prevalent in chronically ill and healthy children but can lead to complications in medical outcomes and increased disability (6). Somatization can be inadvertently encouraged when reporting of physical symptoms (as opposed to emotional distress) garners more attention (7). Illness falsification by children is rare and often is easily recognized. Falsification by the caretaker (Munchausen by proxy) is an insidious form of child abuse that is difficult to detect and can lead to unnecessary treatment, mutilation, and death (8).

The terminal illness and death of a child is a sobering reality of pediatric hospital consultation that provokes significant anxiety in the patient, in families, and in caregivers. Preservation of relationships is crucial. Informing a child that he or she is going to die is difficult, but parents rarely regret sharing this information with their child (9). Depending on their developmental stage, children have differing conceptions or misunderstandings of death. Frank conversations with family or play therapy may help. Comfort care at the end of life is essential, and includes prevention of suffering and treatment of pain, dyspnea, fatigue, and delirium (10).

Many serious illnesses begin in childhood, when they can be more devastating than the same illnesses in adults. As mortality has decreased with advancing technologies, children with serious medical illnesses are now surviving into adulthood. Their illness and treatment when young will have a significant impact on their cognition, behavior, and relationships as adults. How a child will react to illness and to hospitalization will depend on many factors, not limited to just the illness (Table 28.2).

Severe childhood illness presents a set of serious challenges that can be either overwhelming leading to demoralization or fortifying leading to resilience. Nearly one-fifth of American children younger than eighteen years old have chronic illness or special health

Table 28.3 Features of vulnerable child syndrome

- Follows real or perceived threat to child's survival
- Pathological separation difficulties
- Infantilization
- Overly protective, indulgent, or solicitous parents
- Overly dependent, anxious, uncooperative, argumentative child
- Bodily pre-occupation
- Enmeshment
- Fears of growing up and dying
- School under-achievement and expectations of failure

needs, and at least 90% will survive into adulthood. With adaptation to physical illness, outcomes vary widely. Generally, multiple stressors are present before psychiatric disorders arise. Poor adjustment to illness more often reflects the child's caregiver's response to the stress of the child's illness than to the severity of the medical condition. Approximately 20% of children with chronic medical conditions have behavioral and emotional symptoms – twice the rate in the general population.

The hospital or clinic environment can be traumatic for the acutely or chronically ill child. Invasive, painful procedures are highly stressful experiences for children. Painful medical conditions and treatments can interfere with normal pain modulating systems development, provoke anxiety, and amplify later pain sensitivities (11). Consequently, it is critical to intervene whenever possible to reduce discomfort (12). Posttraumatic stress disorder (PTSD) can arise from traumatic injury or frightening hospital experiences. Identifying and easing potentially traumatic situations may decrease the child's stress and improve medical outcomes. Materials for patients, parents, and providers on medical trauma are available at http://www.nctsnet.org (13).

Chronically ill children have difficulty growing up. The impact of their illness depends on how old they are when they become ill, their relationships with family and friends, and their experiences and coping skills. Healthcare providers play a powerful role in the lives of families with a sick child, as trusting parents turn to them for essential medical information and guidance. What providers say often has an enormous impact on parents and their children, with immediate and long-lasting effects. Words matter (14).

The vulnerable child syndrome (VCS) was identified in 1964 to describe a pattern of abnormal relationships and behaviors that follow a real or perceived threat to a child's survival. The cardinal features of VCS include poor sleep in infants or delay starting school because of separation anxiety and subsequent infantilization by overprotective and overly solicitous parents, leading to difficult children and other features. An inability to distinguish mild, self-limited from potentially serious illness can lead to fears of growing up and dying in the child. School underachievement and expectations of failure can evolve (15, 16) (Table 28.3).

Work-up

Children are not little adults. When working with acutely or chronically ill children and adolescents, it is essential to appreciate the variability in normal developmental trajectories and the importance of working with a child's family and its context (Table 28.4). Pediatric psychosomatic medicine consultants typically facilitate coping and adjustment for optimal

Table 28.4 Important skills in working with ill children

- Knowledge of impact of illness on developmental trajectories
- Knowledge of impact of illness on family relationships
- Methods to facilitate coping in children and their families
- Behavioral management techniques to set limits and provide consistency

Table 28.5 Major developmental trajectories

- Physical growth
- Fine and gross motor development
- Language
- Cognition
- Emotions/attachment
- Sexual development

development first, rather than focusing on psychopathology. The consultant must be familiar with developmental trajectories, major developmental milestones, and the view of illness along each (17) (Table 28.5).

The strategic approach to the clinical interview will differ for patients of different ages, presenting family groups, settings, and clinical situations. Meeting with the parents first might elicit mistrust from the child who believes the parents present a negative bias. Interviewing the child first may omit behavioral problems. It's usually best to meet with both child and parent(s) initially, then separately, beginning with the child first. This allows the consultant to observe interactions between the child and the parent(s) and to understand what and how information is shared. This even-handed method saves time and establishes trust with both parent(s) and child.

A hospital room is a difficult setting for an initial psychiatric interview; a flexible approach is needed when working with medically ill children and adolescents. Start by asking about the reasons for hospitalization, and segue into obtaining a medical, developmental, psychiatric, academic, and family history. Most parents can remember when their child first walked and talked and can recall repeated grades or special education services. Detailed information about school, including letter grades and absences, will help in assessment of the child's functioning in his "job" attending school and acquiring new motor, social, and cognitive skills. Additional information on the child's communication skills and ability to form peer relationships is valuable.

Children with medical illness may not develop at the same rate as healthy children because of delayed neurocognitive development, disruptions in education, and limited social experiences. Although children generally pass through similar stages of cognitive development, clinicians cannot assume that chronologic age is equivalent to mental age. Understanding how a child processes information is essential when communicating with him about his disease. Cognitive stage strongly influences children's ability to understand an illness and its causes, treatments, and prognosis. Clinicians frequently overestimate the abilities of young children and underestimate the abilities of older ones to understand medical explanations (Table 28.6).

After asking parents to describe their experiences and understanding, assess the child's understanding of his illness. Simply asking for the child's views is usually the best way to uncover his unique misconceptions and concerns. The pediatric consultant should focus on the child's concerns, not those of the adults. Tailor questions and explanations to the child's

Table 28.6 Developmental stages in chronically ill children and adolescents

Stage of Development [Erikson's Stages] (Piaget's Stages)	Effects of Chronic Illness	Child's Perception of Illness (26)
Infancy (0–1 y) [Trust vs. Mistrust] (Sensory-motor)	• Illness may decrease infant's access to environment. • Parental separation, guilt, anger, and grief may interfere with attachment • Difficulty with trust and possible sense of helplessness	• Little capacity to understand illness
Toddler (2–3 y) [Autonomy vs. Shame and Doubt] (Sensory-motor/pre-operational)	• Motor and language development may be delayed. • Parental reluctance to set limits • Bladder and bowel function may be affected.	• Little capacity and reasoning to understand illness
Preschooler (3–5 y) [Initiative vs. Guilt] (Pre-operational)	• Parental overprotection, regression possible • Initiative may be discouraged.	• Illness can be seen as a punishment for bad behavior.
School Age child (6–12 y) [Industry vs. inferiority] (Concrete operational)	• Possible alienation from peers • Fewer social interactions due to illness • Parents may limit social activities using illness as an excuse. • Illness may hamper normal development of self-esteem and sense of mastery.	• Illness causation is seen as temporal proximity as well as bad behavior. • Older children may understand illness as a result of contact with germs. • Child may understand the internalization of a disease within the body and may also understand role in disease treatment.
Adolescent (13–19 y) [Identity vs. Role Confusion] (Formal Operational)	• Adolescents may be concerned about appearance and medication side effects. • Potential risk taking behavior – i.e., drugs, unprotected sex • Non-compliance with medical regimen	• A greater understanding of the body processes in disease • Greater comprehension of the mind-body connection

understanding to identify and clarify misperceptions. Children frequently believe that illnesses and their treatment are forms of punishment for misdeeds, or they may worry that their disease is contagious. Simple language, frequent repetition, and the use of play, drawing, and story-telling are useful techniques.

Understanding the genetic and environmental contributions of the family is critical for a comprehensive psychiatric consultation. Family structure and relationships and the impact of the child's illness must be explored. Chronic illness can positively or negatively change family dynamics (18). Under the stress of a child's illness, siblings may feel embarrassed, guilty, or jealous. They may be asked to help take care of the house or younger siblings, or may be asked to contribute even more (e.g., blood or tissue donation) (19).

Parents are the legal and financial decision-makers for their children and can choose whether or not to inform a child of a diagnosis. However, the consulting psychiatrist can explore their reasons for non-disclosure and can facilitate communication among the family and between the family and the medical team.

Clinical decision-making and treatment

Although it is natural for parents to indulge a previously well-behaved child who becomes ill, parents should maintain expectations for a child's behavior in and out of the hospital. Otherwise, when the illness improves, parents may have an oppositional child who tantrums to get his way. It is important to intervene quickly to re-establish routine and limits. Although adolescent acting-out may reflect parents who are unable to maintain structure and support, this anger and hostility may also mask anxiety or depression. It is helpful to clarify expectations, identify sources of conflict and stress, confront inappropriate behavior, set limits, provide support, and then address the underlying problem.

It is critical to support the parents' attempts to provide consistent guidance and limit-setting to prevent detrimental emotional and behavioral consequences of childhood illness when the child or adolescent is hospitalized. Similarly, psychiatrists should help parents understand that lack of expectations and overindulgence can lead to low self-esteem, poor problem-solving, and low achievement in the child. The psychiatrist can help parents deepen self-reflection about their parenting styles and improve cooperation with each other in caring for their sick and healthy children.

Psychiatric symptoms are often a manifestation of an underlying medical disorder, and medications may have psychiatric side effects. Identifying the underlying condition and altering the dose of medications may be enough to eliminate symptoms. Psychotropic medications help improve the quality of life of many acutely or chronically ill patients. FDA-approved uses in adult or pediatric patients have not been determined in co-morbid medically ill patients (Table 28.7). Although psychotropic medication use in medically ill populations appears to be common and safe (20), its use is considered "off-label" and should be done judiciously. Start low, go slow, and monitor drug-drug interactions regularly. Children often have more rapid drug metabolism than adults; higher than expected doses may be needed.

Antidepressants are probably the most often used class in medically ill children and adolescents. Selective serotonin reuptake inhibitors target symptoms of depression and/or anxiety. Agents with the least risk of drug-drug interactions, such as citalopram, are preferred for patients on multiple other agents. Mirtazapine is helpful for patients with weight loss and/or nausea and, like other noradrenergic-serotonergic agents, such as duloxetine or the tricyclic antidepressants, may be useful for neuropathic pain. Given the FDA black box warnings of increased risk for suicide ideation with these agents, especially in adolescents, all patients should be carefully assessed for suicide ideation before and during treatment.

Antipsychotics are used to treat delirium and some mood disorders. They relieve nausea and vomiting associated with chemotherapy, and they have a role in palliative care for the terminally ill when mild cognitive impairment in attention and short-term memory may indicate early delirium (21). In general, avoid benzodiazepines in young patients; they may precipitate or exacerbate delirium and over-activation. Intravenous diphenhydramine should be administered very slowly to avoid a sensation of euphoria, which some adolescents may seek.

Table 28.7 Psychotropic medications with FDA-approved uses in children and adolescents

Class	Medication	FDA Labeled Use in Children
Antidepressants	fluoxetine	7–17 y, for depression, OCD
	sertraline	6–17 y, for OCD
	paroxetine	no
	citalopram	no
	escitalopram	12 y and older, for depression
	fluvoxamine	8 y and older, for OCD
	venlafaxine	no
	mirtazapine	no
	bupropion	no
	trazodone	no
	amitriptyline	12 y and older, for depression
	desipramine	12 y and older, for depression
	nortriptyline	6 y and older, for depression
	doxepin	12 y and older, for mixed anxiety and depression
Anxiolytics	clonazepam	up to 10 y or 30 kg, for seizures
	alprazolam	no
	lorazepam	12 y and older, for anxiety, insomnia (oral)
Mood stabilizers	lithium	12 y and older, for bipolar disorder
	valproate	10 y and older, for migraine prophylaxis; pediatric, for epilepsy
	carbamazepine	pediatric, for epilepsy
	oxcarbazepine	2–12 y, for partial seizures, adjunct
	lamotrigine	2 y and older, for partial seizures, Lennox-Gastaut
	gabapentin	3–12 y, for partial seizures, adjunct
Antipsychotics	haloperidol	3 y and older, Tourette's, severe problematic behavior, psychotic disorder, schizophrenia
	risperidone	5–16 y, for irritability in autism 13–17 y, for schizophrenia 10–17 y, for acute mania
	olanzapine	no
	quetiapine	no
	ziprasidone	no
	aripiprazole	13–17 y, for schizophrenia 10–17 y, for acute mania
	droperidol	2 y and older, for postoperative nausea and vomiting prophylaxis
	chlorpromazine	1–12 y, for behavioral syndrome pediatric, for nausea and vomiting, tetanus, pre-surgery for anxiety
	thioridazine	pediatric, for schizophrenia

(cont.)

255

Table 28.7 *(cont.)*

Class	Medication	FDA Labeled Use in Children
Stimulants	methylphenidate	6 y and older, for ADHD and narcolepsy
	dextroamphetamine	6 y and older, for ADHD and narcolepsy
Other	atomoxetine	6 y and older, for ADHD
	clonidine	12 y and older, for hypertension
	guanfacine	12 y and older, for hypertension
	propranolol	pediatric, for hypertension

Key:
ADHD = attention deficit hyperactivity disorder
OCD = obsessive-compulsive disorder

Table 28.8 Tasks of adolescence

- Re-capitulation and resolution of early conflicts
- Independence from parents
- Sexual and personal identity
- Career and financial autonomy
- Personal morality
- Capacity for intimacy
- Adult relationship with parents

Adequate opioid analgesic use is essential for managing pain in ill children and adolescents, as it is in adults, and fear of addiction should not be a deterrent. Inadequate pain control can induce anxiety and depressed mood. Pain scales such as the Wong-Baker Faces have been validated in children and adolescents (22).

Transition from pediatric to adult care

As children with medical problems who might previously have died early are living longer into adulthood, the unanticipated problem of transition from chronically ill child to chronically ill adult now needs to be addressed. A chronic illness adds to the complexity of adolescence. Puberty, autonomy, personal identity, sexuality, education, and vocational choices become more difficult coping tasks for a chronically ill adolescent (Table 28.8). This period may be further complicated by medical setbacks, physical or mental impairments, forced dependence, and perceived poor prognosis (23).

Non-compliance with treatment is frequent in adolescents, and the transitioning patient must have sufficient self-management skills to adapt to the adult healthcare system. Long-term social support may have to be established before the transfer is complete. Pediatric relationships should be sensitively terminated as part of the transition process. A carefully planned transition to adult healthcare should improve self-reliance, enhance autonomy and independence, and support young people in attaining meaningful achievement as adults. Transfer to adult care should be individualized and involves coordination and clear communication with the patient, family, and physicians. This should reduce anxiety for all stakeholders. Two different approaches may be used to plan for the transition: transfer to a specialized center with care focused on pediatric disorders in adults, or transfer to adult disease–specific specialists (24).

As children with serious or chronic illness grow to adulthood, they often have poorer school attendance and lower academic achievement, which typically results in delayed independence, impaired relationships, few marriages, and less permanent employment. Compared with peers, they continue to have elevated use of healthcare services and are more likely to be hospitalized with longer hospital stays (25). Careful attention to their emancipation needs during adolescence may moderate this problem. Eventually, adolescence ends and adulthood begins, even for patients with special healthcare needs.

References

1. Bennett DS. Depression among children with chronic medical problems: a meta-analysis. J Pediatr Psychol. 1994;19:149–69.

2. Phipps S, Srivastava DK. Repressive adaptation in children with cancer. Health Psychol. 1997;16:521–8.

3. Turkel SB, Tavaré CJ. Delirium in children and adolescents. J Neuropsychiatry Clin Neurosci. 2003;15:431–5.

4. Schieveld JN, Leroy PL, van Os J, et al. Pediatric delirium in critical illness: phenomenology, clinical correlates and treatment response in 40 cases in the pediatric intensive care unit. Intensive Care Med. 2007;33:1033–40.

5. Winnick S, Lucas DO, Hartman AL, Toll D. How do you improve compliance? Pediatrics. 2005;115:e718–e724.

6. Shemesh E, Bartell A, Newcorn JH. Assessment and treatment of depression in medically ill children. Curr Psychiatry Rep. 2002;4:88–92.

7. Silber TJ, Pao M. Somatization disorders in children and adolescents. Pediatr Rev. 2003;24:255–64.

8. Stirling J, Committee on Child Abuse and Neglect. Beyond Munchausen syndrome by proxy: identification and treatment of child abuse in a medical setting. Pediatrics. 2007; 119:1026–30.

9. Kreicbergs U, Valdimarsdóttir U, Onelöv E, et al. Talking about death with children who have severe malignant disease. N Engl J Med. 2004;351:1175–86.

10. Wolfe J, Grier HE, Klar N, et al. Symptoms and suffering at the end of life in children with cancer. N Engl J Med. 2000;342:326–33.

11. Fitzgerald M, Beggs S. The neurobiology of pain: developmental aspects. Neuroscientist. 2001;7:246–57.

12. Kain ZN, Caldwell-Andrews A, Wang SM. Psychological preparation of the parent and pediatric surgical patient. Anesthesiol Clin North Am. 2002;20:29–44.

13. National Child Traumatic Stress Network. Medical events and traumatic stress in children and families. 2005. Available from: http://www.nctsnet.org. Accessed December 12, 2005.

14. Pantilat SZ. Communicating with seriously ill patients: better words to say. JAMA. 2009;301:1279–81.

15. Green M, Solnit AJ. Reactions to the threatened loss of a child: a vulnerable child syndrome. Pediatrics. 1964; 34:58–66.

16. Thomasgard M, Metz W. The vulnerable child syndrome revisited. J Dev Behav Pediatr. 1995;16:47–53.

17. Custer JW, Rau RE, Lee CK, eds. The Harriet Lane handbook: a manual for pediatric house officers. 18th ed. St. Louis (MO): Elsevier Science; 2008.

18. Wamboldt MZ, Wamboldt FS. Role of the family in the onset and outcome of childhood disorders: selected research findings. J Am Acad Child Adolesc Psychiatry. 2000;39:1212–9.

19. Sharpe D, Rossiter L. Siblings of children with a chronic illness: a meta-analysis. J Pediatr Psychol. 2002;27:699–710.

20. Clark DB, Birmaher B, Axelson D, et al. Fluoxetine for the treatment of childhood anxiety disorders: open-label, long-term extension to a controlled trial. J Am Acad

Child Adolesc Psychiatry. 2005;44:1263–70.

21. Greenberg DB. Preventing delirium at the end of life: lessons from recent research. J Clin Psychiatry. 2003;5:62–7.

22. Knutsson J, Tíbbelin A, von Unge M. Postoperative pain after paediatric adenoidectomy and differences between pain scores made by the recovery room staff, the parent, and the child. Acta Otolaryngol. 2006;126:1079–83.

23. Blum RW, Garell D, Hodgman CH, et al. Transition from child-centered to adult health care systems for adolescents with chronic conditions. J Adolesc Health. 1993;14:570–6.

24. Tucker LB, Cabral DA. Transition of the adolescent patient with rheumatic disease: issues to consider. Pediatr Clin North Am. 2005;52:641–52.

25. Gledhill J, Rangel L, Garralda E. Surviving chronic physical illness: psychosocial outcome in adult life. Arch Dis Child. 2000; 83:104–10.

26. Koopman HM, Baars RM, Chaplin J, Zwinderman KH. Illness through the eyes of the child: the development of children's understanding of the causes of illness. Patient Educ Couns. 2004; 55:363–70.

Index